Atlas of Implantable Therapies for Pain Management

Timothy R. Deer • Jason E. Pope
Editors

Atlas of Implantable Therapies for Pain Management

Second Edition

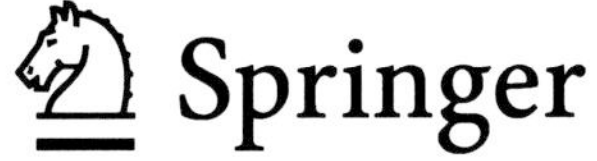

Editors
Timothy R. Deer, MD
The Center for Pain Relief
Charleston, WV
USA

Jason E. Pope
Summit Pain Alliance
Santa Rosa, CA
USA

ISBN 978-1-4939-2109-6 ISBN 978-1-4939-2110-2 (eBook)
DOI 10.1007/978-1-4939-2110-2

Library of Congress Control Number: 2015949703

Springer New York Heidelberg Dordrecht London

Printed on acid-free paper

Springer Science+Business Media LLC New York is part of Springer Science+Business Media (www.springer.com)

To Melissa Deer, my partner in all things and loving wife, who has inspired me for almost 30 years. I look forward to the next 30 years of love and success.

To my children, Morgan, Taylor, Reed, and Bailie, I also dedicate this book. They are my inspiration for life and daily reminders of the blessings I have been given.

To Jane Deer, a wonderful mother and single parent that showed me work ethics and perseverance.

To the memory of my father, Raymond Deer, a tough coal miner who taught me to keep a positive attitude regardless of life's perils.

To Jan Brininstool and the memory of John Brininstool, who accepted me as part of their loving family.

To James Cottrell, MD, who inspired my career, gave me fatherly advice, and was always there.

To Joe Lovett, who provoked my intellectual thought process.

To my current and past CPR medical team: Christopher Kim, MD; Rick Bowman, MD; Doug Stewart, Pa-C; Jeff Peterson; Michelle Miller; Brian Yee, MD; Wil Tolentino, Pa-C; Warren Grace, MD; Sarah King, NP-C; Ashley Comer, NP-C; Rebecca Butcher, NP-C; David Caraway, MD, PhD; Ken McNeil, MD; and Mathew Ranson, MD.

To Robert Levy, MD, PhD, who has been my scientific partner in so many endeavors.

To Nagy Mekhail, MD, PhD, and Stanley Golovac, MD, for advice and guidance during this process.

To Jason Pope, who I enjoy working with on every project. We will have many more, my friend.

This book is dedicated to those who struggle against chronic pain and suffering. The patient–doctor relationship is a special one that touches the soul of the physician, who experiences the success and failure of achieving the desired result.

Most importantly, eternal thanks and glory for all things to God. My daily life is enhanced by my relationship with God, and I know that all success is by his grace.

Timothy R. Deer, MD

To Emily, my wife and partner. Thank you for your unwavering support, grace, and the selflessness you have demonstrated for our family and my career. We are together in all adventures, and I am humbled and thankful we can share this life together.

To my daughter Vivienne, thank you for letting daddy type while we watch cartoons.

To my twins Liam and Olivia, one of our many blessings that came from our tenure in West Virginia: I look forward to our lives together.

To my parents and in-laws, thank you for your unyielding support and advice as I navigate the balance of father, son, husband, and career.

To my twin brother, who always humbles me with his intellect and perspective.

To David Provenzano, Steven Falowksi, and Porter McRoberts for their friendship, candor, guidance, and collaborations.

To my entire past Center for Pain Relief family, thank you for your support, hard work, and stewardship of our patients. A special thanks to those I worked most closely with on a daily basis: Doug Stewart, Jeff Peterson, Diana Tolentino, Danielle Hicks, Neva Terry, Shawn Conley, Stacey Wyatt, Ellen Swanson, Rebecca Butcher, Michelle Miller, Christopher Kim, and Jeff Pack. Thank you for sharing the last few years with me and making them the most enjoyable and influential of my career. You are all truly missed.

To Brad, Lisa, Bria, and Braelyn. Thank you for your friendship and kindness from the start.

To Timothy Deer, my brother, thank you for your friendship, support, advice, and partnership. We will continue to work toward shaping the landscape of pain medicine to improve patient safety and outcomes. We are not victims of circumstance.

To Springer for their continued precision and timeliness in making this second edition a reality.

To the many people who battle chronic pain: you are not alone in this fight—this atlas is an effort to arm your physician partners with more tools in their bag of tricks, improving outcomes and management of your needs.

And finally, thank you to God for making all things possible.

Jason E. Pope

Preface

In this second edition, we refine and expand our teaching in the area of pain treatment using neuromodulation, which we believe is critical to reduce the global epidemic of opioid abuse, societal dysfunction, and the malaise of suffering that so many experience.

Added improvements in this edition include new techniques, new targets, new waveforms, and new concepts in neurostimulation. We also update the brain and spine sections for the neurosurgical treatment of pain via neural bioelectric delivery. The use of intrathecal drug delivery is updated with a focus on safety. We add a section of infection control and reduction of bleeding risks. We have added new drawings, photographs, and tables to further make this a more comprehensive Atlas and to make it more applicable in daily use by our readers.

In the past 5 years, much has evolved in the field of neuromodulation. In addition to pain, we are making great advances in the area of urinary and gastrointestinal health, cardiovascular diseases, Parkinson's disease, inflammatory diseases of the body, and neurological diseases that are life altering and very expensive to society. We expect the third volume of this Atlas in a few years to focus on all of these areas of interest and neuromodulation for the treatment of pain to play a smaller yet important role in a vastly expanding field.

This book is intended to complement fellowship training, peer-to-peer experiences, and hands-on continuing medical education. By giving the visual description of each technique, we intend to improve physician practice and enhance outcomes. The physicians who have collaborated on this book are world class in their research, clinical acumen, and ethics of practice.

We are hopeful that this book becomes a daily reference for students, residents, fellows, and experienced physicians as they strive to help ease suffering.

Charleston, WV, USA — Timothy R. Deer

Contents

Part I Neurostimulation: Spinal Cord

1 **History of Neurostimulation** ... 3
Timothy R. Deer and Jimmy Mali

2 **Patient Selection** ... 7
Corey W. Hunter, Eric T. Lee, Robert Masone, and Timothy R. Deer

3 **Disease Indications** ... 11
Corey W. Hunter, Eric T. Lee, Robert Masone, and Timothy R. Deer

4 **Preoperative Evaluation for Spinal Cord Stimulation** ... 15
Corey W. Hunter, Eric T. Lee, and Timothy R. Deer

5 **Perioperative Precautions for Infection Control** ... 23
David A. Provenzano

6 **Needle Placement for Percutaneous Spinal Cord Stimulation of the Back and Legs** ... 27
Timothy R. Deer, Jason E. Pope, and Louis J. Raso

7 **Physician-Guided Lead Placement: Driving the Lead to the Target Location** ... 33
Timothy R. Deer, Kasra Amirdelfan, Louis J. Raso, and Stanley Golovac

8 **Stimulation of the Spinal Cord by Placement of Surgical-Based Paddle Leads** ... 41
Shivanand P. Lad, Erika Petersen, Andrew Marky, Timothy R. Deer, Robert M. Levy, and Claudio A. Feler

9 **Programming Spinal Cord Stimulation Systems** ... 49
Timothy R. Deer

10 **Anchoring Percutaneous Leads During Permanent Device Placement** ... 57
Timothy R. Deer, Stanley Golovac, and Matthew Kaplan

11 **Tunneling Spinal Cord Stimulation Systems** ... 63
Timothy R. Deer and Jason E. Pope

12 **Pocketing Techniques for Spinal Cord Stimulation and Peripheral Nerve Stimulation** ... 69
Timothy R. Deer and C. Douglas Stewart

13 **Wound Closure** ... 77
Timothy R. Deer and C. Douglas Stewart

14 **Wound Healing** ... 89
Timothy R. Deer and C. Douglas Stewart

15 Complications of Spinal Cord Stimulation 93
Timothy R. Deer and Jason E. Pope

16 Stimulation of the Nervous System to Treat Neuropathic Pain of the Foot 105
Timothy R. Deer and Giancarlo Barolat

17 Sacral Nerve Root Stimulation for the Treatment of Pelvic and Rectal Pain 113
Kenneth M. Alò, Nameer R. Haider, and Timothy R. Deer

18 Selective Nerve Root Stimulation: Facilitating the Cephalocaudal "Retrograde" Method of Electrode Insertion 121
Kenneth M. Alò, Darnell Josiah, and Erich O. Richter

19 Neurostimulation for the Treatment of Anterior Abdominal Pain 129
Nameer R. Haider and Timothy R. Deer

20 Electromyographic/Somatosensory-Evoked Potential Monitoring During Thoracolumbar Spinal Cord Stimulation 135
Erich O. Richter, Marina V. Abramova, Darnell Josiah, and Kenneth M. Aló

21 Electromyographic/Somatosensory Evoked Potential Monitoring During Sacral Neuromodulation 141
Erich O. Richter, Marina V. Abramova, Darnell Josiah, and Kenneth M. Aló

22 The Future of Neurostimulation 145
Timothy R. Deer and Jimmy Mali

23 Spinal Cord Stimulation of the Dorsal Root Ganglion for the Treatment of Pain 151
Greg A. Bara and Timothy R. Deer

24 High-Frequency Stimulation of the Spinal Cord 159
Greg A. Bara and Timothy R. Deer

25 Burst Stimulation: An Innovative Waveform Strategy for Spinal Cord Stimulation 163
Jason E. Pope and Timothy R. Deer

Part II Neurostimulation: Peripheral Nerve and Peripheral Nerve Field

26 Stimulation of the Extraspinal Peripheral Nervous System 171
W. Porter McRoberts, Timothy R. Deer, David Abejon, and Giancarlo Barolat

27 Peripheral Nerve Stimulation for the Treatment of Knee Pain 185
Timothy R. Deer, Jason E. Pope, W. Porter McRoberts, Paul Verrills, and Richard Bowman

28 Neurostimulation of the Upper Extremity by Conventional Peripheral Nerve Stimulation 191
Nameer R. Haider and Timothy R. Deer

29 Ultrasound Guidance for the Placement of Peripheral Nerve Stimulation Devices 197
Mayank Gupta and Timothy R. Deer

30 High-Frequency Electric Nerve Block to Treat Postamputation Pain 205
Amol Soin, Zi-Ping Fang, Jonathan Velasco, and Timothy R. Deer

31 Peripheral Nerve Stimulation Miniaturization 213
Tory McJunkin, Paul Lynch, and Timothy R. Deer

Part III Neurostimulation: The Cranium and the Head

32 Neurostimulation: Stimulation of the Cranium and Head: Stimulation of the Deep Brain for the Treatment of Chronic Pain 225
Shivanand P. Lad, Erika A. Petersen, Andrew Marky, Timothy R. Deer, and Robert M. Levy

33 Stimulation of the Motor Cortex to Treat Chronic Pain 229
Shivanand P. Lad, Andrew Marky, Timothy R. Deer, Robert M. Levy, and Erika A. Petersen

34 Stimulation of the Peripheral Nervous System: Occipital Techniques for the Treatment of Occipital Neuritis and Transformed Migraine 235
Nameer R. Haider and Timothy R. Deer

Part IV Drug Delivery

35 History of Intrathecal Drug Delivery 245
Timothy R. Deer

36 Selection and Indications for Intrathecal Pump Placement 249
Timothy R. Deer and Jason E. Pope

37 Placement of Intrathecal Needle and Catheter for Chronic Infusion 253
Timothy R. Deer, Michael H. Verdolin, and Jason E. Pope

38 Securing and Anchoring Permanent Intrathecal Catheters 263
Timothy R. Deer, Michael H. Verdolin, and Jason E. Pope

39 Tunneling Permanent Intrathecal Catheters 271
Timothy R. Deer, Michael H. Verdolin, and Jason E. Pope

40 Pocketing for Intrathecal Drug Delivery Systems 279
Timothy R. Deer and C. Douglas Stewart

41 Drug Selection for Intrathecal Drug Delivery 287
Karina Gritsenko, Veronica Carullo, Timothy R. Deer, and Jason E. Pope

42 Intrathecal Pump Refills 293
Karina Gritsenko, Veronica Carullo, and Timothy R. Deer

43 Complications of Intrathecal Drug Delivery 301
Karina Gritsenko, Veronica Carullo, and Timothy R. Deer

Index 313

Contributors

David Abejón Hospital Universitario Quirón Madrid, Madrid, Spain

Marina V. Abramova Department of Neurosurgery, Louisiana State University Health Sciences Center, New Orleans, LA, USA

Kasra Amirdelfan IPM Medical Group, Inc., Walnut Creek, CA, USA

Kenneth M. Aló The Methodist Hospital Research Institute, Houston, TX, USA

Greg A. Bara Department of Neurosurgery, University Hospital Dusseldorf, Düsseldorf, Germany

Giancarlo Barolat, MD Barolat Neuroscience, Presbyterian St. Lukes Medical Center, Denver, CO, USA

Richard Bowman, MD The Center for Pain Relief, Charleston, WV, USA

Veronica Carullo Pediatric Pain Management Service, Montefiore Medical Center, Albert Einstein College of Medicine, Bronx, NY, USA

Timothy R. Deer, MD The Center for Pain Relief, Charleston, WV, USA

Zi-Ping Fang Neuros Medical, Inc., Willoughby Hills, OH, USA

Claudio A. Feler Semmes-Murphey Clinic, Memphis, TN, USA

Stanley Golovac Florida Pain, Merritt Island, FL, USA

Karina Gritsenko Montefiore Medical Center, Albert Einstein College of Medicine, Bronx, NY, USA

Mayank Gupta Overland Park Regional Medical Center, Overland Park, KS, USA

Nameer R. Haider, MD Minimally Invasive Pain Institute, Washington, DC, USA

Corey W. Hunter Ainsworth Institute of Pain Management, New York, NY, USA

Darnell Josiah, MD Department of Neurosurgery, West Virginia University Hospitals, Morgantown, WV, USA

Matthew Kaplan Preferred Spine and Pain, Round Rock, TX, USA

Shivanand P. Lad Division of Neurosurgery, Department of Surgery, Duke University Medical Center, Durham, NC, USA

Eric T. Lee Ainsworth Institute of Pain Management, New York, NY, USA

Robert M. Levy Harvey Sandler Department of Neurosurgery, Marcus Neuroscience Institute, Boca Raton, FL, USA

Paul Lynch Arizona Pain Specialists, Scottsdale, AZ, USA

Jimmy Mali Department of Physical Medicine and Rehabilitation, University of North Carolina School of Medicine, Chapel Hill, NC, USA

Andrew Marky Division of Neurosurgery, Department of Surgery, Duke University Medical Center, Durham, NC, USA

Robert Masone Fairfield Medical Center, Lancaster, OH, USA

W. Porter McRoberts Division of Interventional Spine, Pain, and Neurosurgery, Holy Cross Hospital, Fort Lauderdale, FL, USA

Tory McJunkin Arizona Pain Specialists, Scottsdale, AZ, USA

Erika A. Petersen Department of Neurosurgery, University of Arkansas for Medical Sciences, Little Rock, AR, USA

Jason E. Pope Summit Pain Alliance, Santa Rosa, CA, USA

David A. Provenzano Pain Diagnostics and Interventional Care, Pittsburgh, PA, USA

Louis J. Raso Jupiter Interventional Pain Management, Jupiter, FL, USA

Erich O. Richter Department of Neurosurgery, West Virginia University Hospitals, Morgantown, WV, USA

Amol Soin, MD, MBA Greene Memorial Hospital, Wright State University School of Medicine, Centerville, OH, USA

C. Douglas Stewart The Center for Pain Relief, Charleston, WV, USA

Jonathan Velasco Dayton Surgeons Inc., Dayton, OH, USA

Michael H. Verdolin Verdolin Pain Specialists, Chula Vista, CA, USA

Paul Verrills MetroPain Group, Caulfield, South VIC, Australia

Part I

Neurostimulation: Spinal Cord

History of Neurostimulation

1

Timothy R. Deer and Jimmy Mali

1.1 Introduction

When we discuss advances like dorsal root ganglion spinal cord stimulation, high frequency stimulation, burst delivery, MRI compatibility, Bluetooth innovation, and the potential of smart programming, one may ask whether we are already in the future. But Galvani, Volta, Franklin, and Gilbert may have posed the same question as they evolved the field. Interestingly, no matter what advances we see in our daily patient treatment, our phase of the advancement will be viewed as antiquated by those who follow. This is good news; we want to encourage innovation. But at the same time, we need to celebrate the history of the field. The purpose of this chapter is to examine, celebrate, and learn from past thinkers and scientists, and to apply what they have taught us to future thought.

1.2 The Ancient or Classical Age

Many of those involved in neuromodulation say that stimulation began in Mesopotamia with the use of the electric eel to treat foot pain and headache. The ancient history of this discipline is more complex and interesting than simplified version, however.

In Greece, the interest in currents and electrical properties was vast. The Greeks coined the word *elektron* to describe amber, a fossilized resin used to create sparks, and later this term became the modern root of the word *electricity*. Greek physicians were the initial users of current to treat illness, and along with the Mesopotamians, they were credited with the initial sparks that started what is now known as neurostimulation. The first documented use involved the release of electrically charged torpedo fish in clinical footbaths from the Nile to treat prolonged headache. Egyptian physicians called the electric fish "Thunderer of the Nile." The use of electricity continued to develop in both Greece and Rome, and in some communities it was more common than the use of herbs and other medicinal treatments.

1.3 The Dark Ages and Forward

After well-documented use of electrical current in the classical age, the stage went silent for innovation for many centuries. This period has been referred to as the "dark ages" of neuromodulation history. Some use of these concepts may have been made, but documentation was poor, so the ability to teach new pupils and pass on knowledge seemed to evaporate. As time progressed, however, some individuals stepped up to move the field forward:

William Gilbert: This famous seventeenth-century scientist first used the term *electricity* and described the relationship of electromagnetism to the treatment of pain. Gilbert wrote of the use of lodestone, a piece of magnetic iron ore possessing polarity like a magnetic needle. He published reports of using lodestone therapy to treat headache, mental disorders, and marital infidelity. The mechanisms for treating infidelity were never theorized, and the use of electrical current was not well understood.

Ewald Georg von Kleist and *Pieter van Musschenbroek:* These two scientists were both instrumental in inventing the initial methods of harnessing energy via electrical current storage. Eventually their device become known as a Leyden jar, named after the University of Leyden (van Mussenchenbroek's home town). Von Kleist, the bishop of Pomerania, tried to name the device the Kleistian jar, but this name was not adopted. The device was constructed

T.R. Deer, MD (✉)
The Center for Pain Relief, 400 Court Street, Suite 100, Charleston, WV 25301, USA
e-mail: DocTDeer@aol.com

J. Mali
Department of Physical Medicine and Rehabilitation, University of North Carolina School of Medicine, Chapel Hill, NC, USA
e-mail: jmali.md@gmail.com

T.R. Deer, J.E. Pope (eds.), *Atlas of Implantable Therapies for Pain Management*, DOI 10.1007/978-1-4939-2110-2_1

by placing water in a metal container suspended by insulating silk cords, and placing a brass wire through a cork into the water. The process of harnessing electricity was critical to all future work in science and medicine. The work of von Kleist and van Musschenbroek made the development of neuromodulation possible.

Jean Jallabert: The work of von Kleist and van Musschenbroek was critical to the next major development. In 1746, Jallabert used electricity to stimulate muscle fibers. This advancement was used to successfully treat a paralyzed limb, resulting in involuntary contractions, regeneration of muscle, and increased blood flow. Jallabert's success inspired many scientists, and over the following two decades there were several reports of successful treatment of neuromuscular disorders. This work, which seemed highly advanced for that time, led to the theory that electricity was a fluid.

John Walsh: The theory of electricity as a fluid was evaluated by Walsh, who dissected the torpedo fish and explained that the electrical organ of the animal was like the Leyden jar. The torpedo fish, lodestone, Leyden jar, and early muscle experiments were the foundation of neuromodulation that led to the future use of current therapies.

Henry Cavendish: In 1771, Cavendish explained the relationship between electrical force and distance in mathematical theory. This mathematical equation established the groundwork for many future electrical engineering advances.

Alessandro Giuseppe Antonio Anastasio Volta: Volta invented the first battery about 1800. His invention led to the ability to create modern devices.

Luigi Galvani: Galvani may be considered the father of modern neuromodulation. He created what we may term bioelectrics when he first used sparks to move the muscles of frog legs. This simple concept led to the first step of connecting electricity to an animal.

1.4 Neurostimulation First Used in the United States

Benjamin Franklin is important to neuromodulation for two reasons: The development of the lightening rod was an early practical use of electricity, and Franklin was also the first American to use neurostimulation. Franklin's interest in electrical current peaked in 1756, after he learned about the work of Leopoldo Caldani, who reported that discharging a Leyden jar in the vicinity of a mounted and dissected frog's leg could cause it to twitch. Many scientists touted electricity as a miracle cure for many diseases after the presentation of Caldani's work. Especially popular was the hypothesis that paralysis might be cured by this method. Franklin did his own experiments on painful conditions. After discovering that his subjects experienced more discomfort than pain relief, he concluded that these claims were inflated. Unfortunately for Franklin's volunteers, many of whom were desperate and hopeless people, he used high-voltage stimulation that caused injury, pain, and tissue burns.

The first use of neurostimulation in the United States, as Franklin reported to the French Academy of Sciences in Paris, was unsuccessful. This scientific report diminished the interest in electrical treatment in the United States for many years. Considering these issues, Franklin may have harmed the advancement of neurostimulation in the United States, but it is hard to lay blame on such a marvelous figure, who had the type of inquisitive mind that we all strive for. It also makes one wonder which of our current ideas may be off base, harmful, or in need of redirection. Time will tell, as we move forward and seek Food and Drug Administration (FDA) approval for new devices and methods.

1.5 Batteries for Neurostimulation

In 1780, Galvani discovered that touching a frog's leg with a copper wire led to nerve discharge and muscle contraction. He concluded from this experiment that animals had natural electricity that led to movement. This work was predicated on the theory of Isaac Newton that animal fluids had a direct relationship to subtle electrical fields and caused movement.

Twenty years later, Volta published a paper that explained a chemical interaction in animals that led to "animal electricity." His work led to the development of batteries and low-voltage capacitors. Over time, the low-voltage electricity used by Volta was applied to humans; it was much better tolerated by research volunteers than the high-voltage stimulation used by Franklin, and led to progress in pain treatment. The work of both Volta and Galvani led to modern batteries and improved the understanding of electrical current in animals.

1.6 Early Neurostimulation: Failures and Advances

1.6.1 Failures

Unfortunately, the path to the modern use of electricity has not been one of universal success and understanding. Volta felt that the use of electrical current in medicine had no scientific backing. After Jallabert's work became well known, a period of quackery followed, including these misguided efforts:

Magnetism: Franz Mesmer's work on magnetism theorized that the celestial bodies acted upon our bodies by "invisible fluid." He used magnets to channel this fluid and create an electrical field. This "mesmerism" was short-lived in popular acceptance and gave rise to suspicion among the public and the scientific community. Many years later, magnets became a popular alternative treatment, but their relationship to "mesmerism" is unclear.

Infectious disease cures: Elisha Perkins was a questionable scientist who theorized that he could use an electrically charged rod to cure yellow fever. His credibility was highly questioned when he died of the disease after treating himself with the device. After his death, the use of the electrically charged rod fell out of favor in infectious disease treatment.

1.6.2 Advances

Too early for their time: In 1801, electrical currents were used experimentally to resuscitate patients who had suffered cardiac arrest or drowning. This crude technique was an early form of cardioversion. In 1804, a publication titled "The Elements of Galvanism" recommended passing an electrical current through the skin by applying gold leaf to the skin's surface and then attaching a battery source to create an intermittent charge through the body for short intervals. This treatment was applied through the occiput when possible and was used to treat headache, tumors, and generalized pain. Currently occipital nerve stimulation has been found to be successful in treating migraine, headache, and potentially chronic pain.

André-Marie Ampère and *Michael Faraday:* The next steps forward in this field were the result of the work of André-Marie Ampère, who researched the effect of electrical current on magnetic needles. This study led to the understanding that currents can attract or repel each other depending on the flow of current. Faraday, a noted British scientist, advanced this work in 1831, when he described electromagnetic induction. His description was based on the observation that generation of electricity in one wire could "induce" magnetic and electrical effects in a separate wire, based on Ampère's work and his own observations. These descriptions of electromagnetic induction are the critical link to modern neuromodulation in the treatment of pain and movement disorders.

The Magnetic Electrical Machine: E. M. Clarke advanced the field based largely by building on Faraday's work. The Clarke Magnetic Electrical Machine provided a steady supply of induced electricity and led to all future developments in medicine that needed electrical therapy. Initially, it was difficult to apply these therapies to patients because of the strong sensitivity of tissue to direct current. Concepts such as insulation, amplitude, and pulse width were still many years away, but these early developments were critical.

Guillaume-Benjamin-Amand Duchenne (de Boulogne): Duchenne was important in our field because of electropuncture. He used small needles to apply current to the muscle to cause contraction and to assist in muscle mapping, and published these findings in his book, *De l'Electrisation Localisée*. This work led to the development of early prostheses that used surface electrodes to move the body part and eventually to modern rehabilitation stimulation devices. Current conceptual devices are being used to improve motor rehabilitation by applying current to the brain, spinal cord, and nerves of the peripheral extremities.

The first United States patented device: Charles Willie Kent patented the "Electreat" in 1919. This was an early version of transcutaneous electrical stimulation. The work was based largely on an 1871 publication by Beard and Rockwell, which explained how the Faradic current principles might be applied to pain relief.

1.7 High-Frequency Stimulation and Voltage Alterations

The focus now is on the potential for high-frequency stimulation to treat patients in a paresthesia-free method of current delivery. This seems to be a new concept, but high frequency has a long history, at least in theory. The French physiologist d'Arsonval found that the application of high-frequency current caused less pain. He used 10,000 oscillations per second, which was increased further by Hertz in 1890, when he was able to achieve 1,000,000,000 oscillations per second without stimulating tissue in a painful manner. This initial stimulation was at a low voltage that was eventually increased by Hertz's spark gap resonator, a device that allowed the use of a gap in the otherwise complete electrical circuit to discharge current at a prescribed voltage. This increase in voltage control along with high frequency led to successful treatment of arthritis, pain, and tumors. The developments of d'Arsonval and Hertz remain critical for modern stimulation programming platforms. As we review these historical figures, the reader can put together each step and the impact it has had on current devices and delivery.

1.8 Modern Neurostimulation: 1960 to the Present

The use of neurostimulation as we clinically know it today really had its start in the 1960s. Critical developments included basic and bench science research. Woolsey used electrical stimulation to map the animal cortex and subcortex. Melzack and Wall further increased our understanding of pain perception with a 1965 publication in *Science*, which provided the basic groundwork for the clinical application of neurostimulation. The gate control theory described inhibitory and excitatory relationships in the nervous system, particularly in pain pathways.

At the University Hospitals of Cleveland, Case Western Reserve, Norman Shealy described the use of electrical current to modulate the nervous system and change the perception of pain and suffering. Dr. Shealy worked with an engineering student, Thomas Mortimer, to develop a stimulating lead that would work on the dorsal columns of the spinal cord. They used a crude platinum electrode design with a positive and negative electrode to treat a 70-year-old man with thoracic pain from inoperable bronchogenic carcinoma. The generator was an external cardiac device with the lead placed in the intrathecal space. Although the target was not ideal and the patient was not one that would be considered appropriate today, the outcome was excellent during the test stimulation, which lasted 1½ days. An account of this landmark achievement was published as a case report in 1967.

This work ignited the field and led to multiple projects that stimulated advancement. Shealy and others, such as William Sweet at Massachusetts General Hospital, modified the technique over the next few years to stimulate the epidural space. Sweet and Wepsic applied the concept of neurostimulation to the peripheral nervous system in a 1968 paper, "Treatment of chronic pain by stimulation of fibers of primary afferent neuron." This work was an early example of taking work in the central nervous system and applying it to different targets.

The first device company to achieve FDA approval for an implantable neuromodulation device was Medtronic (Minneapolis, Minnesota) in 1968. These early devices required radiofrequency communication between the electrodes and power source. Earl Bakken, the founder of Medtronic and inventor of the wearable pacemaker, became a critical figure in neurostimulation, committed to advancing the field.

Yoshio Hosobuchi was another great pioneer in this field. He discovered that these devices could be used in the deep brain to treat facial pain. His 1973 paper, "Chronic thalamic stimulation for the control of facial anesthesia dolorosa," was the birth of deep brain stimulation. Many patients were treated over the ensuing 4 years, but the use of electrical delivery to the brain was restricted in 1977, when the FDA determined that the use of these devices for pain was safe and effective but that they should not be used for other indications until further blinded, prospective research was performed.

Takashi Tsubokawa advanced this work further in 1991, when he showed that stimulation of the motor cortex alleviated pain of central origin. This was the origin of motor cortex stimulation, which was less invasive, easier to apply, and had fewer apparent risks. Eventually, deep brain stimulation was approved for the treatment of movement disorders in Parkinson's disease and dystonia. Several studies of deep brain and motor cortex stimulation are currently ongoing, involving pain, depression, obsessive compulsive disorder, traumatic brain injury, Alzheimer's disease, and obesity.

The past 5 years have shown more promising advances than the previous 20. Significant advances have included dorsal root ganglion spinal cord stimulation, high-frequency stimulation, burst stimulation, MRI compatibility, and new lead and programming platforms that could change the field and enhance people's lives for many years forward.

Suggested Reading

Beard GM, Rockwell AD. A practical treatise on the medical and surgical uses of electricity; including localized and central galvanization, franklinization, electrolysis and galvano-cautery. New York: Wood; 1871.

Cameron T. Safety and efficacy of spinal cord stimulation for the treatment of chronic pain: a 20 year literature review. J Neurosurg. 2004;100:254–67.

Deer T. Current and future trends in spinal cord stimulation for chronic pain. Curr Pain Headache Rep. 2001;5:503–9.

Henderson J. Peripheral nerve stimulation for chronic pain. Curr Pain Headache Rep. 2008;12:28–31.

Hosobuchi Y. Subcortical electrical stimulation for control of intractable pain in humans. Report of 122 cases (1970–1984). J Neurosurg. 1986;64:543–53.

Hosobuchi Y, Adams JE, Rutkin B. Chronic thalamic stimulation for the control of facial anesthesia dolorosa. Arch Neurol. 1973;29:158–61.

Kumar K, Nath R, Wyant G. Treatment of chronic pain by epidural spinal cord stimulation: a 10 year experience. J Neurosurg. 1991;75:402–7.

Levy RM, Deer TR, Henderson J. Intracranial neurostimulation for pain control: a review. Pain Physician. 2010;13:157–65.

Melzack R, Wall PD. Pain mechanisms: a new theory. Science. 1965;150:971–9.

North RB, Kidd DH, Farrokhi F, Plantadosi SA. Spinal cord stimulation versus repeated lumbosacral spine surgery for chronic pain: a randomized, controlled trial. Neurosurgery. 2005;56:98–107.

Shealy CN, Mortimer JT, Reswick JB. Electrical inhibition of pain by stimulation of the dorsal columns: preliminary clinical report. Anesth Analg. 1967;46:489–91.

Sweet WH, Wepsic JG. Treatment of chronic pain by stimulation of fibers of primary afferent neuron. Trans Am Neurol Assoc. 1968;93:103–7.

Tsubokawa T, Katayama Y, Yamamoto T, Hirayama T, Koyama S. Chronic motor cortex stimulation for the treatment of central pain. Acta Neurochir Suppl (Wien). 1991;52:137–9.

Patient Selection

2

Corey W. Hunter, Eric T. Lee, Robert Masone, and Timothy R. Deer

2.1 Introduction

When contemplating neuromodulation as the next potential step, the treatment paradigm in the pain care algorithm, careful attention must be paid to the patient's potential to respond to the therapy. There are a number of factors (both disease- and patient-specific) one must consider when selecting patients for this treatment modality to maximize the change of a successful outcome. Data suggest that particular disease states are more likely to respond to spinal cord stimulation (SCS) than others (*e.g.*, radicular pain versus phantom limb).

This chapter delineates the criteria to consider when assessing a patient's candidacy for an implantable SCS system. Importantly, the goal of this chapter is not to dogmatically and inclusively describe selection criteria, but rather to give guidance and insight for potential refinement of patient selection.

2.2 Indications

The indications for neuromodulation through SCS are growing every day, owing in large part to steadily improving technology, new devices, and the devoted efforts by clinicians to responsibly explore novel uses for this modality, thus expanding its seemingly limitless utility. Particular disease states that were once considered "low probability for success," such as those that may contribute to axial low back pain, are now showing great promise. The same is true for groin pain, phantom limb pain, and chest wall pain. This improvement in outcomes may change the entire thought process for patient selection. The advent of new lead arrays, new structural targets, and new waveform and frequency delivery has paved the way for continued successes. At the time of this writing, multiple prospective randomized studies are now ongoing in both the United States and abroad that will further define these candidates.

Analysis of available data regarding potentially successful outcomes lends a degree of predictability when selecting candidates. This section outlines which criteria tend to predict a greater likelihood of sustainable positive results.

The indications for SCS that are best supported by the literature include radicular pain after spinal surgery, Complex Regional Pain Syndrome (CRPS) types I and II, peripheral nerve injury, painful neuropathies, lumbar radiculopathy, and cervical radiculopathy (Table 2.1). Vascular diseases, such as refractory angina with no correctable lesions, ischemic pain, and pain related to other peripheral vascular diseases, also appear to have a great potential for response.

A number of studies over the past 30 years suggest that SCS has preferential success for common pain characteristics. In 1998, Kumar et al. reported that the five most common etiologies for treatment with SCS were Failed Back Surgery Syndrome (FBSS), peripheral vascular disease, peripheral neuropathy, multiple sclerosis (MS), and CRPS. The largest percentage of successful response to SCS was noted in peripheral neuropathy (73 %) and reflex sympathetic dystrophy (100 %). FBSS had a success rate of 52 %, likely secondary to its mixed neuropathic and nociceptive nature. Kumar went on to say that patients without surgical procedures prior to implant typically responded better, and if a surgical history was present, having a shorter transition time to implant improved the outcome. In summary, he found SCS most successful in intractable angina and ischemic pain, as well as CRPS and neuropathic pain after spinal surgery.

C.W. Hunter • E.T. Lee
Ainsworth Institute of Pain Management,
115 E. 57th Street #1210, New York, NY 10022, USA
e-mail: chunter@ainpain.com; elee@ainpain.com

R. Masone
Fairfield Medical Center, 3999 Lancaster Thornville Road N, Lancaster, OH 43130, USA
e-mail: rmasone@sbcglobal.net

T.R. Deer, MD (✉)
The Center for Pain Relief, 400 Court Street, Suite 100, Charleston, WV 25301, USA
e-mail: DocTDeer@aol.com

T.R. Deer, J.E. Pope (eds.), *Atlas of Implantable Therapies for Pain Management*, DOI 10.1007/978-1-4939-2110-2_2

North et al. reported that SCS was successful in producing pain relief in up to 60 % of patients with arachnoiditis secondary to failed back surgery. Additional work showed that SCS could be superior to reoperation in patients randomized to one of these treatment arms.

In the past two decades, significant advances in both hardware and software for these devices appear to have significantly improved the outcome for FBSS (Table 2.2). Specifically, data for new, advanced multicolumn paddle leads, percutaneous paddle lead arrays, high-frequency 10,000 kHz stimulation, and burst stimulation offer new promise to these patients that may reduce the burden of failed treatment and, if successful, may offer alternatives to additional back surgery or increasing opioids.

It has been suggested that SCS is most effective in the setting of sympathetically mediated pain states, with success rates approaching 70 %. Kemler and colleagues produced peer-reviewed, high-level evidence that SCS was superior to conservative treatment for CRPS. In addition to sympathetic pain, evidence of effectiveness for pain of vasculopathic origin is also mounting. Many studies have shown improved pain, better function, and, perhaps most importantly, improved limb salvage in settings where the distal extremity ischemic lesion measures less than 3 cm.

The development of novel systems to perform dorsal root ganglion (DRG) stimulation within the neuroaxis may result in improved outcomes in neuropathic groin and extremity pain owing to the ability to target specific abnormal pain fibers that were traditionally very challenging with SCS.

Table 2.1 Likelihood of success with spinal cord stimulation

High probability
Chronic radicular pain
Neuropathic pain
Peripheral neuropathy
Ischemic pain
Refractory angina pectoris (not amenable to surgery)
Sympathetically mediated pain
Peripheral vascular disease
Failed Back Surgery Syndrome with radicular components
Complex Regional Pain Syndrome (CRPS), types I & II
Moderate probability
Visceral pain
Multiple sclerosis–induced nerve pain
Cancer-related pain syndromes such as radiation neuritis, chemotherapy-induced neuropathy
Low probability
Deafferentation pain
Spinal cord injury pain
Central/post-stroke pain
Cancer pain without nerve component
Nociceptive pain
Nerve root avulsion

Table 2.2 New technology producing outcome changes

New technology	Technical aspect	Disease states impacted
High-frequency 10 kHz	Similar to current systems Technical software advancement	Axial back pain, patients who do not like or respond to paresthesia, salvage for failed SCS
Burst stimulation	Similar to current systems, different waveform Technical software advancement	Axial back pain, patients who do not like or respond to paresthesia, salvage for failed SCS
Percutaneous paddles	Requires epidural sheath Technical hardware advancement	Axial back pain, complex pain patterns
Dorsal root ganglion spinal cord stimulation (DRG-SCS)	Technical advancement of both hardware and software	Expands the field: phantom pain, chest wall pain, groin pain, foot pain
MRI compatibility	Hardware advancement	Expands the field for those who need serial MRI

2.3 Exclusion

Even as SCS has preferential success for some pain types, its failure in others has been reported in a number of studies. It should be noted that many of the unsuccessful outcomes previously reported may have been a product of shortcomings of the technology employed, and in its current form, may be more responsive. That being stated, the following data reference the disease states and pain states that have been shown to be historically resistant to SCS.

Patients at higher risk of failure include those with spinal cord injury, thalamic stroke pain or pain of any origin within the brain, complete nerve root avulsion, and aching nociceptive pain of the limb secondary to arthritis. Other factors that may have negative predictive value includes cauda equina syndrome, paraplegia, primary bone pain, deafferentation syndrome, and cancer pain secondary to tissue invasion.

2.4 On the Horizon

Traditionally, pelvic, rectal, or anal pain has been characterized as somewhat resistant to SCS with a risk for failure, but a number of studies referencing retrograde and sacral lead placements report promising results. In 2011, Hunter et al. published their successes in treating these regions of pain with lead placements over the conus and the high thoracic region (Table 2.3).

Another pain syndrome that has shown resistance to traditional tonic SCS is discogenic low back pain. Conventionally placed leads over the dorsal columns in the epidural space have met with disappointing results. In recent European and Australian studies, Deer et al. have described some success in treating discogenic low back pain with a radicular component by placing leads over the dorsal root ganglion at various levels, most commonly at L2.

The need for neuroaxial imaging after placement of SCS is very rare, but recent MRI compatibility advancements have broadened the scope of neuromodulation to include patients who require serial MRIs for disease surveillance. Among these patients are those with MS, intracranial tumors or malignancy, and neurodegenerative diseases.

Table 2.3 Novel lead placements with reports of success for pain states traditionally resistant to spinal cord stimulation

Disease type	Lead placements with reported success
Pelvic pain	High thoracic (T6-7), over the conus, or sacrally via hiatus or retrograde approach
Discogenic pain	Dorsal root ganglion
Postherpetic neuralgia	Dorsal root ganglion, dorsal column at corresponding level with or without peripheral nerve lead
Axial low back pain	Newer paddle arrays via laminotomy or percutaneous approach New current delivery
Phantom limb pain	Dorsal root ganglion
Groin pain	Dorsal root ganglion at T12 or L1

Suggested Reading

Al-Kaisy A, Van Buyten JP, Smet I, Palmisani S, Pang D, Smith T. Sustained effectiveness of 10 kHz high-frequency spinal cord stimulation for patients with chronic, low back pain: 24-month results of a prospective multicenter study. Pain Med. 2012. doi:10.1111/pme.12294.

Cameron T. Safety and efficacy of spinal cord stimulation for the treatment of chronic pain: a 20-year literature review. J Neurosurg. 2004;100:254–67.

de la Porte C, Siegfried J. Lumbosacral spinal fibrosis (spinal arachnoiditis). Its diagnosis and treatment by spinal cord stimulation. Spine. 1983;8:593–602.

De Ridder D, Vanneste S, Plazier M, van der Loo E, Menovsky T. Burst spinal cord stimulation: toward paresthesia-free pain suppression. Neurosurgery. 2010;66:986–90.

Deer TR, Raso LJ. Spinal cord stimulation for refractory angina pectoris and peripheral vascular disease. Pain Physician. 2006;9:347–52.

Deer T, Grigsby E, Weiner R, Wilcosky B, Kramer J. A prospective study of dorsal root ganglion stimulation for the relief of chronic pain. Neuromodulation. 2013;16:67–72.

Henderson JM, Schade CM, Sasaki J, Caraway DL, Oakley JC. Prevention of mechanical failures in implanted spinal cord stimulation systems. Neuromodulation. 2006;9:183–91.

Hunter C, Davé N, Diwan S, Deer T. Neuromodulation of pelvic visceral pain: review of the literature and case series of potential novel targets for treatment. Pain Pract. 2013;13:3–17.

Kemler MA, de Vet HC, Barendse GA, van den Wildenberg FA, van Kleef M. Effect of spinal cord stimulation for chronic complex regional pain syndrome Type I: five-year final follow-up of patients in a randomized controlled trial. J Neurosurg. 2008;108(2):292–8.

Kumar K, Toth C, Nath RK, Laing P. Epidural spinal cord stimulation for treatment of chronic pain—some predictors of success. A 15-year experience. Surg Neurol. 1998;50:110–21.

Kumar K, Hunter G, Demeria D. Spinal cord stimulation in treatment of chronic benign pain: challenges in treatment planning and present status, a 22-year experience. Neurosurgery. 2006;58:481–96.

Liem L, Russo M, Huygen FJ, Van Buyten JP, Smet I, Verrills P, et al. A multicenter, prospective trial to assess the safety and performance of the spinal modulation dorsal root ganglion neurostimulator system in the treatment of chronic pain. Neuromodulation. 2013;16:471–82. doi:10.1111/ner.12072.

Meglio M, Cioni B, Rossi GF. Spinal cord stimulation in management of chronic pain: a 9-year experience. J Neurosurg. 1989;70:519–24.

North RB, Wetzel FT. Spinal cord stimulation for chronic pain of spinal origin: a valuable long-term solution. Spine. 2002;27:2584–91.

Ohnmeiss D. Patient satisfaction with spinal cord stimulation for predominant complaints of chronic, intractable low back pain. Spine J. 2001;1:358–62.

Shealy CN, Mortimer JT, Reswick JB. Electrical inhibition of pain by stimulation of the dorsal columns: preliminary clinical report. Anesth Analg. 1967;46:489–91.

Turner JA, Loeser JD, Deyo RA, Sanders SB. Spinal cord stimulation for patients with failed back surgery syndrome or complex regional pain syndrome: a systematic review of effectiveness and complications. Pain. 2004;108:137–47.

3 Disease Indications

Corey W. Hunter, Eric T. Lee, Robert Masone, and Timothy R. Deer

3.1 Introduction

Treating the proper patient with the proper device at the proper time is the essential key to medicine and extends to a successful neurostimulation experience. This chapter focuses on disease states that best lend themselves to a good outcome.

An analysis of peer-reviewed data suggests that particular disease states are more likely to be responsive to spinal cord stimulation (SCS) than others. An example may be a patient with chronic lumbar or cervical radicular pain who in general is an excellent candidate for conventional tonic SCS, as compared to a patient with phantom limb pain who has been traditionally unlikely to respond. Interestingly, success has been seen recently in this complex phantom and stump pain group with the use of dorsal root ganglion spinal cord stimulation (DRG-SCS).

3.2 Indications

The appropriate indications for neurostimulation are expanding rapidly. This is due in large part to steadily improving technology, a rapid innovation cadence, new devices, and devoted efforts by clinicians to explore new and novel uses for this modality, thus expanding its seemingly limitless utility. Particular disease states that were once considered "low probability for success," such as those that may contribute to axial low back pain, are now considered viable candidates. The advent of new lead arrays, new programming software, and enhanced screening has paved the way to continued successes.

Analysis of available data regarding potentially successful outcomes lends a degree of predictability when selecting candidates. This section outlines what criteria tend to predict a greater likelihood of sustainable positive outcomes.

The indications for SCS that are best supported by the literature include burning or shooting pain in the extremity after lumbar or cervical spinal surgery, Reflex Sympathetic Dystrophy (RSD)/Complex Regional Pain Syndrome (CRPS), types I and II, peripheral nerve injury, painful neuropathies, refractory angina with no correctable lesions, ischemic pain, and pain related to peripheral vascular disease.

A number of studies over the past 30 years suggest that SCS has preferential success for common pain characteristics. In 1998, Kumar et al. [1] reported the five most common etiologies for treatment with SCS were failed back surgery syndrome (FBSS), peripheral vascular disease, peripheral neuropathy, multiple sclerosis (MS), and CRPS. The largest percentage of successful response to SCS was noted in peripheral neuropathy (73 %) and reflex sympathetic dystrophy (100 %). FBSS had a success rate of 52 %, likely secondary to its mixed neuropathic and nociceptive nature. Kumar et al. [1] went on to describe that patients without surgical procedures prior to implant typically respond better and, if a surgical history was present, having a shorter transition time to implant improved the outcome.

It has been suggested that SCS is very efficacious in the setting of sympathetically driven pain states, with success rates approaching 70 %. In 1989, Meglio et al. [2] reported that SCS was most effective in vasculopathic pain, low-back pain, and post-herpetic neuralgia. North et al. [3] reported that SCS was successful in producing pain relief in up to 60 % of patients with arachnoiditis. He further proposed that

C.W. Hunter • E.T. Lee
Ainsworth Institute of Pain Management,
115 E. 57th Street #1210, New York, NY 10022, USA
e-mail: chunter@ainpain.com; elee@ainpain.com

R. Masone
Fairfield Medical Center,
3999 Lancaster Thornville Road N, Lancaster, OH 43130, USA
e-mail: rmasone@sbcglobal.net

T.R. Deer, MD (✉)
The Center for Pain Relief, 400 Court Street, Suite 100,
Charleston, WV 25301, USA
e-mail: DocTDeer@aol.com

T.R. Deer, J.E. Pope (eds.), *Atlas of Implantable Therapies for Pain Management*, DOI 10.1007/978-1-4939-2110-2_3

SCS had success rates as high as 88 % in FBSS, suggesting it may even be superior to reoperation. He found it most successful in intractable angina and ischemic pain, as well as CRPS and neuropathic pain after spinal surgery.

With the advent of new technology and ideas, peer-reviewed publications are now reporting successes in treating axial low back pain. Some of these advances include DRG-SCS at L2, high frequency SCS at 10 kHz, hybrid systems with epidural and peripheral leads, and burst SCS. In addition to enhancing outcomes with axial back pain, these new therapies have expanded the chance of success with chest wall pain, groin pain, visceral pain, and other conditions once thought unlikely to be successful.

3.3 Exclusion

Whereas SCS has preferential success for some pain types, its failure in others has been reported in a number of studies. It should be noted that many of the unsuccessful outcomes previously reported may have been a product of technological shortcomings of the time or possibly resulting from a lack of accessibility to the more advanced product lines currently available. Notwithstanding, the following data reference those disease/pain states that have been shown to be historically resistant to SCS.

Patients at higher risk of failure include those with spinal cord injury, thalamic stroke pain, or pain of any origin within the brain, complete nerve root avulsion, and aching nociceptive pain of the limb. With additional analysis of some of the longest-standing prospective data sources, one can surmise that other areas of potentially increased failure rates include cauda equina syndrome, primary bone pain, pain from dystonia and paraplegia, extensive arachnoiditis, deafferentation pain, and cancer pain

3.4 On the Horizon

Traditionally, pelvic, rectal, and anal pain has been characterized as somewhat resistant to SCS with a risk for failure; however, a number of studies referencing retrograde and sacral lead placements report promising results. More recently in 2011, Hunter et al. [4] published their successes in treating these regions of pain with lead placements over the conus and the high thoracic region. This work is encouraging, as is work by Kapural et al. [5] on SCS to treat abdominal pain and diseases of the viscera.

Congestive heart failure is another exciting area in development and shows great promise in both animal models and human pilots. The next decade could prove to be a time of digital medicine that changes and saves patient lives.

Another pain syndrome that has shown resiliency to SCS is discogenic low back pain, as conventionally placed leads over the dorsal columns in epidural space have met with disappointing results. Recently, Liong et al. described some success in treating discogenic low back pain with a radicular component by placing leads over the dorsal root ganglion at the affected levels.

Table 3.1 shows the probability of success with conventional SCS. Table 3.2. shows common lead targets for pain distributions and potential enhanced outcomes with new technology.

Table 3.1 Disease bias With SCS

High probability	Chronic radicular pain Neuropathic pain Peripheral neuropathy Visceral pain Ischemic pain Sympathetically driven pain Peripheral vascular disease Multiple sclerosis Refractory angina pectoris (not amenable to surgery) Painful ischemic peripheral vascular disease Failed back surgery syndrome Complex regional pain syndrome (CRPS), types I and II
Low probability	Deafferentation pain Spinal cord injury pain Central/post-stroke pain Cancer pain Nociceptive pain Nerve root injury

Table 3.2 Novel lead placements with reports of success for pain states traditionally resilient to SCS

Disease type	Lead placements with reported success
Pelvic pain	High thoracic (T6-7), over the conus, or sacrally at S1, S2, S3 via hiatus or retrograde approach
Discogenic pain	Dorsal root ganglion, multi-contact paddles at T8, T9, HF 10 kHz at T8, T9. Burst SCS at T8, T9, T10
Post-herpetic neuralgia	Dorsal root ganglion, or hybrid with epidural and subcutaneous leads
Axial low back pain	Dorsal root ganglion, multi-contact paddles at T8, T9, HF 10 kHz at T8, T9. Burst SCS at T8, T9, T10
Phantom limb pain	Dorsal root ganglion
Groin pain after hernia repair	Dorsal root ganglion or hybrid SCS plus PNS
Congestive heart failure	T1, T2, T3

References

1. Kumar K, Toth C, Nath RK, Laing P. Epidural spinal cord stimulation for treatment of chronic pain—some predictors of success. A 15-year experience. Surg Neurol. 1998;50:110–21.
2. Meglio M, Cioni B, Rossi GF. Spinal cord stimulation in management of chronic pain, a 9-year experience. J Neurosurg. 1989;70:519–24.
3. North RB, Wetzel FT. Spinal cord stimulation for chronic pain of spinal origin: a valuable long-term solution. Spine. 2002;27:2584–91.
4. Hunter C, Davé N, Diwan S, Deer T. Neuromodulation of pelvic visceral pain: review of the literature and case series of potential novel targets for treatment. Pain Pract. 2013;13:3–17.
5. Kapural L, Deer T, Yakovlev A, Bensitel T, Hayek S, Pyles S, et al. Technical aspects of spinal cord stimulation for managing chronic visceral abdominal pain: the results from the national survey. Pain Med. 2010;11(5):685–91.

Suggested Reading

Al-Kaisy A, Van Buyten J-P, Smet I, Palmisani S, Pang D, Smith T. Sustained effectiveness of 10 kHz high-frequency spinal cord stimulation for patients with chronic, low back pain: 24-month results of a prospective multicenter study. Pain Med. 2014;15:347–54.

Cameron T. Safety and efficacy of spinal cord stimulation for the treatment of chronic pain: a 20-year literature review. J Neurosurg. 2004;100(3 Suppl Spine):254–67.

Deer T, Grigsby E, Weiner R, Wilcosky B, Kramer J. A prospective study of dorsal root ganglion stimulation for the relief of chronic pain. Neuromodulation. 2013;16:67–72.

Dela Porte C, Seigfried J. Lumbosacral spinal fibrosis spinal arachnoiditis: its diagnosis and treatment by spinal cord stimulation. Spine. 1983;8:593 603.

De Ridder D, Vanneste S, Plazier M, van der Loo E, Menovsky T. Burst spinal cord stimulation: toward paresthesia-free pain suppression. Neurosurgery. 2010;66:986–90.

Henderson JM, Schade CM, Sasaki J, et al. Prevention of mechanical failures in implanted spinal cord stimulation systems. Neuromodulation. 2006;9:183–91.

Kumar K, Hunter G, Demeria D. Spinal cord stimulation in treatment of chronic benign pain: challenges in treatment planning and present status, a 22-year experience. Neurosurgery. 2006;58:481–96.

Liem L, Russo M, Huygen FJPM, et al. A multicenter, prospective trial to assess the safety and performance of the spinal modulation dorsal root ganglion neurostimulator system in the treatment of chronic pain. Neuromodulation. 2013;16:471–82.

Ohnmeiss D. Patient satisfaction with spinal cord stimulation for predominant complaints of chronic, intractable low back pain. Spine J. 2001;1:358–63.

Shealy C, Mortimer J, Reswick JB. Electrical inhibition of pain by stimulation of the dorsal columns: preliminary clinical report. Anesth Analg. 1967;46:489–91.

Turner JA, Loeser JD, Deyo RA, Sanders SB. Spinal cord stimulation for patients with failed back surgery syndrome or complex regional pain syndrome: a systematic review of effectiveness and complications. Pain. 2004;108:137–47.

Preoperative Evaluation for Spinal Cord Stimulation

4

Corey W. Hunter, Eric T. Lee, and Timothy R. Deer

4.1 Introduction

Preoperative evaluation and clearance is imperative to any surgical procedure. Due diligence must be paid to ensure the lowest chance of complication and the highest likelihood of success. This includes managing the patient's expectations of the device and managing the procedure for its safe implementation. Tonic stimulation therapies require lead placement location optimization and intraoperative cogent patient feedback, highlighting the importance of optimizing preoperative education and expectations. In addition, optimization of disease comorbidities and procedural hematological and infectious risk avoidance are of equal importance. Given this unique set of considerations, one can see the preoperative assessment for spinal cord stimulation (SCS) has several distinctive components.

This chapter reviews the preoperative evaluation for SCS as it pertains to (1) ensuring patient safety by minimizing risks (known and theoretical), (2) identifying the intended entry point, pathway, and position for final lead placement while safeguarding that these are feasible and impose minimal risk, and (3) maximizing the possibility for a positive outcome (pain relief).

4.2 Procedural Considerations

Before any surgical procedure, a proper history and physical examination should always be performed. This will be the time to identify any comorbidities that may impact the procedure itself and give the physician time to follow through on any suboptimal health concerns. It is equally important to elucidate any new information—especially changes or appearance of new symptoms—that may adversely affect the procedure itself such as neurological changes, fevers, skin lesions, or other significant health changes.

4.3 History

4.3.1 Infection

Despite the minimally invasive nature of SCS, infection is still a concern. Any type of infection can pose a serious risk to the patient; however, an epidural abscess can be a particularly devastating complication in even the healthiest of patients (Fig. 4.1). Therefore, careful attention should be paid to any perioperative illnesses or conditions that may suppress the immune system. The skin in and around the intended entry point(s) should be carefully inspected for any signs of recent infection. Even with diligent skin sterilization technique, if pathogens are present within the skin from a lesion of some sort, the needle has potential to carry these pathogens directly into the epidural space leading to infection. One should inquire about any history of methicillin-resistant *Staphylococcus aureus*. If so, the physician may wish to take additional precautions such as preoperative bathing with chlorhexidine, intranasal bactobran, and preoperative vancomycin. In complex cases, additional consultation may be needed.

Systemic infections should be treated and under good control prior to moving forward. If any evidence of potential bacteremia exists, the benefit of the stimulation system should be carefully weighed prior to moving forward. In the case of local infections such as cellulitis, the case should be delayed until proper evaluation and treatment can be arranged. This danger should be considered when the patient has had a recent infection in the area of needle insertion. This is not an uncommon concern when considering SCS as part

C.W. Hunter • E.T. Lee
Ainsworth Institute of Pain Management,
115 E. 57th Street #1210, New York, NY 10022, USA
e-mail: chunter@ainpain.com; elee@ainpain.com

T.R. Deer, MD (✉)
The Center for Pain Relief, 400 Court Street, Suite 100,
Charleston, WV 25301, USA
e-mail: DocTDeer@aol.com

T.R. Deer, J.E. Pope (eds.), *Atlas of Implantable Therapies for Pain Management*, DOI 10.1007/978-1-4939-2110-2_4

of an algorithmic process for the treatment of intractable disorders. It is for these reasons, the authors advocate getting a basic complete blood count (CBC) prior to implant. Urinalysis may also be helpful in those patients with a history of urinary tract diseases or risks.

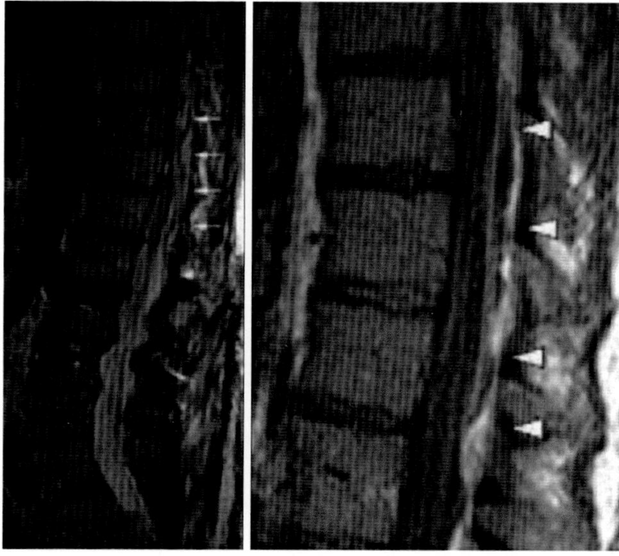

Fig. 4.1 Sagittal T2-weighted MRI of an epidural abscess (*arrows*, *arrowheads*) from an SCS trial

4.3.2 Coagulopathy

Bleeding is a concern in any surgical procedure, but probably none more so than in any case in which epidural access is involved. An epidural hematoma is a tragic and catastrophic complication. In a healthy, uncomplicated patient, the incidence is as low as 1 in 40,000. Given the plethora of data as they pertain to epidural hematomas, there is a predictability of sorts as to when the risk may be higher at certain points than others (Fig. 4.2). As a result, guidelines are now in place that give some safeguards to lower the risk.

The patient should have no untreated bleeding disorders. Prior to implanting the device the patient should be questioned concerning diseases that affect clotting, liver function, and platelet activity. A preoperative workup would include a CBC including a platelet count.

- **International Normalized Ratio (INR)**—the most predictive of potential complication
- **Prothrombin time/partial thromboplastin time (PT/PTT) and bleeding times**—not as reliable, but may be helpful as general sources of information.
- **Platelet function assay studies**—a new test area that may lend information for patients on drugs that affect platelet function.

Special attention should be paid to assess whether the patient is taking any medication that may put she or he at risk for increased bleeding. The guidelines of the American Society of Regional Anesthesia (ASRA) on bleeding and medication should be reviewed when doing a patient evaluation (Table 4.1). If it is discovered the patient is taking a medication listed on the ASRA guidelines that may affect bleeding, the prescribing physician should be consulted to determine if he or she can safely discontinue those medications for the appropriate length of time prior to invading the epidural space. At this point, this is the best available guidance, but it was not designed for neuromodulation devices. It would be preferable in the future to have guidance directly applicable to this field.

In permanent implants, the drugs may be restarted a few days after the leads are surgically secured. The number of days required off of these drugs is controversial and will vary from one medication to the next. New classes of drugs are being developed that are much more potent than the currently available products and may result in new risks for patients undergoing invasive procedures. The implanting physician should ask the prescribing physician to recommend a time course in which the blood clotting should be back to a normal baseline, but in many cases, this may be difficult to determine.

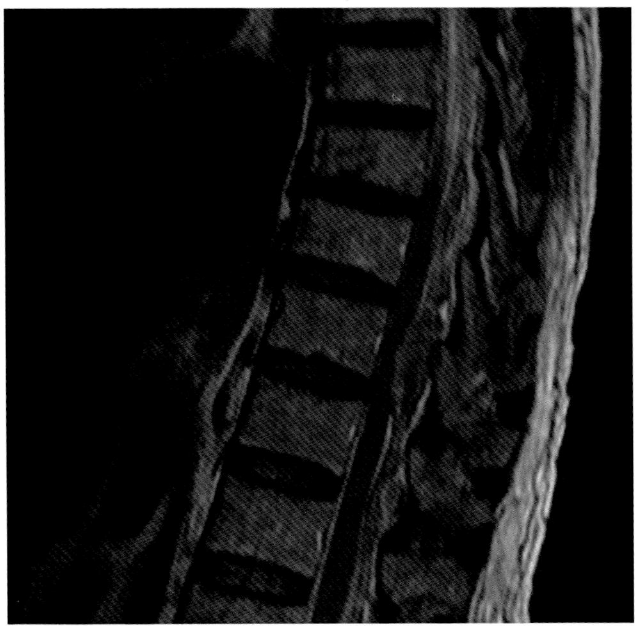

Fig. 4.2 Sagittal T2-weighted MRI of an epidural hematoma following spinal cord stimulator implant

Table 4.1 American Society for regional anesthesia consensus guidelines on anticoagulation and neuraxial blocks 2010

Antiplatelet medications	
Nonsteroidal anti-inflammatory drugs (NSAIDs) or cyclooxygenase-2 (COX-2) inhibitors	May continue
Aspirin (low dose)	Preferably stopped 2–3 d prior for thoracic and cervical epidurals, may be continued in lumbar epidurals.
Thienopyridine derivatives	
Clopidogrel (Plavix)	Discontinue for 7 d
Ticlopidine (Ticlid)	Discontinue for 14 d
Prasugrel	Discontinue for 7–10 d
Glycoprotein IIb/IIIa inhibitors	
Abciximab (ReoPro)	24–48 h
Eptifibatide (Integrilin)	8 h
Tirofiban (Aggrastat)	8 h
The above are the times suggested until normal platelet aggregation is regained. Neuraxial techniques should be avoided until platelet function is recovered	
Warfarin (coumadin)	
Check INR (coagulation response time) INR should be normalized	
2003 Guidelines stated INR <1.5	

Table 4.1 (continued)

Heparin	
Subcutaneous heparin	No contraindication (dosing twice daily and <10,000 U total daily dose)
Block should be performed before the injection is given	
If frequency is 3 times a day or >10,000 U, safety has not been established	
Intravenous heparin	Wait 2–4 h after last dose of IV heparin
Wait a minimum of 1 h after neuraxial block to restart IV heparin	
Low-molecular-weight heparin (LMWH)	
LMWH preoperative—wait time from last dose	
Enoxaparin (Lovenox) 0.5 mg/kg BID (prophylactic dose)	12 h
Enoxaparin (Lovenox) 1 mg/kg BID (prophylactic dose)	24 h
Enoxaparin (Lovenox) 1.5 mg/kg QD	24 h
Dalteparin (Fragmin) 120 U/kg BID	24 h
Dalteparin (Fragmin) 200 U/kg QD	24 h
Tinzaparin (Innohep) 175 units/kg QD	24 h
LMWH postoperative—time to wait after procedure before restarting	
Twice-daily dosing	24 h
Once-daily dosing	6–8 h
Patients with epidural catheter on LMWH	
Enoxaparin (Lovenox) 0.5 mg/kg: remove the catheter ≥12 h after last dose	
Enoxaparin (Lovenox) 1–1.5 mg/kg, dalteparin (Fragmin), or tinzaparin (Innhop): remove the catheter ≥24 h after last dose	
The catheter should be removed as soon as possible	
Restart the LMWH ≥2 h after catheter removal	
Specific Xa inhibitor: fondaparinux (arixtran)	
No definitive recommendations	
If neuraxial performed: recommend single-needle atraumatic placement or alternate thromboprophylaxis, avoid indwelling catheter	
Fibrinolytic/thrombolytic drugs	
Absolute contraindications	
Thrombin inhibitors	
No definitive recommendations	
Herbal therapy	
Neuraxial block not contraindicated for single herbal medication use	
The following are the times to normal hemostasis owing to anticoagulant effect:	
Garlic:	7 d
Ginkgo:	36 h
Ginseng:	24 h
The guidelines are the same for the placement and removal of epidural catheters	

4.3.3 Cardiac Issues and Hypertension

Patients with extensive cardiac history must be carefully evaluated in conjunction with their cardiologist. Cardiac clearance should be considered based on guidance from the anesthesiologist involved in the care. Recently SCS has been cleared for use concurrently with pacemaker devices in many settings. The physician should obtain clearance from the treating cardiologist and have the devices checked in the perioperative period. In the case of a patient with a documented history of hypertension, pressures should be well controlled at the time of the implant.

4.3.4 Diabetes Mellitus

Diabetes is another common condition that has significant impact on patient's outcome and health. Uncontrolled sugars or disease management can lead to increased infection risk and poor healing. Coordination with the primary care physician and/or endocrinologist managing the patient's condition should ensue. Whereas "blood sugar" is an easy value to test, hemoglobin A1c (HgA1c)) is particularly helpful to gauge and assess for degree of control over the previous 3 months. Although no specific value may determine proceeding with trial, poorly controlled diabetic patients would most likely have increased risk of infection in a population that already has increased risk nearly twice as high as the general population—9 to 4 % according to an evaluation published by Mekhail et al. in 2011 [1]. Interestingly, in cases of successful SCS, the increased ability to function can lead to improved exercise, weight loss, and better control of diabetes.

4.3.5 Allergies and Dermatological Diseases

Cutaneous allergic reactions, although uncommon, can be a complicating factor. There are reports in the literature in which patients have developed reactions and inflammatory dermatitis at the concordant insertion site as well as that of the dressings. Heightened awareness should be present in people with a history of contact dermatitis/allergies to any materials used in the equipment used, from cleansing agents, to contrast, to metals, to bandaging and products containing latex (Fig. 4.3).

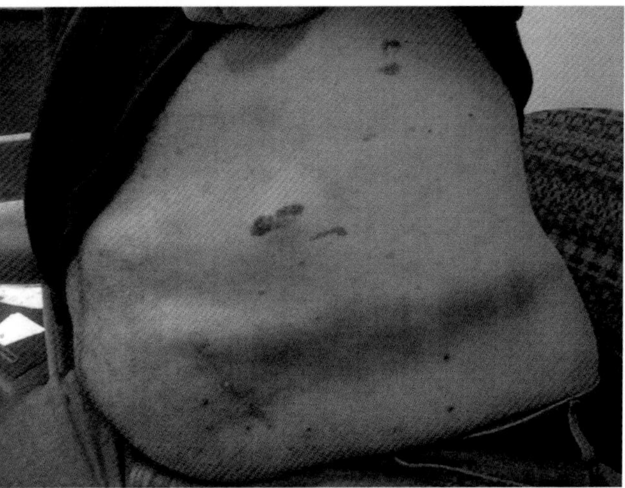

Fig. 4.3 Erythematous rash on the abdomen and flank primarily overlying lead extension

4.4 Physical

As with any preoperative workup, a thorough physical examination is a staple mark of good medicine. One should pay careful attention to and focus on neurological components such as manual motor testing and sensory elements (allodynia, hyperalgesia, and paresthesia). Special consideration should be given to gait and balance because it has been suggested that falls pose an increased risk for lead migration and damage, which obviously hinder the outcomes and increase complication rates.

4.5 Radiological Evaluation

Anatomy and imaging is commonplace for SCS workups. In the process of selecting a patient for SCS, the region of a patient's pain is carefully mapped. This will guide the physician to carefully choose an area of the nervous system to apply neuromodulation; as it pertains to stimulation of the dorsal columns, this will involve the introduction of leads into the spine. Magnetic resonance imaging (MRI) offers visualization of the spine and its corresponding anatomy in high detail. In cases in which MRI is either unavailable or the patient has a contraindication to it (e.g., body habitus, stents, implanted metal), computed tomography (CT) is an acceptable alternative. CT myelogram is another option that many physicians feel is more reliable than any other imaging study. Some authors have recommended the consideration of epidurography prior to introducing a lead, but there is no evidence this option would add benefit.

In cases in which the intended lead placement is the cervical spine, concerns of available space are even more paramount. Because the anatomy of cervical spine is smaller than the lumbar, imaging can be utilized to evaluate the safety of introducing a foreign object (the lead). In cases of potential critical stenosis, a consultation with neurosurgery may be warranted prior to going forward. Keeping the patient conversant during lead placement can also improve safety.

Additional considerations and potential complications may be elucidated with preoperative imaging. Congenital abnormalities (scoliosis and stenosis) can occur throughout the spine that can increase the difficulty of a procedure and potentiate risk.

4.6 Special Considerations

The previously iterated considerations reference guidelines that will help to maximize the precision and safety of the placement of the lead itself while minimizing the risk (Table 4.2). However, one may follow these recommendations in the most typical patient for SCS and still not meet with a positive outcome. The uniqueness of SCS lies in making sure the candidate can optimally perceive the potential benefit of this particular modality. Analysis of the available literature has shown that some predictability of success can be made in advance of trialing the patient for a stimulation system. These criteria should be considered in addition to those outlined previously.

Table 4.2 Preoperative considerations for SCS that predict safety and success with SCS

Procedure-specific considerations	SCS-specific considerations
Absence of infection at site of implant or signs of systemic infection	Absence of aberrant opioid-related drug use behavior suggesting opioid abuse or diversion
Absence of bleeding diathesis	Lost prescriptions
No history of bleeding disorders or platelet abnormalities	Dose escalation without practitioner's approval
No history of nosebleeds, easy bruising, or difficulty controlling bleeding	Requests for frequent refills
Discontinue all medications affecting hemostasis (NSAIDs, antiplatelet drugs, anticoagulants)	Evidence of drug diversion
Absence of uncontrolled hypertension	Obtaining opioids from multiple prescribers or other sources
Absence of uncontrolled blood sugars	Absence of psychiatric/psychological co-morbidities
Awareness of any history of contact dermatitis or potential allergic complications	Untreated mood disorders (anxiety, depression)
If dermatological reaction is predicted, consider alternatives or prophylaxis	Untreated psychosis
Radiological review to ensure the epidural space can accommodate the lead	Personality disorders
	Appropriate understanding of the risks and benefits of SCS

4.6.1 Prescription Medications

The ideal candidate should have no untreated or unmanaged drug addiction problems; this includes prescription and illicit drugs. A patient may be taking opioids for pain as long as these are properly prescribed and managed by a physician. Patients who arbitrarily dose escalate without their physician's approval or instruction frequently request early refills owing to excessive consumption or lost prescriptions or display other signs of drug seeking should be considered for treatment of the underlying addiction problem first. After the patient is successfully treated and considered stable, one may wish to reconsider trialing him or her.

4.6.2 Psychiatric and Psychological

It is well stated in the literature that psychiatric and psychological conditions can adversely affect outcomes with SCS. As part of the standard workup, a patient must typically undergo psychiatric or psychological clearance. This can be of great benefit—not just in determining the obvious of whether or not the patient is of sound mind and judgment (*see* Sect. 4.6.3) but can aid in identifying those with underlying psychiatric/psychological comorbidities that may undermine the potential for a successful outcome.

Many patients afflicted with chronic pain also suffer from conditions like depression and anxiety. Outcome studies have shown the presence of these problems does not adversely affect the likelihood of success as long as they are considered stable. Like with addiction, once the problem has been addressed and managed, the trial can proceed. Screening for depression or anxiety can be difficult. Work by Doleys and Brown [2] showed that the Minnesota Multiphasic Personality Inventory (MMPI) is not predictive of an adverse outcome even if the patient's scores indicated high levels of depression and anxiety. In this analysis, the patients with the worst scores on this inventory had excellent outcomes and showed a major improvement in repeat testing. Absolute contraindications to SCS are schizophrenia and delusional disorders.

Because of the complexity of this issue, if the implanting doctor is concerned about the issue, she or he should consult a psychologist or psychiatrist well versed in the relationship between pain and depression and familiar with SCS. The other area of concern is personality disorders. Whereas several personality disorders can lead to functional disabilities, the diagnosis of borderline personality disorder should be seen as a relative contraindication to moving forward with an implant. Antisocial personality disorder is another worrisome problem and these patients should also be viewed with caution.

4.6.3 Cognition

The patient should have appropriate cognitive ability to understand the procedure, the risks, and expectations of the therapy. The patient must also understand the use of the equipment and the technical responsibilities of having the device implanted. Cognitive functioning can be diminished because of neurological disease or medical illnesses or from a baseline level of intelligence that does not allow for implanting. A psychologist, psychiatrist, or neurologist may be helpful in determining competence when the implanting doctor has doubts. In these settings a non-rechargable device with simple programming is often ideal. Family support can be critical to a good outcome in this complex group.

4.6.4 Education

The preoperative period is an ideal time for patient education and discussion. Several studies have suggested that preprocedure education improves the likelihood of a positive outcome. This includes aspects of coping, understanding their condition, and the goals and expectations of the procedure. Material such as videos, DVDs, and patient education booklets can be a great supplement to patient discussion.

References

1. Mekhail N, Mathews M, Nageeb F, Guirguis M, Mekhail N, Cheng J. Retrospective review of 707 cases of spinal cord stimulation: indications and complications. Pain Pract. 2011;11:148–53.
2. Doleys D, Brown J. MMPI Profile as an outcome "predictor" in the treatment of non cancer pain patients utilizing intraspinal opioid therapy. Neuromodulation. 2001;4:93–7.

Suggested Reading

Brook A, Georgy B, Olan WJ. Spinal cord stimulation: a basic approach. Tech Vasc Interv Radiol. 2009;12:64–70.

Burton A, Fukshansky M, Brown J, Hassenbusch III SJ. Refractory insomnia in a patient with spinal cord stimulator lead migration. Neuromodulation. 2004;7:242–5.

Campbell C, Jamison R, Edwards R. Psychological screening/phenotyping as predictors for spinal cord stimulation. Curr Pain Headache Rep. 2013;17:307.

Celestin J, Edwards R, Jamison R. Pretreatment psychosocial variables as predictors of outcomes following lumbar surgery and spinal cord stimulation: a systemic review and literature synthesis. Pain Med. 2009;10:639–53.

Chaudhry ZA, Najib U, Bajwa Z, Jacobs WC, Sheikh J, Simopoulos T. Detailed analysis of allergic cutaneous reactions to spinal cord stimulator devices. J Pain Res. 2013;6:617–23.

Levy R, Henderson J, Slavin K, et al. Incidence and avoidance of neurologic complications with paddle type spinal cord stimulation leads. Neuromodulation. 2011;14:412–22.

North R, Kidd D, Wimberly R, Edwin D. Prognostic value of psychological testing in patients undergoing spinal cord stimulation: a prospective study. Neurosurgery. 1996;39:301–10.

Oakley J. Spinal cord stimulation: patient selection, technique, and outcomes. Neurosurg Clin N Am. 2003;14:365–80.

Ohnmeiss D. Patient satisfaction with spinal cord stimulation for predominant complaints of chronic, intractable low back pain. Spine J. 2001;1:1358–63.

Shealy C, Mortimer J, Reswick JB. Electrical inhibition of pain by stimulation of the dorsal columns: preliminary clinical report. Anesth Analg. 1967;46:489–91.

Sparkes E, Raphael J, Duarte R, LeMarchand K, Jackson C, Ashford R. A systemic literature review of psychological characteristics as determinants of outcome for spinal stimulation therapy. Pain. 2010;150:284–9.

Villavicencio A, Burneikiene S. Elements of the pre-operative workup. Case examples. Pain Med. 2006;7 Suppl 1:S35–46.

5 Perioperative Precautions for Infection Control

David A. Provenzano

5.1 Introduction

Surgical site infections (SSIs), which represent approximately 22 % of all healthcare-related infections, are associated with significant healthcare costs and medical morbidity. When an SSI occurs, direct inpatient medical costs typically double. Infection rates for implantable pain therapies (spinal cord stimulation and intrathecal drug delivery) have been reported in the range of 2–8 %. Recently, substantial emphasis has been placed on reducing the incidence of SSIs. Although SSIs may occur at any location, most infections related to implantable pain therapies occur at the generator site or the intrathecal pump pocket.

It is imperative that implanting physicians understand the risk for SSIs, their causative factors, and methods to decrease their rate of occurrence. Because research specific to the prevention of SSIs in implantable pain therapy is limited, evidence-based processes and well-developed infection control practices that are known to reduce the incidence of SSIs must be extrapolated from other surgical fields. In this chapter, infection control strategies and risk reduction methods are divided into the three stages of the perioperative period: preoperative, intraoperative, and postoperative (Table 5.1).

Table 5.1 Methods to decrease the rate of surgical site infections in implantable pain therapy [1]

Preoperative
Identification of patient risk factors
Optimizing immune and nutritional status
Optimizing medical comorbidities such as diabetes, immunosuppression, and dental disease
Preoperative screening and decolonization for *Staphylococcus aureus* carriers
Appropriate selection of intravenous antibiotic prophylaxis based on hospital pathogens
Weight-based dosing of antibiotics
Appropriate hair removal
Evaluation for skin lesions or areas of local infection
Intraoperative
Selecting appropriate agent for skin antisepsis
Wide prep and drape
Laminar flow and HEPA filters for operating room
Limiting traffic in operating room
Adequate hemostasis
Limiting tissue trauma and avoiding electrocautery at tissue surface
Vigorous wound irrigation
Careful tissue approximation and attention to wound closure
Limiting surgical time
Postoperative
Occlusive dressing for at least 48 h
Attention to tape allergies and skin irritants
Continuing to optimize comorbidities
Education regarding fever and warning signs of early infection
Close wound surveillance
Consulting with an infectious disease specialist if any signs or warning signals of infection are present

HEPA high-efficiency particulate air

D.A. Provenzano
Pain Diagnostics and Interventional Care,
Pittsburgh, PA, USA
e-mail: davidprovenzano@hotmail.com

T.R. Deer, J.E. Pope (eds.), *Atlas of Implantable Therapies for Pain Management*, DOI 10.1007/978-1-4939-2110-2_5

5.2 Preoperative Practices

Before an implantable pain therapy procedure, it is important to identify and (if possible) modify known patient risk factors for the development of SSIs, including altered immunity (*e.g.*, HIV/AIDS or corticosteroid use), malabsorption syndrome, poor dental hygiene, diabetes, obesity, remote infection, and tobacco use. If hair removal is required, it should be performed immediately before surgery, using electrical clippers.

Because a majority of SSIs are caused by *Staphylococcus aureus* (the leading nosocomial pathogen globally), it is important to preoperatively identify carriers of both methicillin-sensitive *S. aureus* (MSSA) and methicillin-resistant *S. aureus* (MRSA). More than 80 % of healthcare-associated *S. aureus* infections have an endogenous origin. In one review examining infection for implantable pain therapies, *S. aureus* was the most commonly identified organism. Preoperative decolonization protocols for known carriers of *S. aureus* (both MSSA and MSRA), which include mupirocin nasal ointment and chlorhexidine soap, have been shown to reduce the risk of postoperative *S. aureus* infections in other populations receiving implantable devices (*i.e.*, total joint arthroplasty).

Prophylactic antibiotic therapy with weight-based dosing (Table 5.2) has been shown to reduce the incidence of wound infection by 50 %, independent of surgery type. Weight-based dosing is important in order to achieve tissue and serum minimum inhibitory concentrations. Furthermore, failure to optimize antimicrobial therapy has been shown to increase the risk of infection by twofold to sixfold. Intravenous antibiotics should be administered within 1 h prior to surgical incision, or within 2 h when vancomycin is used. Additional studies have indicated a further reduction in SSIs when antibiotics (excluding vancomycin) are given within 30 min before incision. A study examining risk factors for infection following spinal surgery demonstrated a 3.4-fold increased risk of SSI if antibiotics were given after surgical incision.

Table 5.2 Preoperative weight-based dosing of antibiotics [2]

	≤80 kg	81–160 kg	≥160 kg
Cefazolin	1 g	2 g	3 g
Clindamycin[a]	600 mg	900 mg	1200 mg
Vancomycin[b]	20 mg/kg	20 mg/kg (max 2500 mg)	3000 mg

[a]Clindamycin may also be used in individuals with a beta-lactam allergy
[b]Vancomycin use should be reserved for the following indications: (1) MRSA colonization; (2) institutionalized patients; (3) procedure performed in a facility with a recent outbreak of MRSA; and (4) beta-lactam allergy

5.3 Intraoperative Practices

One of the most important intraoperative practices is the appropriate selection of skin antisepsis. The two solutions most commonly used for skin preparation are based on povidone-iodine or chlorhexidine. Povidone-iodine is an iodophor, a complex of iodine and organic carrier compounds. These complexes destroy microbial protein and DNA, and are active against a wide spectrum of bacteria and fungi. Specifically povidone-iodine is a complex of bactericidal iodine with the polymer polyvinylpyrrolidone. In order for iodophors to have significant bactericidal activity, two minutes of contact is required to release free iodine. The free iodine is responsible for the antimicrobial activity. In vitro data have demonstrated significant residual bacterial counts when exposure time is limited. The antimicrobial effects of iodophors may be inhibited or neutralized by an organic compound such as blood. In addition, some *S. aureus* has been shown to be resistant to the antimicrobial effects of povidone-iodine. Adverse reactions to povidone-iodine include contact dermatitis and impaired wound healing secondary to its cytotoxic effects on fibroblasts and keratinocytes (the predominant cell type in the epidermis).

Chlorhexidine gluconate is active against a broad spectrum of gram-positive and gram-negative bacteria, yeasts, and molds. Its mechanism of action includes the disruption of cytoplasmic membranes. Chlorhexidine-based products are superior to iodophors as a result of their residual antimicrobial effects, rapid activity, high binding to the skin, and lack of negative inhibitory effects by organic compounds. Studies examining SSI rates in individuals prepped with products based on either povidone-iodine or chlorhexidine demonstrated a substantial reduction in the overall rate of SSIs in the chlorhexidine group. Skin irritation and erythema have been documented with chlorhexidine-based products. Isopropyl alcohol, an effective bactericidal agent that disorganizes cell membrane lipids and denatures cellular proteins, is often added to increase antimicrobial activity.

Although the practice of double gloving has not been conclusively demonstrated to reduce SSIs, it is recommended because it has been shown to reduce the perforation rates of the inner gloves.

It is important to control and optimize the operating room by limiting traffic, keeping the operating room doors closed, and maintaining positive pressure ventilation. In an effort to prevent intraoperative contamination, the C-arm cover (*i.e.*, sterile drape) should not be considered sterile, and surgical personnel should avoid contact. Previous research has demonstrated significant intraoperative contamination of the C-arm cover during the course of a surgical procedure, with the upper portions of the image intensifier exhibiting the greatest rate of bacterial contamination. SSIs have also been associated with surgical case order, with surgeries performed later in the day carrying a higher risk for a postoperative infection. Extended operative time is a known independent risk factor for SSIs, so the surgeon and surgical team should try to optimize operating room efficiency.

Prior to wound closure and placement of the generator or intrathecal pump into the pocket, the wound should be irrigated to assist in the removal of foreign material, debris, and blood clots. Although many practitioners often add antibiotics to the irrigation, this practice has not conclusively been shown to positively influence infection rates compared with normal saline irrigation without antibiotics. In addition, surgical technique should emphasize minimizing tissue damage and eradicating dead space.

5.4 Postoperative Practices

An occlusive dressing should be used to protect the surgical incision for a minimum of 24–48 h. If dressing changes are required during the early recovery process, hand washing and sterile technique are recommended. Appropriate education on the signs and symptoms of infection should be provided to the patient and appropriate caregivers. It is also important to have appropriate follow-up, which includes wound surveillance.

If an infection is suspected, a diagnostic workup and consultation with an infectious disease specialist should be initiated. Laboratory tests including white blood count, C-reactive protein (CRP), and erythrocyte sedimentation rate (ESR) may be helpful in defining the occurrence of an SSI. It is important to remember that CRP and ESR are markers of inflammation and are not specific for infection. CRP is a quantitative test that exhibits more consistent and predictable kinetics in the postoperative period and therefore may be more helpful in determining the existence of a postoperative infection. The postoperative decrease in ESR is slow, and the ESR may remain elevated for up to 1 year after spinal surgery.

In some patients, superficial infections can be treated effectively with antibiotics. If this treatment method is chosen, close surveillance is required to monitor for the spread of the infection to deeper structures. If the infection has spread to deeper structures, then surgical incision, drainage, and removal of the devices is required. An MRI can be performed to determine if the infection has spread to the neuraxis. Reimplantation may be considered once the infection has been effectively treated and the infectious disease specialist has provided surgical clearance.

Conclusions

It is of paramount importance for pain physicians who manage implantable pain therapies (spinal cord stimulation and intrathecal drug delivery systems) to have a strong understanding of SSI prevention and control. When appropriate steps are taken during all three stages of the perioperative process, the risk of infection can be significantly reduced. Even when all measures are followed, however, SSIs may still occur, so appropriate follow-up is mandatory.

References

1. Deer TR, Provenzano DA. Recommendations for reducing infection in the practice of implanting spinal cord stimulation and intrathecal drug delivery devices: a physician's playbook. Pain Physician. 2013;16:E125–8.
2. Alexander JW, Solomkin JS, Edwards MJ. Updated recommendations for control of surgical site infections. Ann Surg. 2011;253:1082–93.

Suggested Reading

Biswas D, Bible JE, Whang PG, Simpson AK, Grauer JN. Sterility of C-arm fluoroscopy during spinal surgery. Spine (Phila Pa 1976). 2008;33:1913–7.

Bowater RJ, Stirling SA, Lilford RJ. Is antibiotic prophylaxis in surgery a generally effective intervention? Testing a generic hypothesis over a set of meta-analyses. Ann Surg. 2009;249:551–6.

Chen AF, Wessel CB, Rao N. Staphylococcus aureus screening and decolonization in orthopaedic surgery and reduction of surgical site infections. Clin Orthop Relat Res. 2013;471:2383–99.

Darouiche RO, Wall Jr MJ, Itani KM, Otterson MF, Webb AL, Carrick MM, et al. Chlorhexidine-alcohol versus povidone-iodine for surgical-site antisepsis. N Engl J Med. 2010;362:18–26.

Follett KA, Boortz-Marx RL, Drake JM, DuPen S, Schneider SJ, Turner MS, et al. Prevention and management of intrathecal drug delivery and spinal cord stimulation system infections. Anesthesiology. 2004;100:1582–94.

Mangram AJ, Horan TC, Pearson ML, Silver LC, Jarvis WR. Guideline for prevention of surgical site infection, 1999. Hospital Infection Control Practices Advisory Committee. Infect Control Hosp Epidemiol. 1999;20:250–78.

Matar WY, Jafari SM, Restrepo C, Austin M, Purtill JJ, Parvizi J. Preventing infection in total joint arthroplasty. J Bone Joint Surg Am. 2010;92 Suppl 2:36–46.

Mok JM, Pekmezci M, Piper SL, Boyd E, Berven SH, Burch S, et al. Use of C-reactive protein after spinal surgery: comparison with erythrocyte sedimentation rate as predictor of early postoperative infectious complications. Spine (Phila Pa 1976). 2008;33:415–21.

6 Needle Placement for Percutaneous Spinal Cord Stimulation of the Back and Legs

Timothy R. Deer, Jason E. Pope, and Louis J. Raso

6.1 Introduction

Needle placement is one of the most important procedural tasks in placing a percutaneous spinal cord stimulation device, yet it is often overlooked in regard to its impact on the overall outcome and ease of the procedure. Needle placement sets the tone for the ease of placing the lead, the angle of lead placement, and the potential for complications. It is often viewed as a simple procedure, yet it is a technique that should be performed with vigilance and planning (Table 6.1). Prior to placing the needle, the patient must be prepared and positioned, and a fluoroscopic scout film is taken to evaluate the best route to use when placing the needle. If the patient has had instrumentation or has scoliosis or congenital spinal defects, a recent plain film should be reviewed prior to going to the operating room. If stenosis is a concern, the clinician should consider an MRI or CT scan prior to moving forward, to ensure that there is adequate room in the epidural space.

Table 6.1 Checklist prior to needle placement

1. Understand the anatomy at the location of planned needle entry
2. Review the skin integrity for lesions or local infection
3. Review recent plain films if there is concern about barriers to needle placement
4. Review recent CT or MRI images if significant stenosis is a concern
5. Plan the angle of approach for the needle, including the paramedian angle and needle-to-spine angle (as illustrated in this chapter)

T.R. Deer, MD (✉)
The Center for Pain Relief, 400 Court Street, Suite 100, Charleston, WV 25301, USA
e-mail: DocTDeer@aol.com

J.E. Pope
Summit Pain Alliance,
392 Tesconi Court, Santa Rosa, CA 95401, USA
e-mail: popeje@me.com

L.J. Raso
Jupiter Interventional Pain Management,
2141 South Alternate A1A #110, Jupiter, FL 33477, USA
e-mail: ljraso@gmail.com

T.R. Deer, J.E. Pope (eds.), *Atlas of Implantable Therapies for Pain Management*, DOI 10.1007/978-1-4939-2110-2_6

6.2 Technical Overview

After proper patient preparation, the physician should develop a strategy for needle placement. This strategy should include level of entry, angle of entry, side of entry, and method of identifying the epidural space. The physician should also plan the site for the placement of the needle tip at the time of epidural space entry in relation to bony landmarks. Once the route of entry is determined, a local anesthetic injection is given (Fig. 6.1). At this point, a #15 blade is used to make a small stab wound to place the needle. This step allows for an easier entry into the tissues and may reduce the risk of introducing infection into the epidural space from skin pathogens. The needle is then ideally placed at an angle of 30–45° and advanced until it contacts the lamina of the vertebral body caudal to the planed interlaminar space entry. It is then advanced and "walked off" cephalad into the ligament (Fig. 6.2). In some patients, anatomical variants may require modification of the needle angle to increase the ease and safety of access. In addition, the body habitus of the patient must be accommodated: If the patient is obese, a more caudal skin entry site is required to ensure maintenance of the desired needle angle of entry, whereas a more cephalad skin entry site is needed for very thin patients. Once the needle is established in the ligament, the stylet is removed and the needle is advanced carefully, using the loss of resistance or hanging drop technique (Figs. 6.3 and 6.4). Some have described a method of using a wire to identify the entry into the epidural space, but this technique is not well established or uniform and should be used only if the implanter is trained in this approach. In some settings, such as in the upper thoracic spine, the anatomy makes entry into the epidural space at a reasonable angle difficult. In these settings, the use of a curved-tip needle may be helpful. An example of this type of needle is seen in Fig. 6.4.

The angle of the needle approach will determine the end point of the tip when entering the epidural space. In most cases, this point will be just below the spinous process on an anterior-posterior view, and it will be in the posterior epidural space on a lateral view (Figs. 6.5, 6.6, and 6.7). At this time, the needle is ready for lead placement (Fig. 6.8).

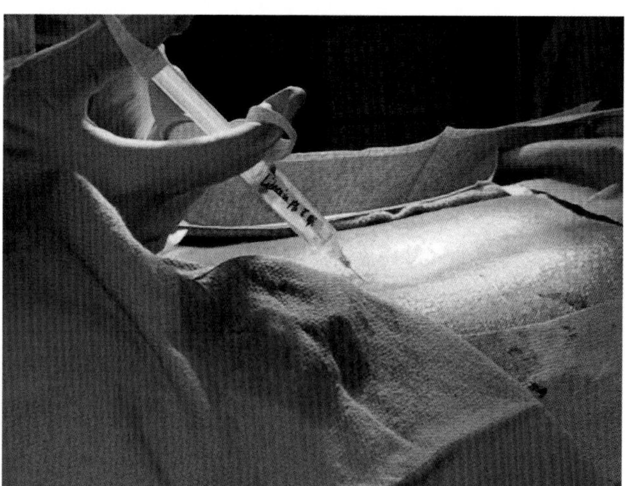

Fig. 6.1 Local anesthetic should be applied in the same plane that is planned for the needle placement. The local anesthetic should be placed in the skin and subsequent tissues to the level of the supraspinous ligament. If the needle is advanced aggressively into the spine, injection of local anesthetic into the spinal fluid can lead to an accidental spinal block

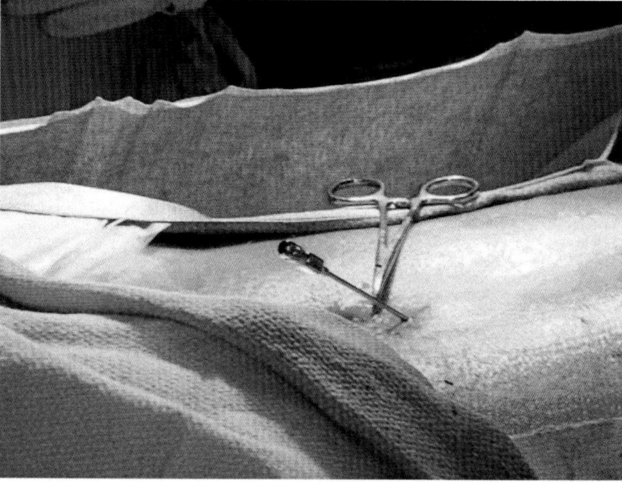

Fig. 6.2 The angle of needle placement should be between 30° and 45° when possible. In some cases, the patient's anatomy will not lend itself to that angle and adjustments must be made accordingly

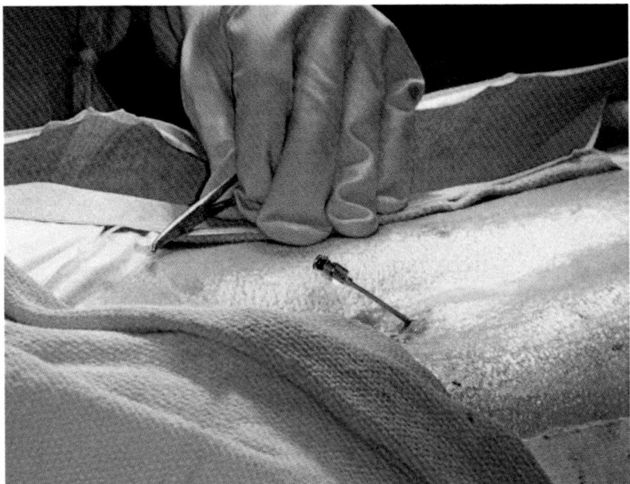

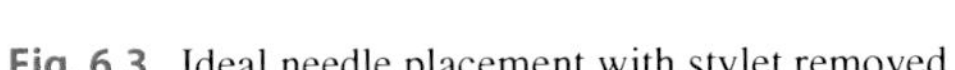

Fig. 6.3 Ideal needle placement with stylet removed

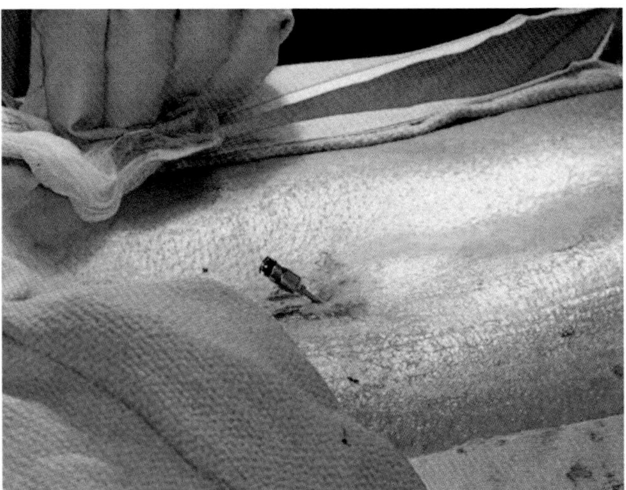

Fig. 6.5 Needle placement in the epidural space

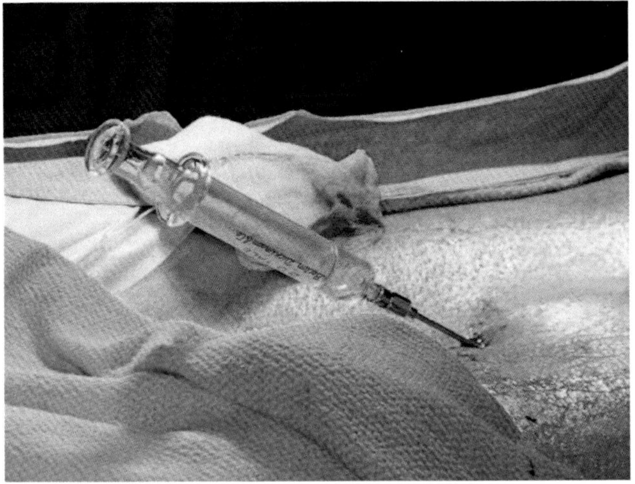

Fig. 6.4 The confirmation of needle placement is performed by loss of resistance or hanging drop technique. The use of contrast occasionally is needed, but it should be avoided if possible

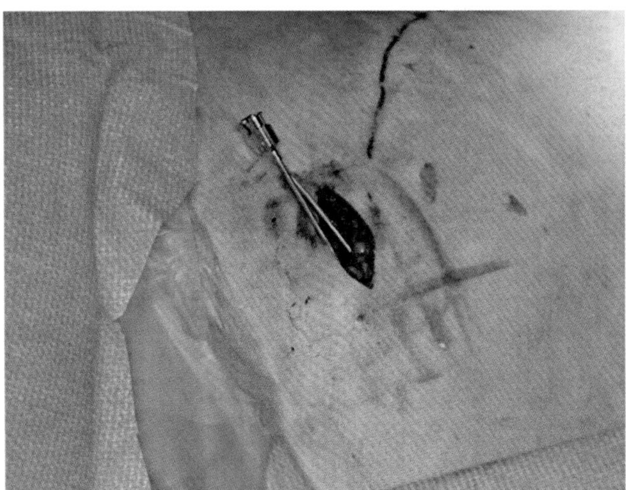

Fig. 6.6 In morbidly obese patients, a cutdown may be needed to achieve a safe angle. The physician must weigh the risks of the cutdown with the risk of a sharper angle, which can lead to wet tap or nerve injury

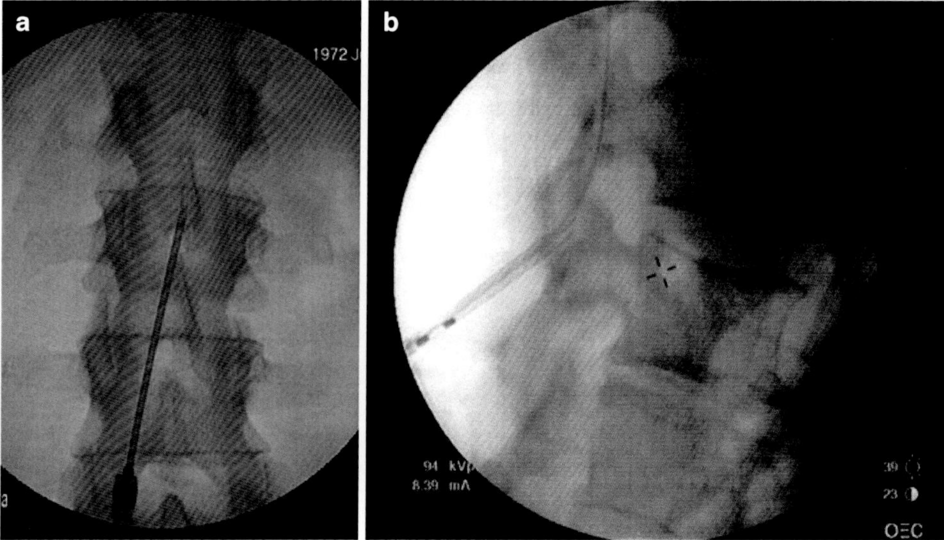

Fig. 6.7 Fluoroscopic guidance is critical for placement. Anterior-posterior and lateral images are needed to confirm needle placement

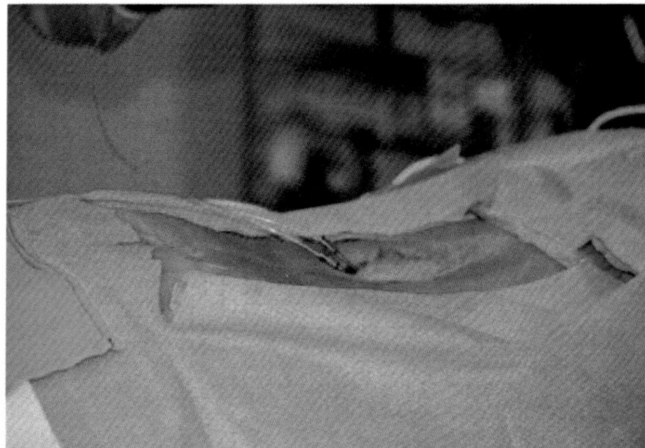

Fig. 6.8 Once the needle position is acceptable, the leads are placed to the proper target

6.3 Risk Avoidance

Several types of risk accompany needle placement: infection of the skin, tissues, or epidural space; epidural bleeding or hematoma; nerve injury; and post–dural puncture headache. These risks can be minimized by care in following risk-avoidance procedures.

6.3.1 Risk of Infection

Do a thorough presurgical workup of coexisting diseases that may increase patient risks and determine whether the risks are acceptable. Primary care physicians and other specialists should be consulted to ensure that all systems are optimally controlled prior to implant. Choose a sterile operating area, prep widely, drape widely, use prophylactic antibiotics as directed, make a skin entry puncture, and use sterile dressings.

6.3.2 Bleeding Risks

Assess preoperative risks of bleeding and determine whether the risks are acceptable. Consult with primary care or a cardiovascular specialist regarding drugs that affect platelet function, bleeding times, or other areas of hemostasis, and determine whether the patient can be removed from those medications for an acceptable period prior to needle placement. Consult with primary care regarding disease states that affect bleeding, such as leukemia or other diseases of the hematological system. If the platelet function is below 50,000, the physician should be hesitant to proceed without the written consent of the treating physician assessing the patient's bleeding status.

6.3.3 Risk of Nerve Injury

The ability to harm a patient by introducing a large needle into the neuroaxis is a substantial worry. Fortunately, despite this potential harm, significant injury is rare. Several steps are critical to avoid nerve injury: (1) Keep the patient alert and responsive during needle placement even when using monitored anesthesia care or conscious sedation; (2) Keep the needle angle at 45° or less; (3) If paresthesia is elicited, remove the needle immediately and enter the spine at a different location once the paresthesia dissipates; (4) If the patient complains of a stabbing or lancinating pain during needle placement, consider giving intravenous steroids as a method of reducing neuritis. The decision to give steroids (e.g., dexamethasone, at a dose of 2–12 mg) should be weighed against the risks of steroids for other disease states.

6.3.4 Headache Risk

The risk of dural puncture is low with the placement of spinal cord stimulation leads. The risks can be reduced by proper positioning, proper fluoroscopic imaging, needle angle of 45° or less, and careful advancement of the needle through the ligaments with image guidance as the needle is advanced. Needle placement should be confirmed by x-ray, hanging drop, loss of resistance, or in rare cases, the use of contrast. Once a dural puncture has been identified, the patient's risk of headache may be reduced by increasing intravenous fluids, using abdominal binders to change intra-abdominal pressure, giving caffeine, and limiting activity. The use of a blood patch should be reserved for situations in which a severe post–dural puncture headache is not resolved with conservative measures.

Conclusions

The placement of a needle into the epidural space is seen by many clinicians as a simple portion of the implant of a spinal cord stimulation device, but needle placement should be viewed as a critical portion of the procedure and should be carefully planned and executed. By following the recommendations of this chapter, the chance of a successful outcome should be enhanced.

Suggested Reading

Deer T. Current and future trends in spinal cord stimulation for chronic pain. Curr Pain Headache Rep. 2001;5:503–9.

Falowski S, Celii A, Sharan A. Spinal cord stimulation: an update. Neurotherapeutics. 2008;5:86–99.

Krames E. Implantable devices for pain control: spinal cord stimulation and intrathecal therapies. Best Pract Res Clin Anaesthesiol. 2002;16:619–49.

Slavin KV, Hsu FPK, Fessler RG. Intrathecal opioids: intrathecal drug-delivery systems. In: Burchiel KJ, editor. Surgical management of pain. New York: Thieme; 2002. p. 603–13.

Physician-Guided Lead Placement: Driving the Lead to the Target Location

7

Timothy R. Deer, Kasra Amirdelfan, Louis J. Raso, and Stanley Golovac

7.1 Introduction

The placement of spinal cord stimulation (SCS) systems has several important components. For tonic stimulation requiring therapeutic paresthesia overlying the patient's pain, placement of the device within the epidural space is paramount. Lead placement is important because the ability to delivery energy in the correct location and the flexibility to change the array of stimulation are dependent on the lead location. In the past few are shared in this chapter. In successfully placing leads the physician must choose a patient with acceptable anatomy for placement, properly insert a needle, and pick a target for the desired lead location for proper stimulation. In many patients the most difficult component of the procedure is guiding the lead from the needle to the end location. Multiple factors will influence the ease in which this task is completed. By modifying the technique, the physician can maximize the ease in which the lead is guided to the target.

T.R. Deer, MD (✉)
The Center for Pain Relief, 400 Court Street, Suite 100, Charleston, WV 25301, USA
e-mail: DocTDeer@aol.com

K. Amirdelfan
IPM Medical Group, Inc., 450 N. Wiget Lane, Walnut Creek, CA 94598, USA
e-mail: DoctorA@ipmdoctors.com

L.J. Raso
Jupiter Interventional Pain Management, 2141 South Alternate A1A #110, Jupiter, FL 33477, USA
e-mail: ljraso@gmail.com

S. Golovac
Florida Pain, 4770 Honeyridge Lane, Merritt Island, FL 32952, USA
e-mail: sgolovac@mac.com

7.2 Technical Overview

In some clinical settings guiding a lead is technically very simple. The needle is placed at an angle of 40° or less from a paramedian approach, both in the sagittal plane and from the surface of the skin, into an area of the spine with excellent anatomy and the lead advances to the posterior epidural space without any obstructions. Unfortunately, in some patients the lead placement and guidance is very difficult. In these settings the clinician must make proper adjustments to the technique to optimize the procedure and improve the chances for a good outcome. In each setting physicians should go through a checklist of issues in their mind to improve success.

Prior to placing the lead the physician should evaluate and optimize needle placement. This includes proper needle angle, bevel orientation, and approach off the midline in a paramedian approach (Fig. 7.1a, b).

Once the needle has been addressed, the next component to examine should be the lead itself. Issues to consider are the type of stylet (Fig. 7.2a), length of lead, and whether the position is ideal for initial exit from the needle to start on a correct path toward the target. Initially in most cases the curved stylet is the initial starting point for lead placement. In situations in which the lead is advancing too far laterally, a change to a straight stylet (Fig. 7.2b) may allow the lead to correct toward the midline. In some clinical settings the physician may need to alternate between a curved and a straight stylet several times to maneuver the lead to the desired location. The need to exaggerate the curve in the stylet is rare, but in some cases the physician may create an exaggerated curve creating a "hockey stick" angle that is needed to drive the lead toward midline when it is tracking laterally. In cases in which an exaggerated stylet is used, the physician should reconfirm placement of the lead with both fluoroscopy and computer screening once the stylet is removed to detect a "rebound movement" that results in lead movement once the rigidity of the stylet is removed. Lead issues are reviewed in Table 7.1. New stylets with polymer coatings may allow for

T.R. Deer, J.E. Pope (eds.), *Atlas of Implantable Therapies for Pain Management*, DOI 10.1007/978-1-4939-2110-2_7

easy lead placements and stylet removal without lead contour changes. Despite this advance the lead can still be difficult to place.

Epidural obstructions can be frustrating and potentially dangerous when attempting to successfully place a lead. These obstructions can be caused by several factors (Table 7.2) and can lead to a failure of the procedure. All manufacturers include a wire coil in their typical lead deployment kit. This coil wire can be used to create a pathway or channel in the epidural space to help with lead advancement. These wire inserts can be helpful, but they can also lead to complications and should be used with caution. The authors prefer a different method for overcoming this issue. That is to use a technique of finesse and a gentle approach to avoid trauma. In this method the lead is advanced to the point of obstruction and then repeatedly advanced forward. Each time an obstruction is felt, the lead is withdrawn, and then advanced only during exhalation. In many cases this method will lead to an ability to advance the lead without traumatizing the tissue. Other options include using the curved and straight stylet to "drive" around the obstructive structure. In the event that these methods are unsuccessful, a different intralaminar level of entry should be considered. If difficulty persists past a reasonable number of attempts, the procedure should be aborted and a surgical laminotomy approach should be considered, even for the trial phase.

Once the lead is driven to the desired target, hand-held computer screening can be used to ensure that the patient has the desired response. In the event the response is not optimal, additional modifications may be needed. Trolling of the lead can be used to optimize placement. In this method the lead is activated to the sensory threshold and then adjusted in the epidural space until optimal placement is achieved. When the clinician is satisfied with the placement, a fluoroscopic image should be taken on lateral and anteroposterior views and saved for future comparisons if there are any concerns about lead migration.

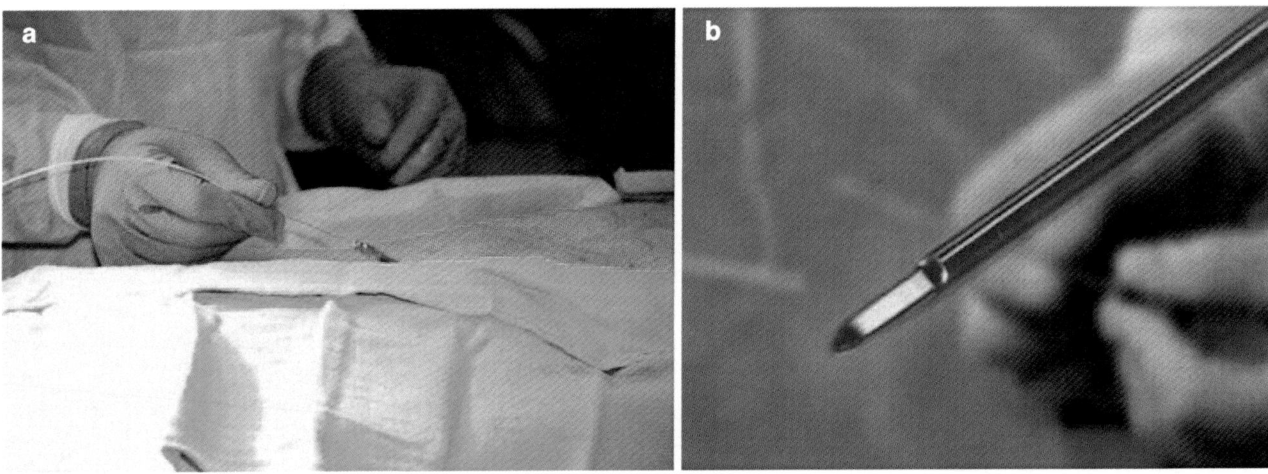

Fig. 7.1 The bevel of the needle should be cephalad (**b**) and the lead should be introduced with the goal of placement within the posterior epidural space (**a**)

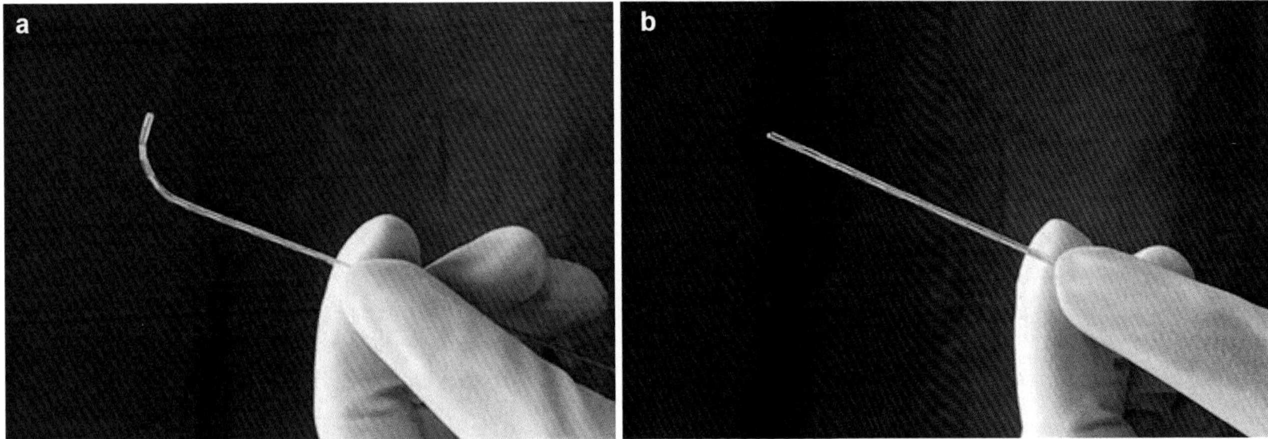

Fig. 7.2 (**a**) Curved stylet; (**b**) Straight stylet

Table 7.1 Lead issues

Lead issue	Options
Lateral lead movement	Rotate the lead using a curved stylet
Obstruction to movement	Gently reposition the lead alternating the curved and straight stylets
	Gently tap the lead against the obstruction on multiple rapid attempts, withdrawing slightly each time
	Use the wire coil to pass the obstruction (use caution and stop if pain occurs)
Failure to achieve stimulation despite optimal X-ray placement	Troll with the lead to find an area responsive to stimulation, try different programming arrays including a guarded cathode
High impedance of the lead	Reposition the lead cephalad or caudad

Table 7.2 Causes of obstructions

Epidural fibrosis
Epidural vessels
Fascial bands
Spinal stenosis
Disc protrusions compressing the canal
Postsurgical scarring

7.3 Risk Assessment

1. The risk of nerve injury should be considered when guiding a lead to the target zone. The lead may contact a nerve root or dorsal root entry zone and lead to an injury to the neural structures.
2. The lead can rent the dura and lead to a chronic cerebrospinal fluid leak. This can produce a chronic post–dural puncture headache.
3. The lead can dissect an epidural vessel and cause a bleed that may create an epidural hematoma and subsequent neural injury.
4. The lead may be guided to the lateral or anterior position in the epidural space that can cause a motor nerve stimulation that can be very painful and stressful to the patient.

7.4 Risk Avoidance

1. To avoid nerve injury the clinician should keep the patient conversant and alert during the time of lead placement. An alert patient can warn of paresthesia and result in a change in practice for the implanter.
2. To avoid the risk of dural tear or rent, the lead should be advanced only when resistance is minimal and the lead should not be forced to advance past an obstruction. When using the wire coil device, caution should be exercised to avoid excessive force.
3. Drugs that affect the bleeding function of the patient can lead to severe complications if not stopped prior to implant. The decision to stop warfarin, clopidogrel (Plavix), and other drugs should be made by the treating physician for the affliction for which these drugs are being prescribed. The risk versus the benefit of stopping these drugs should be considered prior to moving forward. Proper laboratory values that may have an impact on bleeding should be considered prior to moving forward.
4. It is important to obtain an anteroposterior film and a lateral film to ensure the lead is not positioned near a nerve root or ventral fiber area. The evaluation of only one view can lead to a miscalculation of lead placement.
5. The use of a shallow needle angle for entry into the epidural space is important for risk avoidance. This maneuver will improve the ease of passing the lead, help with directing the lead, and lower the incidence of lead migration over time.

Conclusions

The ability to drive a lead into a proper target zone can vary in difficulty. The physician can have a great impact on this process by making modifications noted in this chapter. The process of guiding a lead is essential to the procedure.

7.5 Supplemental Images

See Figs. 7.3, 7.4, 7.5, 7.6, 7.7, 7.8, and 7.9.

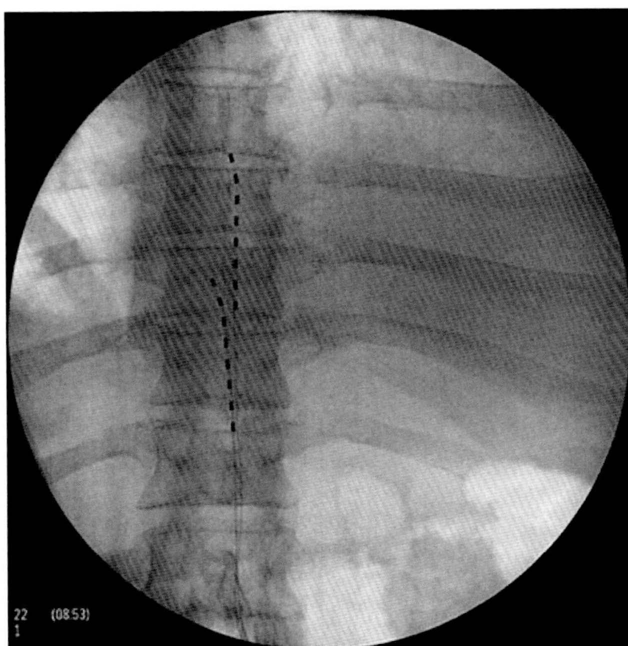

Fig. 7.3 Percutaneous leads covering the T8–10 vertebral bodies

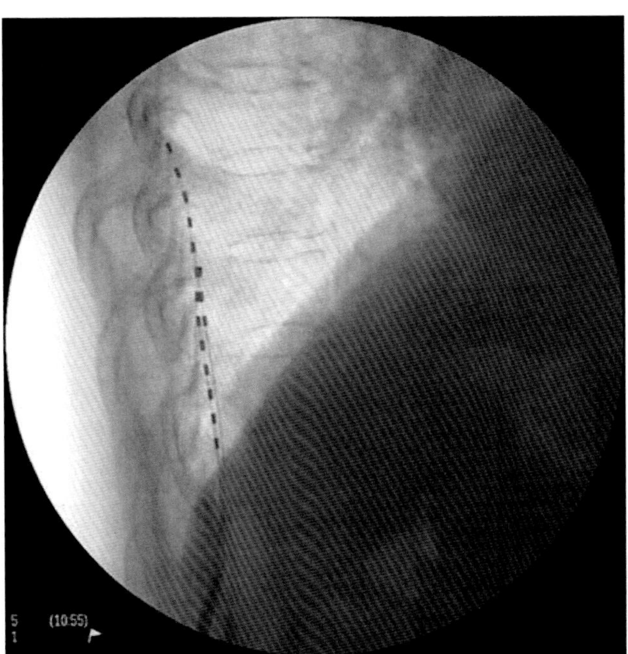

Fig. 7.5 Lateral view showing correct lead placement for thoracic implantation of SCS systems

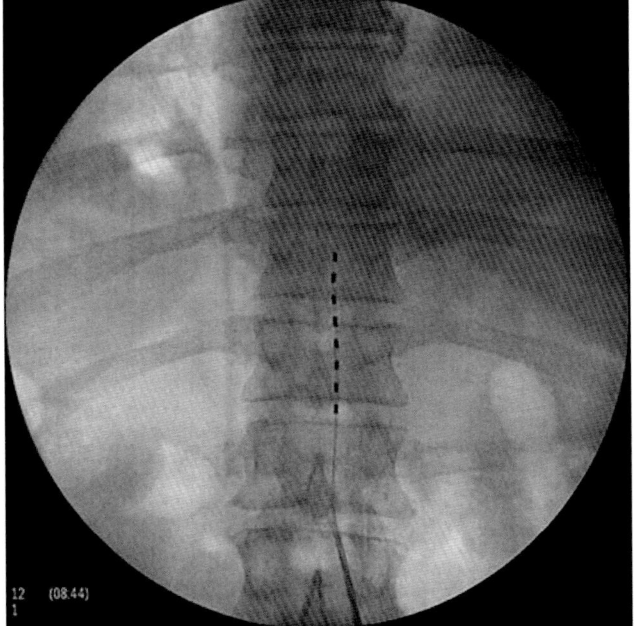

Fig. 7.4 Percutaneous lead covering T10 and T11 off THE midline to provide unilateral coverage

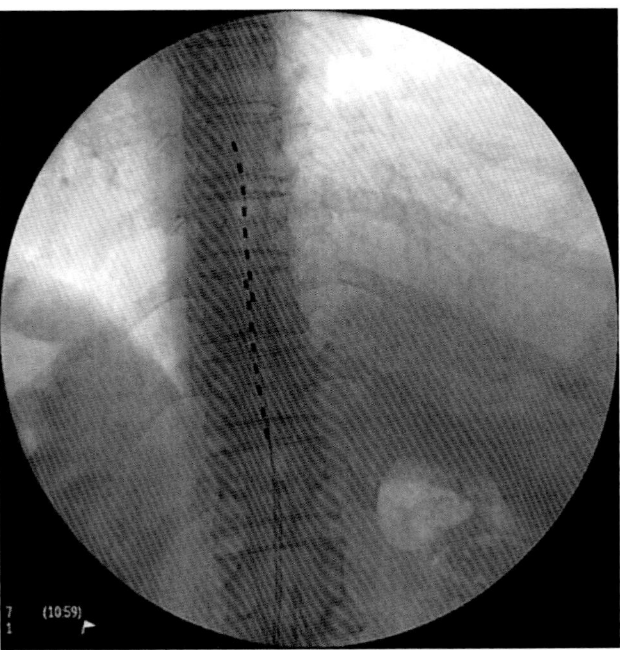

Fig. 7.6 Staggered percutaneous array covering T8–11

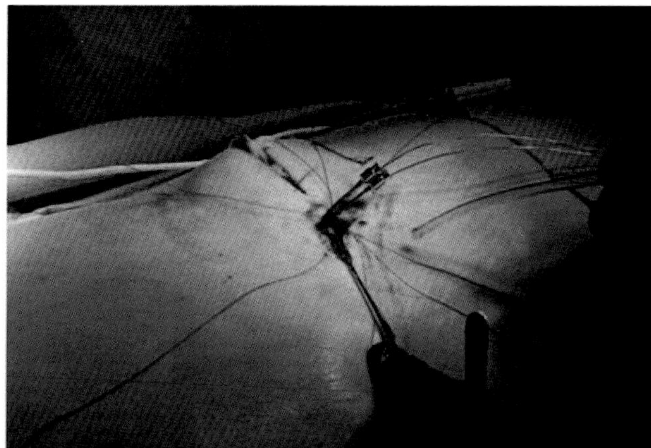

Fig. 7.7 Once the leads are confirmed on x-ray, a cutdown is performed, anchoring stitches are placed, and a pocket is made to implant the generator

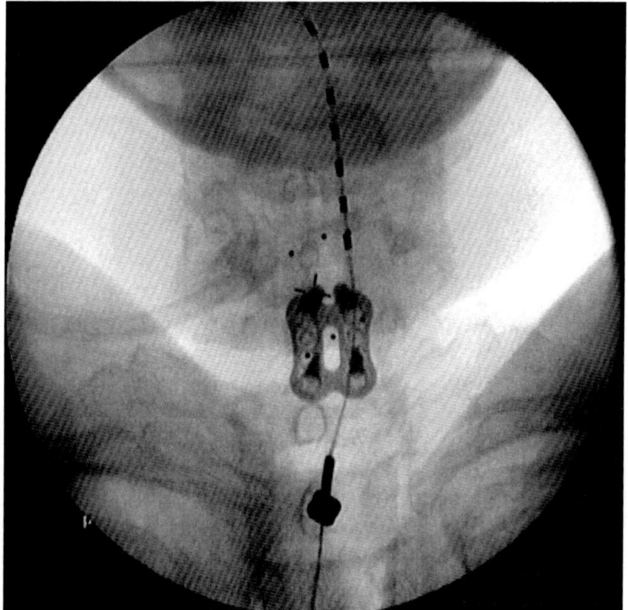

Fig. 7.8 Percutaneous placement of a cervical lead in a patient with a history of anterior fusion

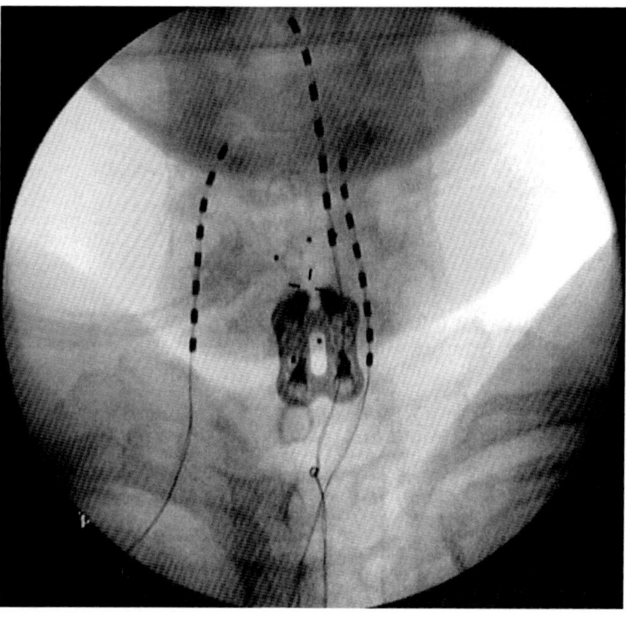

Fig. 7.9 Combined stimulation of percutaneous and peripheral leads for the treatment of axial and radicular and cervical pain

Suggested Reading

Bradley K. The technology: the anatomy of a spinal cord and nerve root stimulator: the lead and the power source. Pain Med. 2006;7 Suppl 1:S27–34.

North RB, Kidd DH, Olin JC, Sieracki JM. Spinal cord stimulation electrode design: prospective randomized, controlled trial comparing percutaneous and laminectomy electrodes—part I: technical outcomes. Neurosurgery. 2002;51:381–90.

8 Stimulation of the Spinal Cord by Placement of Surgical-Based Paddle Leads

Shivanand P. Lad, Erika Petersen, Andrew Marky, Timothy R. Deer, Robert M. Levy, and Claudio A. Feler

8.1 Introduction

Spinal cord stimulation can be achieved through various methods. One of the least invasive and most popular options is percutaneous lead placement via a needle in the epidural space and passing a cylindrical lead into the desired epidural location, producing circumferential modulation of surrounding structures of the neuroaxis. Percutaneous implantation of leads is favored by the majority of interventional pain physicians and is a common method of performing most trials and many permanent implants. An increasingly common method of placing the permanent spinal cord stimulation leads is via an open surgical technique in which a small laminotomy is performed, allowing a ribbon-type surgical or paddle lead to be placed in an antegrade or retrograde fashion into the epidural space under direct visualization. The paddle lead allows for a more efficient, unidirectional lead that may offer more stability. Paddle leads are indicated based on surgeon preference as well as other clinical factors detailed in Table 8.1.

Table 8.1 Indications for paddle lead placement

Indications
Surgeon prefers paddle lead
Surgeon not skilled in percutaneous technique
Difficult needle access to the spine because of anatomical characteristics
Epidural fibrosis
Revision because of lead migration
Inadequate power with percutaneous leads
Positional stimulation

S.P. Lad
Division of Neurosurgery, Department of Surgery, Duke University Medical Center, Durham, NC, USA
e-mail: nandan.lad@duke.edu

E. Petersen
Department of Neurosurgery, University of Arkansas for Medical Sciences, 4301 West Markham #507, Little Rock, AR 72205, USA
e-mail: eapetersen@uams.edu

A. Marky
Division of Neurosurgery, Department of Surgery, Duke University Medical Center, Durham, NC, USA
e-mail: andrew.marky@duke.edu

T.R. Deer, MD (✉)
The Center for Pain Relief, 400 Court Street, Suite 100, Charleston, WV 25301, USA
e-mail: DocTDeer@aol.com

R.M. Levy
Harvey Sandler Department of Neurosurgery, Marcus Neuroscience Institute, 800 Meadows Road, Boca Raton, FL, USA
e-mail: rlevy@brrh.com

C.A. Feler
Semmes-Murphey Clinic, 6325 Humphreys Boulevard, Memphis, TN 38120, USA
e-mail: claudiofeler@gmail.com

T.R. Deer, J.E. Pope (eds.), *Atlas of Implantable Therapies for Pain Management*, DOI 10.1007/978-1-4939-2110-2_8

8.2 Technical Overview

The placement of a paddle electrode requires additional surgical skills as compared with the percutaneous placement of stimulation leads. Unlike the percutaneous cylindrical lead implantation, it does not require the ability to place a needle in the epidural space and to drive a lead. Placing a paddle lead through the open approach requires the surgical skills to safely dissect, expose the spinolaminar junction, and perform a small laminotomy, which allows for direct visualization while placing the lead (Fig. 8.1). A variety of anesthetic choices are available including general anesthesia with neuromonitoring or awake placement with local/mac or spinal anesthesia, the latter two of which still allow appropriate paresthesia mapping. While the patient is upright prior to surgery, it is important to determine the appropriate location for the future pulse generator by marking the patient's belt line and seat line and placing the pulse generator such that it does not interfere with either. The procedure is initiated by properly positioning the patient in the prone or the semilateral position and ensuring all standard surgical precautions are taken to optimize patient safety. Once the patient is positioned, fluoroscopy is utilized to identify the appropriate interspace (e.g., T9–10).

An incision is planned over the appropriate interspinous process. This area, as well as the gluteal pocket, is shaved, prepared, and draped in the usual sterile fashion (Fig. 8.2). After infiltration of local anesthetic, the thoracic incision is opened with a 10-blade scalpel. Subperiosteal dissection is performed and retractors are placed. A small laminotomy is performed (using a combination of Leksell rongeurs, Kerrison punches, and diamond drill). An adequate opening is made for the placement of the paddle lead (Fig. 8.3). Selection of the appropriate paddle lead depends on a number of factors including choice of trial system, selection of active contacts during the trial stimulation (close or wide spacing), epidural anatomy, and size of laminotomy. A paddle lead is advanced under fluoroscopic guidance such that the middle of the lead is positioned over where the patient had most adequate stimulation during the trial procedure (Fig. 8.4).

Next, the gluteal incision is opened. A pocket is made for the pulse generator and a subcutaneous pass is then made from the gluteal area to the thoracic incision. The paddle lead extension wires are brought through from top to bottom. The distal ends of the extensions are then inserted into the pulse generator and the set screws are tightened. Electronic analysis of the neurostimulator system is then performed with electrode selectability, cycling, output modulation, impedance, and compliance tested and found to be in an acceptable range.

As stated previously, some surgeons perform an awake test stimulation with a goal of obtaining paresthesias in the desired painful areas; other surgeons work under general anesthesia confirming placement using a combination of x-ray guidance and evoked potential stimulation. A typical stimulation occurs to 4–6 Hz at a pulse width of 300–350 μs with increases in amplitude until electromyographic signal changes are detected. If the goal is to achieve bilateral lower extremity stimulation, central lead placement is usually desired. In some cases, the fluoroscopic and anatomical midlines vary and the stimulation is more accurate. In cases of unilateral limb pain, the goal is to stimulate the midline and the area just off the midline to the side of pain generation.

Options for paddle lead configurations include single, dual, tripolar, or pentapolar configurations, variability in number of leads placed, spacing of electrodes, curve of the paddle, and overall shape of the lead(s). The complexity of the lead, variation in programming, and hours of stimulation result in a marked variability in the amount of energy required by the pulse generator.

A strain-relief loop is also placed in the thoracic area and anchored down to the interspinous ligament. The extension is coiled beneath the pulse generator that is placed in the pocket. At the conclusion of the lead placement, a final x-ray confirmation is made to document position for future reference (Fig. 8.5). Both incisions are irrigated copiously with bacitracin irrigation and closed in multiple layers.

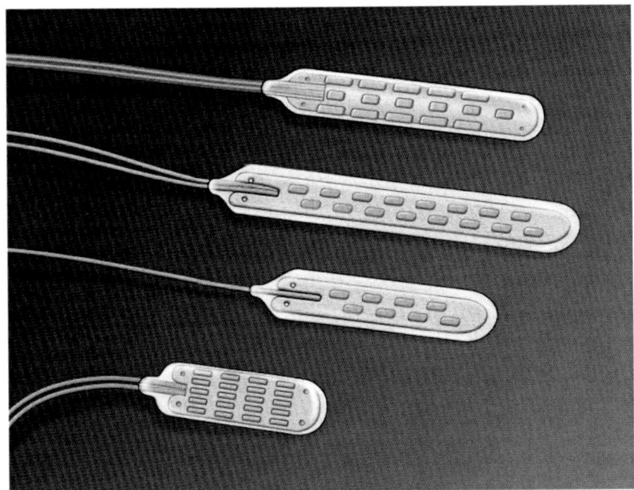

Fig. 8.1 Types of paddle leads

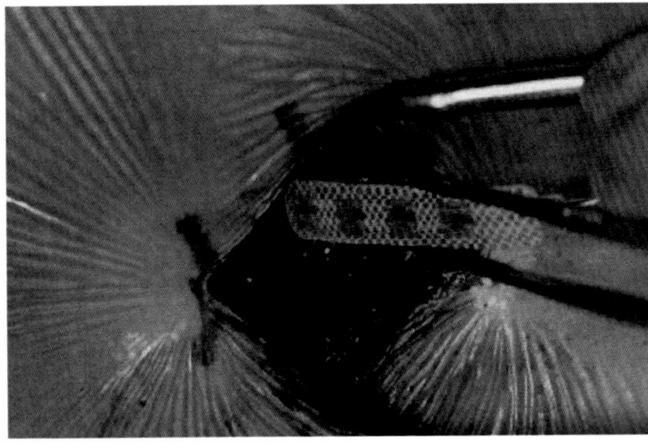

Fig. 8.4 Lead placement into the epidural space

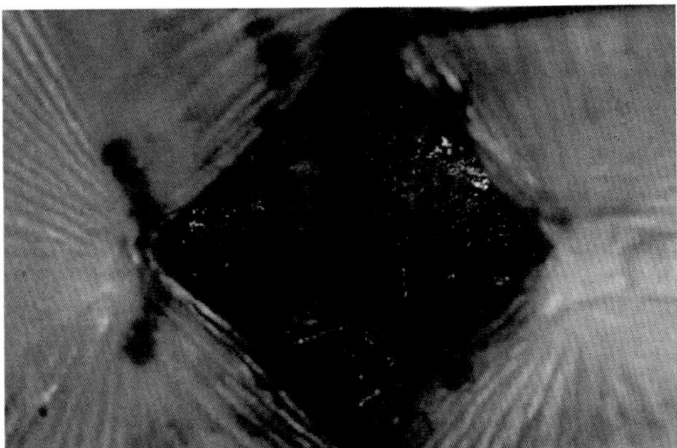

Fig. 8.2 Exposure for lead placement

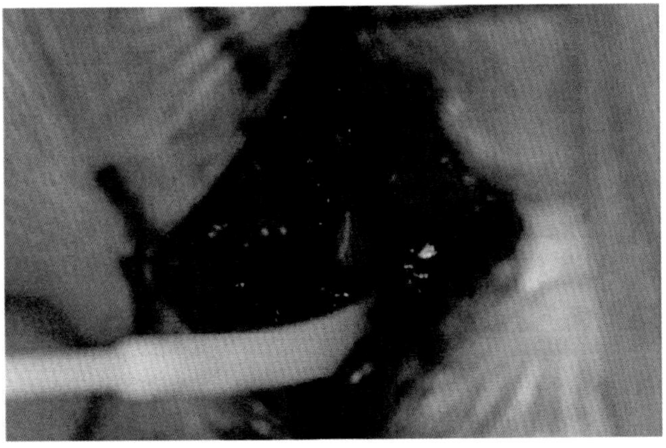

Fig. 8.3 Preparation of the epidural space

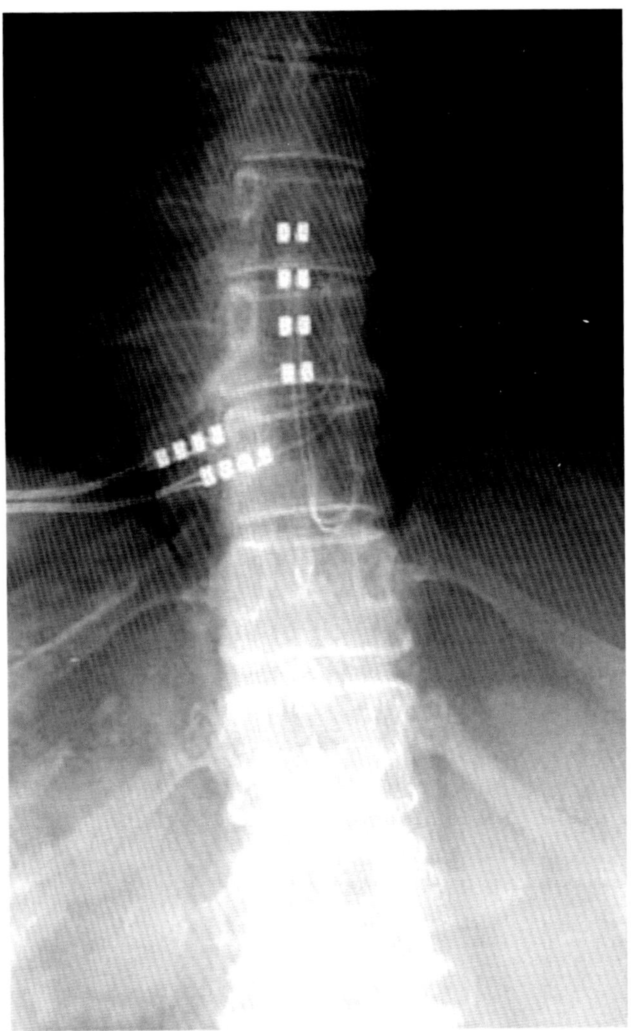

Fig. 8.5 Fluoroscopic confirmation of lead placement

8.3 Risk Assessment

1. The placement of a paddle lead requires bone removal and tissue disruption. This leads to the risk of epidural bleeding and possible epidural hematoma.
2. Infection is a concern and possible complications include osteomyelitis, epidural abscess, meningitis, sepsis, and death. The most common complication is superficial wound infection.
3. Paddle leads are considered much more stable than percutaneous leads. Possible system failures include lead fracture, lead migration, and current leak from abnormalities of the wire covering or insulation.
4. Epidural fibrosis develops below and around the leads and may cause a change in the stimulation parameters and could change the overall success of the procedure.

8.4 Risk Avoidance

1. The risk of bleeding can be minimized by optimizing the patient's health prior to implant. The physician should review laboratory values that have an impact on the bleeding function. Medications that affect bleeding function should be reviewed by the patient's family doctor or cardiologist and modified to reduce bleeding risk if possible. If the patient cannot come off drugs that affect platelets and bleeding function for an acceptable period of time prior to implant because of medical risks, the procedure should not be performed for concern of epidural hematoma. The patient and the caregivers should be informed to monitor postoperative symptoms to identify bleeding early and allow immediate treatment.
2. Prior to surgery, the physician should review the patient's planned incision sites for infection or lesions in the surgical area. The surgery should be delayed if there is any doubt about the safety of moving forward.
3. Preoperative antibiotics, intraoperative antibiotic irrigation, and postoperative oral antibiotics may reduce the risk of infectious complications. This should be coupled with careful attention to detail of preparing, draping, and wound closure to reduce the risk of contamination. In patients with a history of immune system compromise such as human immunodeficiency virus/acquired immunodeficiency syndrome (HIV/AIDS), cancer, poorly controlled diabetes mellitus, and primary immune dysfunction, a consultation with an infectious disease specialist or primary care doctor should be considered.
4. Prior to placing a paddle lead, the surgeon should consider the amount of room in the spinal canal and determine whether there is adequate room for the volume of the lead. This can be determined by a preoperative magnetic resonance imaging (MRI) or computed tomography (CT) myelogram. The implanter may also decompress the spinal canal at the time of implant by performing more extensive bony removal at the stenotic levels.
5. Careful attention to lead position, strain-relief loop at the incision site, and avoidance of pressure on the lead can reduce the risk of fracture and electrical system disruption. Over the past few years, the quality of lead manufacturing has also reduced this risk.

Conclusions

The paddle lead option is often a very good solution to treating difficult pain problems. This method can be chosen because of the preference of the surgeon or can be an option based on clinical scenarios that develop based on patient needs and anatomy. Unidirectional current, efficient energy delivery, and enhanced lead stability are all reasons to consider the paddle lead approach in treating patients with difficult pain syndromes. Device selection may continue to evolve as the availability of first-generation percutaneous paddles, new paresthesia-free devices and mechanisms such as high-frequency and burst stimulation, and new targets such as the dorsal root ganglion continue to be added to the neuromodulation armamentarium. These new offerings may reduce the need for surgical paddles, but thus far, the extent of this paradigm shift has not been determined.

8.5 Supplemental Images

See Figs. 8.6 and 8.7.

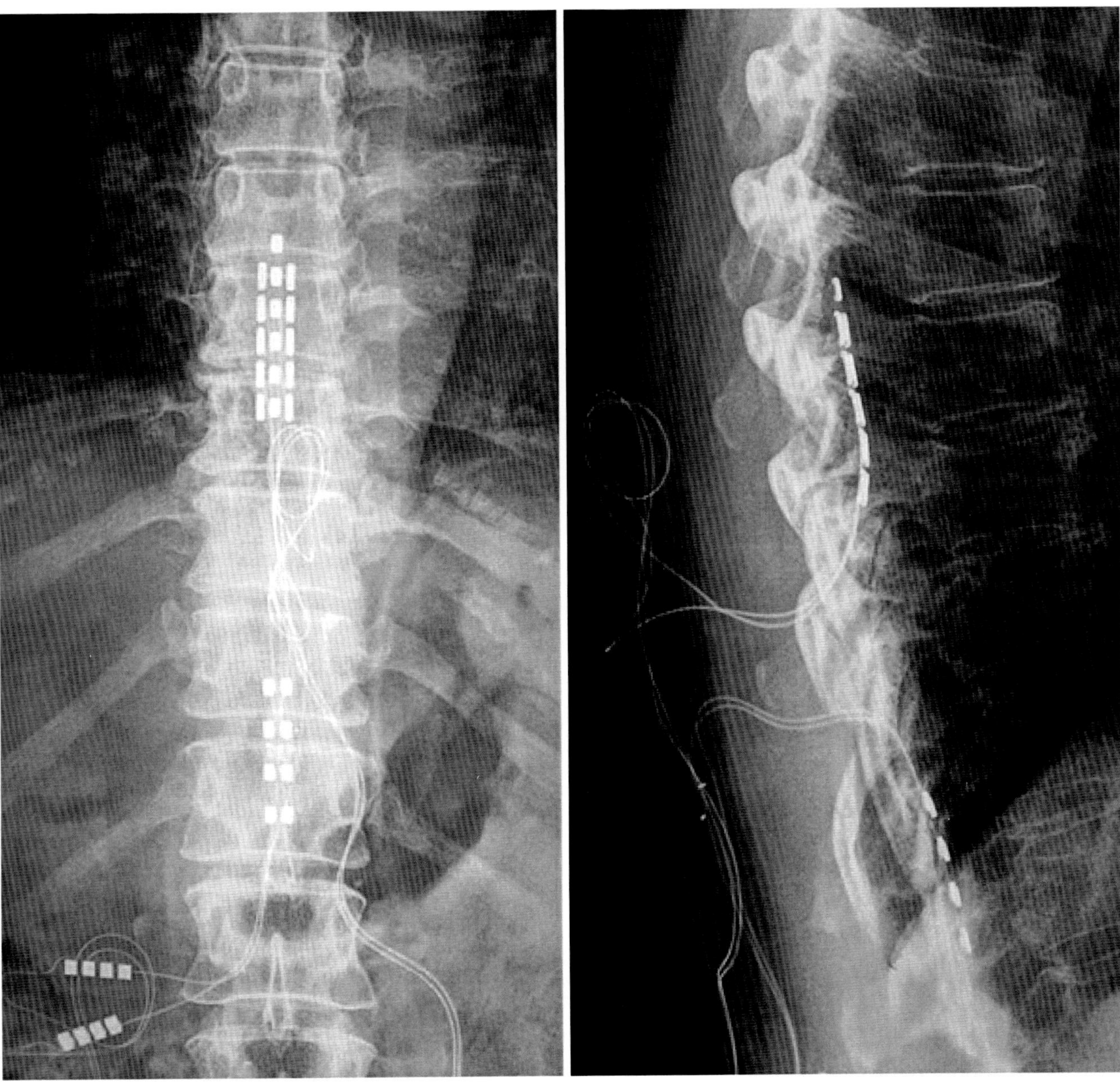

Fig. 8.6 Dual paddle leads to treat axial and foot pain

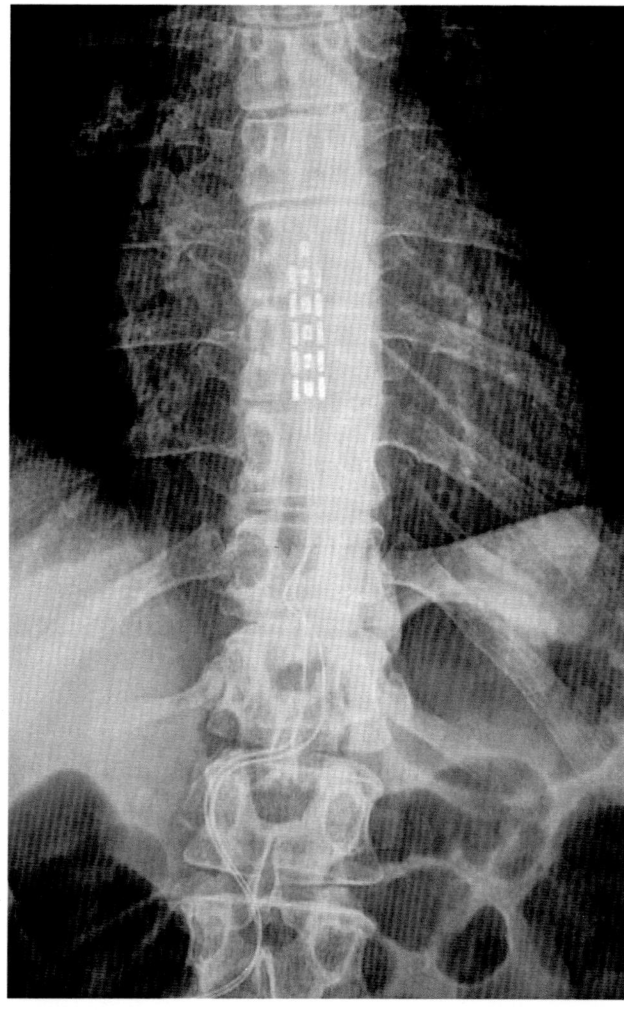

Fig. 8.7 Proper placement of paddle for lumbar radiculopathy

Suggested Reading

Buvanendran A, Lubenow T. Efficacy of transverse tripolar spinal cord stimulator for the relief of chronic low back pain from failed back surgery. Pain Physician. 2008;11:333–8.

Falowski S, Celii A, Sharan A. Spinal cord stimulation: an update. Neurotherapeutics. 2008;5:86–99.

North R, Olin KD, Sieracki J. Spinal cord stimulation electrode design: prospective, randomized, controlled trial comparing percutaneous and laminectomy electrodes-Part I: Technical outcomes. Neurosurgery. 2002;51:381–90.

Oakley J, Prager J. Spinal cord stimulation: mechanisms of action. Spine. 2002;27:2574–83.

9 Programming Spinal Cord Stimulation Systems

Timothy R. Deer

9.1 Introduction

The placement of a lead into the epidural space is an accomplishment that is essential to performing spinal cord stimulation. Once the lead is in place, the clinician must program the device to deliver current to change the way the spine modulates neural signals. Each device manufacturer has significant intellectual property design that makes their programming unique. The goal of this chapter is to give a noncommercial look at general programming principles. The physician should have a good understanding of electrical properties that are critical in achieving an overall acceptable outcome. The first perception the physician must comprehend is the lead target for ideal stimulation (Table 9.1). The targets are a starting point for programming, but they may vary based on patient-specific anatomy. The basic concepts of programming involve the understanding of amplitude, pulse width, and frequency (Fig. 9.1). Amplitude involves the intensity of the electrical field. Increasing the amplitude changes the size of the electrical field. Pulse width is the length of time the nerve target is exposed to an impulse. Frequency is the number of exposures that occur per minute of stimulation.

Table 9.1 Targets for lead placement

Cathode placement	Stimulation target
Cervical	
C2	Face, below the maxillary region
C2–C4	Neck, and shoulder to hand
C4–C7	Forearm to hand
C7–T1	Anterior shoulder
Thoracic	
T1–T2	Chest wall
T5–T6	Abdomen
T7–T9	Back and legs
T10–T12	Leg limb
Lumbar/sacral	
L1	Pelvis
T12, L1	Foot
L5, S1	Foot, lower limb
S2 to S4	Pelvis, rectum
Sacral hiatus	Coccyx

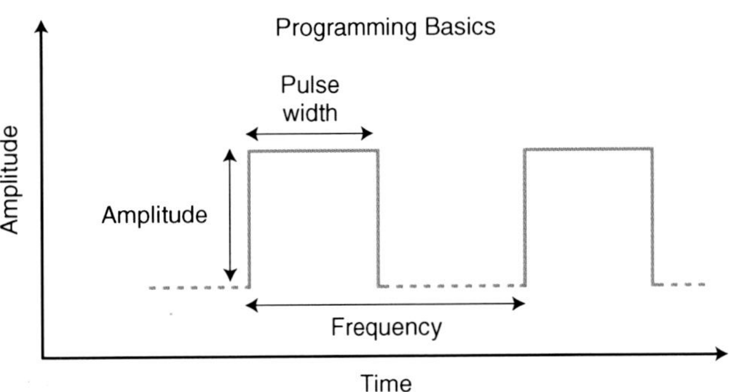

Fig. 9.1 Programming basics

T.R. Deer, MD
The Center for Pain Relief, 400 Court Street, Suite 100, Charleston, WV 25301, USA
e-mail: DocTDeer@aol.com

T.R. Deer, J.E. Pope (eds.), *Atlas of Implantable Therapies for Pain Management*, DOI 10.1007/978-1-4939-2110-2_9

9.2 Technical Overview

The basic concept of using electrical current to modulate the neurotransmission of pain signals involves creating an electrical field that changes synaptic connections. Thinking of membrane as an uneven capacitor, application of a charge can create a membrane potential change. This results in a cathode-driven depolarization, and an anode-driven hyperpolarization (Fig. 9.2). This strategy of using cathodes and anodes concurrently allows the clinician to shape the current to achieve the desired therapeutic stimulation, as previously described by Holsheimer. Using a paddle lead configuration, we can illustrate the vertical and horizontal mapping that can form the patient response created by changing the number and position of positive and negative contacts (Fig. 9.3).

To shape the field, the clinician must understand several components:

1. Where is the lead position? The target location of the lead will determine the stimulation possibilities. The implanter should review the anterior-posterior view and the lateral view to determine the patient's response to changes in lead activation.
2. How many contacts are on the lead? An octipolar lead will allow many more possible combinations of programming than a quadripolar lead. A paddle lead with multiple contacts may allow lead screening in both vertical and horizontal orientations.
3. How many leads or contacts are in the spine? By adding a second or third percutaneous lead, the number of programming options will increase dramatically. This is also true for changing from a simple quadripolar surgical lead to a more complex tripolar or pentapolar paddle lead. These increased contact systems lead to an exponential improvement in possible electrode combinations to shape the field.
4. The system must contain one cathode to drive current. A single cathode drives current to that area of the system. The addition of cathodes to the system leads to dispersion of the current. A general rule is that the number of cathodes is directly proportional to the concentration of current in an area of neural tissue. In some peripheral nerve tissues, the addition of multiple cathodes will result in current being spread through the area, increasing the number of small nerve fibers exposed to the current.
5. The system must contain one anode to create a field along with the cathode. Anodes may be used to guard a cathode to isolate the negative charge, or they may be used to shape current based on multiple cathode and anode combinations.
6. The amplitude of stimulation will determine the strength of the stimulation delivered to the patient. In some settings, increasing the amplitude will result in increased radicular fiber recruitment and perception of a spread of the impulse to additional areas in the extremity or axial region.
7. The frequency of stimulation will determine the number of impulses provided to the nerve tissue per minute. Some patients prefer a low frequency; others prefer the frequency to be very high. The use of high-frequency stimulation has been found to be helpful in some conditions (*e.g.*, complex regional pain syndrome) that may fail low-frequency stimulation.
8. The pulse width determines the amount of time the nerve tissue is exposed to the current. Increasing pulse width can change the area of stimulation in a limb. In some settings, pulse width adjustment has no effect on the perception of stimulation.

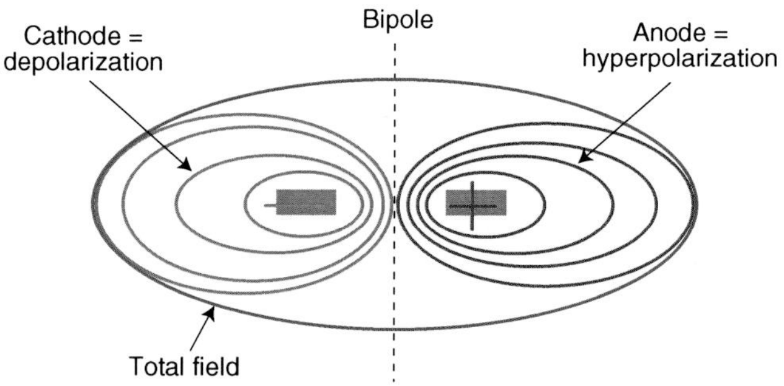

Fig. 9.2 Depolarization/hyperpolarization

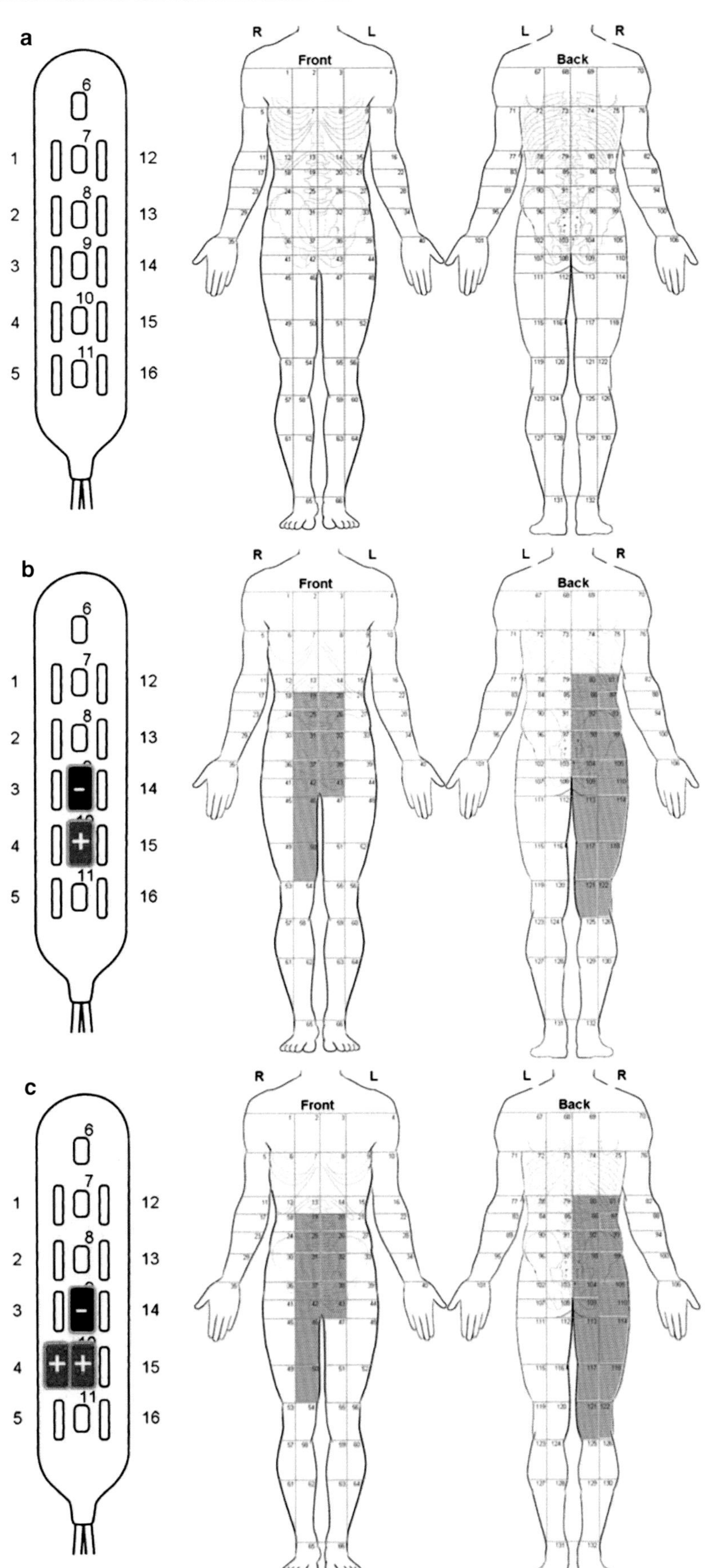

Fig. 9.3 (**a**) Clinical example of programming, array off. (**b**) Bipolar array. (**c**) Dual anode with cathode. (**d**) Staggered array. (**e**) Dual matched cathode/anode. (**f**) Staggered array. (**g**) Shifting of the field. (**h**) Lateral array (Reprinted with permission of St. Jude Medical; all rights reserved)

Fig. 9.3 (continued)

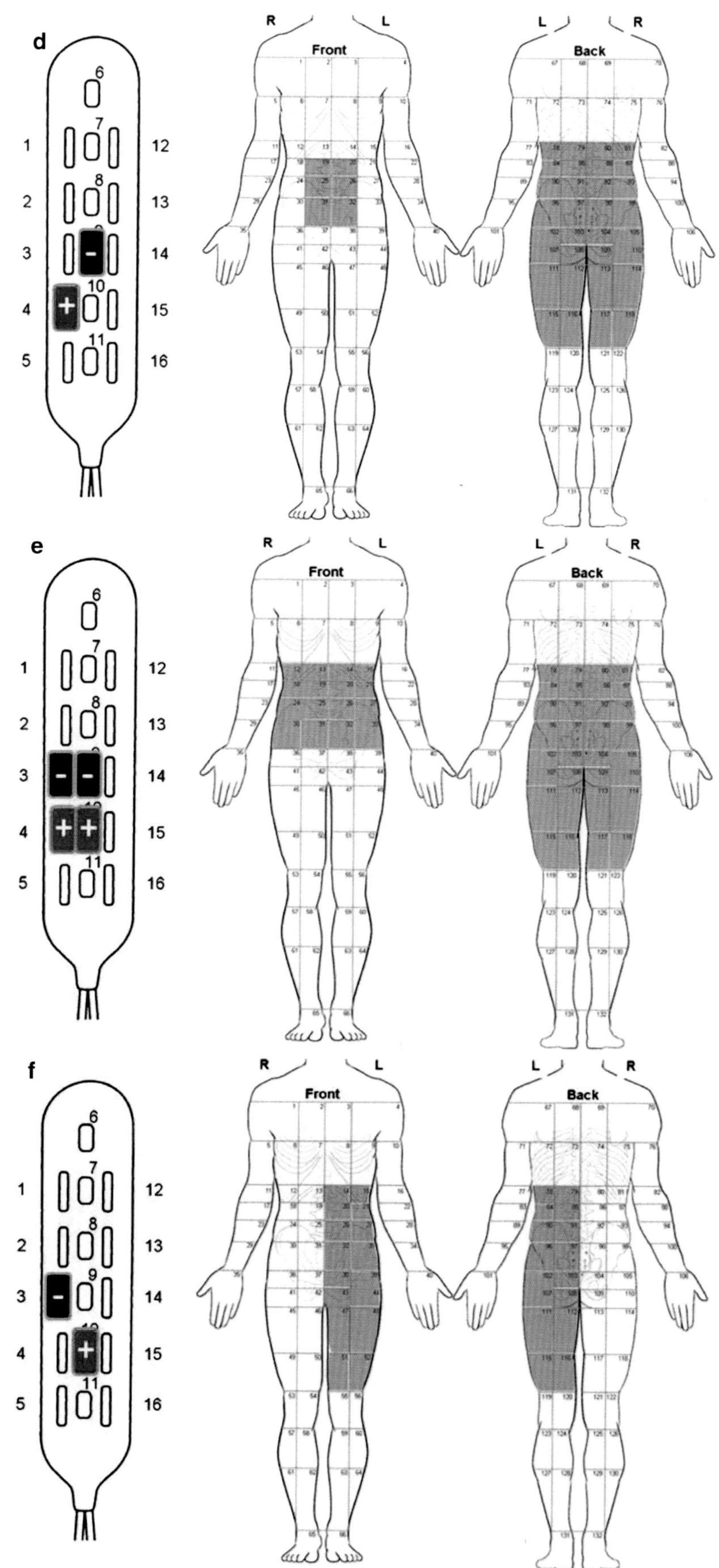

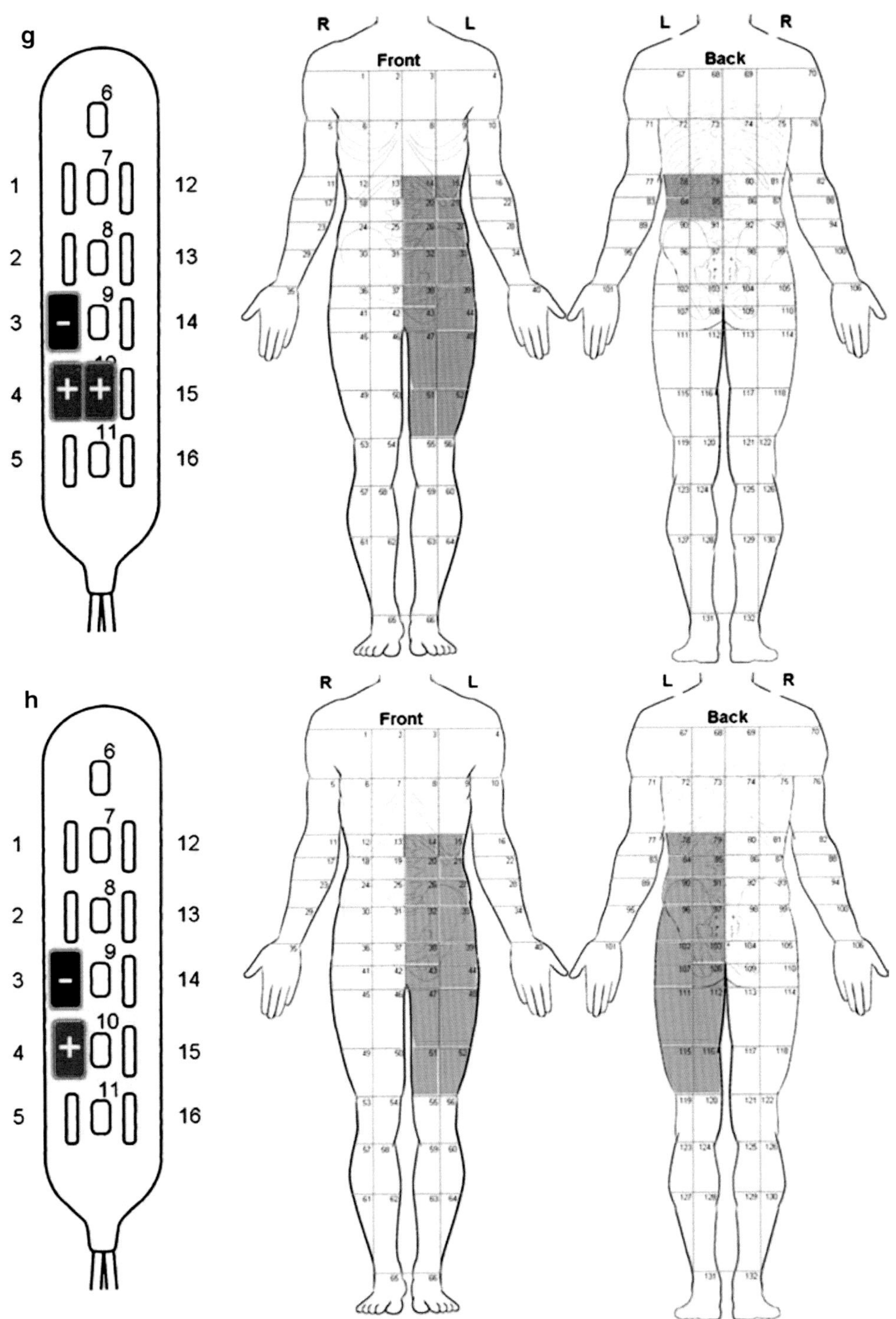

Fig. 9.3 (continued)

9.3 Risk Assessment

Several programming pitfalls can stand in the way of achieving a successful spinal cord stimulation system:

- The placement of leads into an improper anatomical location will make it difficult to achieve proper programming, even in the best of hands or with the ideal technology.
- Prior to programming the system, the implanter and the programmer should identify the electrode contact position. Activating a contact that is in the wrong position can lead to painful paresthesias. Electrodes in the far lateral or anterior epidural space can result in motor activation when programmed.
- Improper understanding of programming can lead to a failed trial or permanent implant even in the setting of a proper candidate, good lead placement, and good surgical technique.
- If the lead is positioned on top of epidural adipose tissue, a large blood vessel, or epidural scar or fibrosis, conduction from the lead to neural tissue may be poor, causing the system to fail.
- Improper contacts at the generator or at a connector location will lead to poor electrical current transfer and a failed or inefficient system.
- Patients may require different programs based on activity; for example, the patient may require low amplitudes and simple programming while at rest, but may require much different parameters during walking or other activity.

9.4 Risk Avoidance

Care in implantation and programming can minimize the pitfalls:

- Before attempting to program the system, the clinician should ensure that the leads are in proper position based on the target of stimulation. Lateral views should also confirm the lead in the proper posterior epidural space.
- The electrodes may vary in orientation, with some contacts more lateral than others. The programming is based on the physician's activating the proper contact and deciding on ideal anode and cathode positions.
- During the implant of trial leads and the subsequent permanent implant, the clinician should strive for lead placement that allows for ideal coverage at the center of the lead. This is true for single and dual percutaneous leads and for surgical paddle leads.
- "Dead zones" (areas of minimal or no stimulation) are identified by high impedance on attempted programming or failure to elicit a paresthesia despite high amplitudes. This problem can be avoided during the trial phase and at the time of permanent implantation by repositioning the lead. Once the lead is in place, the problem can be addressed by programming alternate contacts, increasing the ratio of cathodes to anodes to drive current, programming the other lead in dual-lead systems, or by surgical revision to change the lead position. In cases of epidural fibrosis, a revision to a paddle lead may be necessary to increase current strength.
- High impedance can be a sign of improper contacts within the system. This can occur at the generator or at extensions or connectors when used. At the time of surgery, it is important to clean the contacts and ensure that the system is dry, with no fluid in the connections. Once the system is implanted, this problem usually will require programming of alternative contacts; in some patients, reoperation is needed to explore the connections for fluid or damage.
- New, advanced systems allow multiple program selections, which the patient can control when doing different activities. This ability can be helpful to stimulate different dermatomes, to cycle programs to give a sensation of broader coverage, or to treat patients whose pain pattern changes with varying activity, such as those with spinal stenosis.

9.5 Future Trends

Commonly, spinal cord stimulation employs a frequency of 40–60 Hz. New current waveform applications have been developed that use high-frequency stimulation, with research suggesting pain reduction without the need for therapeutic paresthesia coverage overlying the typical painful area.

Traditional tonic stimulation with 40 Hz stimulates the lateral path of pain perception. It appears that high-frequency stimulation at 5000–10,000 Hz stimulates the medial path, most commonly involved with the affective component of pain (Fig. 9.4).

Studies suggest that lead placement is less confined to the Barolat coverage mapping described in Table 9.1, and may be less positional and offer an option for patients not responsive to tonic stimulation. Burst stimulation delivers a 40 Hz burst with five spikes at 500 Hz per burst and engages the medial and lateral pathway, which may affect not only the brain's quantitative assessment of pain but also the qualitative awareness and attention to pain, potentially employing the best of both tonic and high-frequency stimulation concurrently.

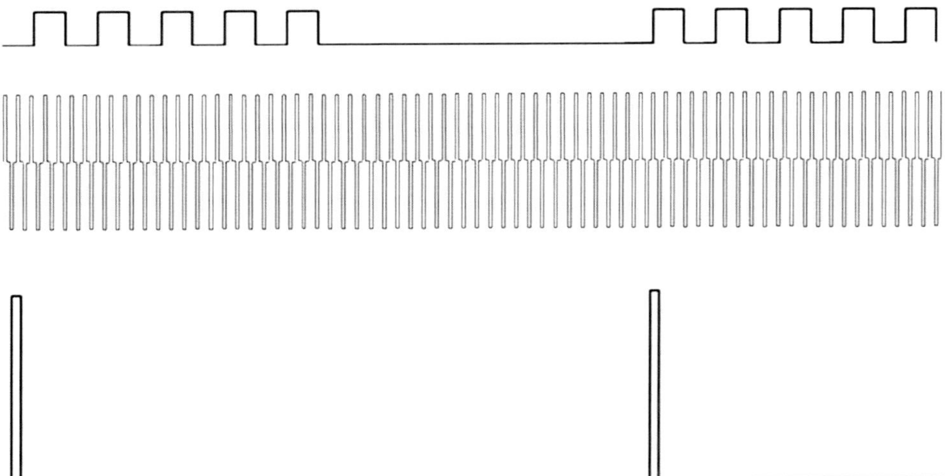

Fig. 9.4 Waveform innovations. Burst stimulation (*top*), high frequency stimulation at 10,000 Hz (*middle*), and tonic stimulation at 40 Hz (*bottom*)

Conclusions

Many physicians spend hours training to implant leads, place generators, and connect systems. These surgical concerns must be addressed, and competence is part of the core skills of an implanter, but it is also important for the physician to understand electrophysiology and how programming can impact the success of a system. This understanding is important for lead placement, troubleshooting, changing pain patterns, and overall patient care. The competent implanter should have a good understanding of the concepts in this chapter and be prepared to instruct technicians and nurses who assist in the programming.

Suggested Reading

De Ridder D, Plazier M, Kamerling N, Menovsky T, Vanneste S. Burst spinal cord stimulation for limb and back pain. World Neurosurg. 2013;80:642–9.

Falowski S, Celii A, Ashwini S. Spinal cord stimulation: an update. Neurotherapeutics. 2008;5:86–99.

Harke H, Gretenkort P, Ulrich Ladleif H, Koester P, Rahman S. Spinal cord stimulation in postherpetic neuralgia and in acute herpes zoster pain. Anesth Analg. 2002;94:694–700.

Krauss JK, Weigel R, Blahak C, Bäzner H, Capelle HH, Grips E, et al. Chronic spinal cord stimulation in medically intractable orthostatic tremor. J Neurol Neurosurg Psychiatry. 2006;77:1013–6.

Kumar K, Hunter G, Demeria D. Spinal cord stimulation in treatment of chronic benign pain: challenges in treatment planning and present status, a 22-year experience. Neurosurgery. 2006;58:481–96.

Schlaier JR, Eichhammer P, Langguth B, Doenitz C, Binder H, Hajak G, et al. Effects of spinal cord stimulation on cortical excitability in patients with chronic neuropathic pain: a pilot study. Eur J Pain. 2007;11:863–8.

Tiede J, Brown L, Gekht G, Vallejo R, Yearwood T, Morgan D. Novel spinal cord stimulation parameters in patients with predominant back pain. Neuromodulation. 2013;16:370–5.

Anchoring Percutaneous Leads During Permanent Device Placement

10

Timothy R. Deer, Stanley Golovac, and Matthew Kaplan

10.1 Introduction

In many settings, the education and training of an implanting physician for spinal cord stimulation (SCS) focuses on the preoperative evaluation, needle placement, lead direction and location, and overall surgical technique as critical parts of a good long-term outcome. In the best of hands, all of these issues are important, but the procedure is made durable with the action of properly anchoring the lead. This chapter focuses on this component of SCS placement.

Even with meticulous attention to anchoring, lead migration can occur and is generally the complication most often reported at 1 year after implantation. New anchors, methods, and technology may reduce this problem to a negligible issue.

10.2 Technical Overview

The procedure for preoperative assessment, positioning, needle placement, and lead location and selection is completed in the usual fashion. The angle of the needle may affect the ease of anchoring. In general, the angle should be at 45° or less, if possible based on the anatomy. This low angle allows for less torque on the lead when placing the anchor (Figs. 10.1, 10.2, and 10.3). An incision to the fascia and ligament may be made either prior to lead placement (Fig. 10.4) or after the needle is in position. The clinician should dissect the fatty tissue from the area surrounding the needle so that fascia and ligament are easily visible (Fig. 10.5). The fascia has a shiny appearance that should be visualized around the lead entry, and the ligament resembles leather. Anchoring sutures are then placed in the desired location to properly align the lead to reduce torque on the structure and to allow a strain relief loop.

Anchoring can be a challenge in some patients who tend to be more technically difficult. Patients in this category may include those with uncontrolled diabetes, morbid obesity, a history of multiple spine surgeries, or poor tissue health secondary to cachexia. Attention to detail will be critical in this patient group.

When the needle and stylet are removed, careful attention should be given to maintaining the lead position. This portion of the procedure should be confirmed with fluoroscopic views taken before and after the needle and stylet have been removed to ensure that the position remains consistent. At this point, an anchor is moved over the lead to the entry point of the lead into the fascia or ligament (Fig. 10.6). The anchor should be brought forward so that no slack exists between the anchor and the lead. In some settings, the physician can improve this situation by making an incision around the needle before removing it. This incision will allow the anchor to slide into the ligament. At this time, additional sutures may be placed, based on the type and manufacturer of the anchor chosen. Some clinicians prefer a single suture, whereas others prefer multiple sutures to avoid lead movement. New anchoring methods are available for those who have challenges in suturing or who prefer uniformity in suture spacing. In addition to securing the anchor to the tissue, it is important to secure the lead to the anchor, which can be done by using surgical ties (or preferably mechanical anchors) to secure the lead (Fig. 10.1).

Some anchor models are equipped to mechanically lock onto the lead to prevent the lead from moving despite a

T.R. Deer, MD (✉)
The Center for Pain Relief, 400 Court Street, Suite 100, Charleston, WV 25301, USA
e-mail: DocTDeer@aol.com

S. Golovac
Florida Pain, 4770 Honeyridge Lane, Merritt Island, FL 32952, USA
e-mail: sgolovac@mac.com

M. Kaplan
Preferred Spine and Pain, 1250 South AW Grimes Boulevard, Round Rock, TX 78664, USA
e-mail: kaplan.matthew@yahoo.com

T.R. Deer, J.E. Pope (eds.), *Atlas of Implantable Therapies for Pain Management*, DOI 10.1007/978-1-4939-2110-2_10

secure, immovable anchor. The Clik™ anchor (Boston Scientific, Natick, MA) is a locking anchor that is placed over the lead (Figs. 10.7 and 10.8). The company recommends first securing the lead to the fascia before locking the lead in place. This lead has a screw lock system, which is tightened using a screwdriver until it "clicks." The lead can be locked and unlocked by turning the screw. Medtronic (Minneapolis, MN) has introduced two new compression-fit anchors (Injex®), which come as either a bi-wing design (Fig. 10.9) or a bumpy design (Fig. 10.10). The lead comes preloaded on a dispenser tool (Fig. 10.11). The anchor and dispenser tool are placed over the lead, the anchor slides into place, and the dispenser tool locks the anchor onto the lead. The anchor and lead are then secured to the fascia. St. Jude Medical (St. Paul, MN) has introduced the Swift-Lock™ anchor. This is a cigar-shaped anchor that is placed over the lead. The anchor is then secured to the fascia. Using either fingers or hemostats, the anchor is rotated until two triangles line up to indicate that the anchor is locked to the lead. The anchor can be unlocked by reversing the twist direction (Fig. 10.12). When using these systems, attention must be paid to avoid tension on lead components that can damage and eventually fracture the lead. When using these types of anchors, it is also important to carefully secure the anchor to the tissue so that the anchor itself will not shift.

In addition to mechanical anchoring, the physician can do things to reduce the severity of complications associated with minor lead migrations. The physician should pay careful attention to the stimulation pattern of the lead(s) when obtaining optimal stimulation. The ideal lead orientation involves obtaining optimal stimulation patterns using electrodes in the center of the lead. This allows for correction of small lead distance migrations with programming changes rather than surgical revisions. Excellence in anchoring involves more than technical skill; it also involves a good understanding of the concept of spinal neurostimulation programming.

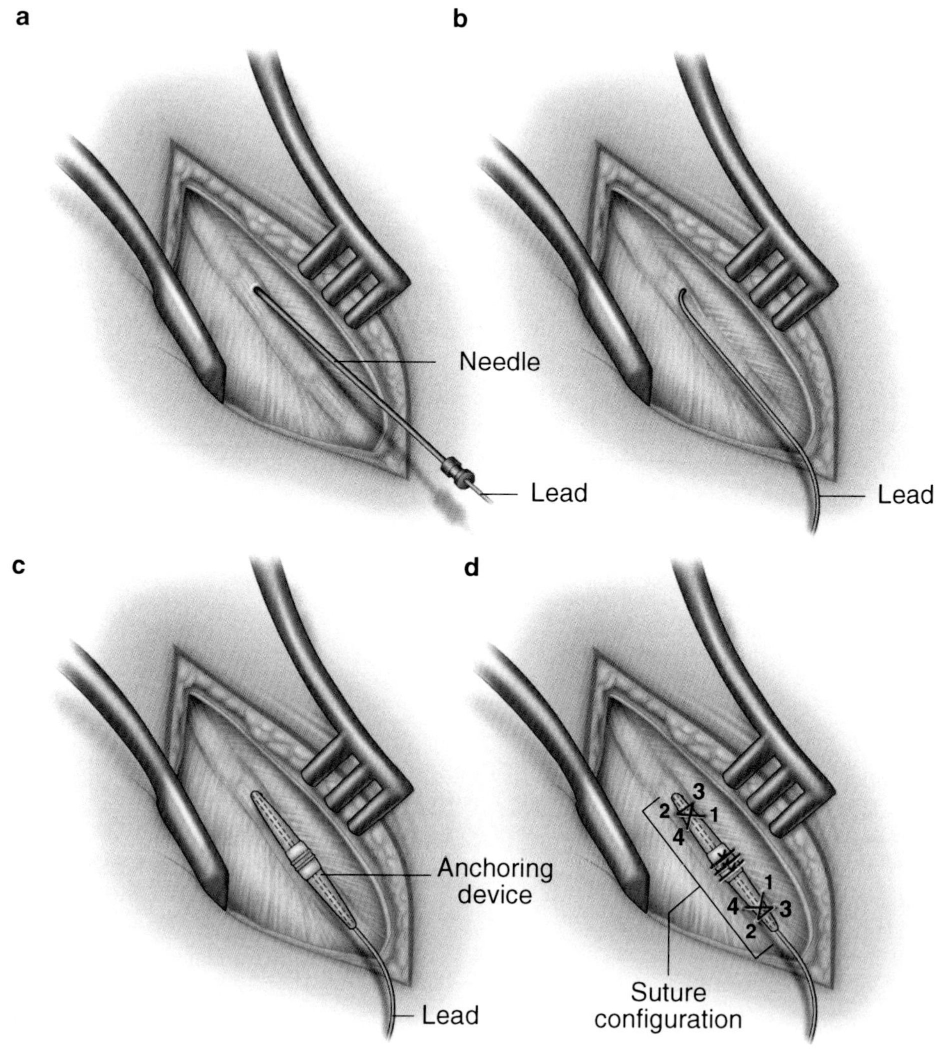

Fig. 10.1 Anchoring and suturing technique. Proper needle placement (**a**). Proper placement of the surgical lead (**b**). Proper placement of the anchoring device at the fascia entry point (**c**). Suturing of the anchoring device (**d**) employing the Deer-Stewart suturing technique, showing three interrupted sutures in the middle of the anchor and figure-of-eight sutures at the distal and proximal anchor ends. The figure-of-eight sutures are numbered based on needle entry

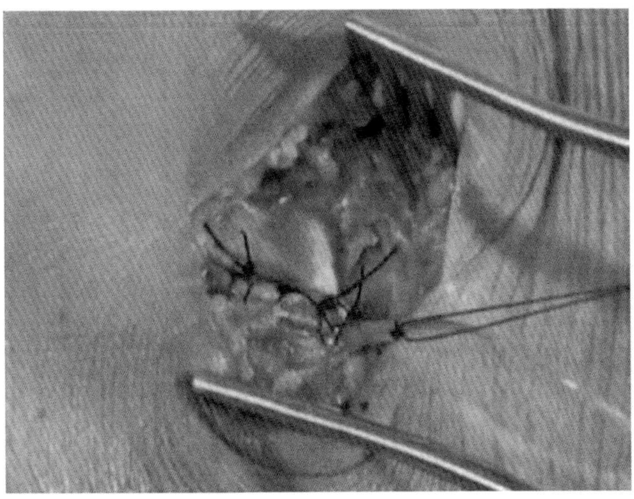

Fig. 10.2 Anchoring to fascia and ligament

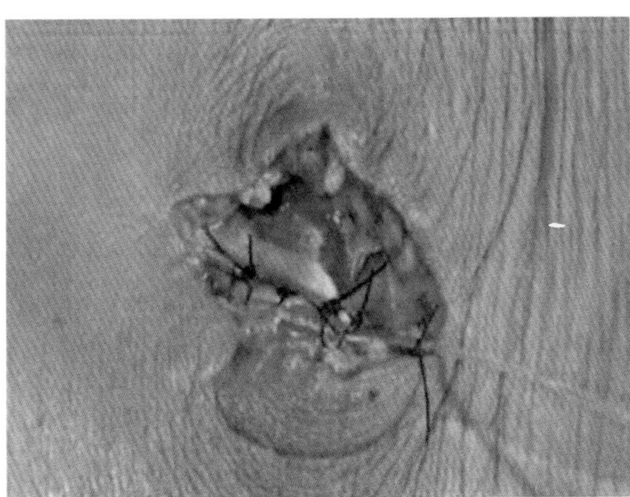

Fig. 10.3 Anchoring to the fascia and ligament

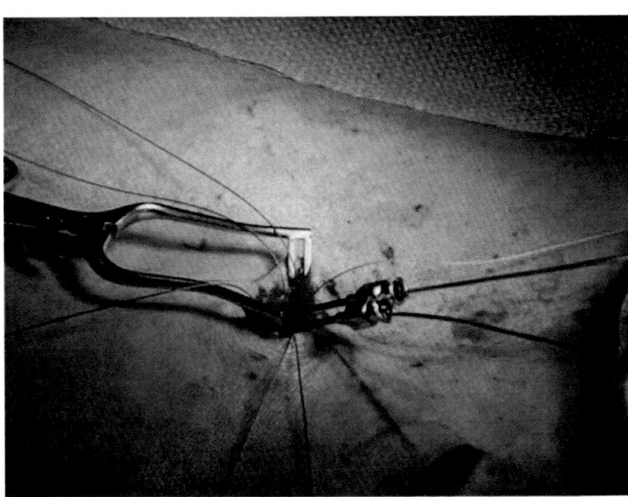

Fig. 10.4 Sutures may be placed in the fascia and ligament prior to removing the needles, in order to protect the leads

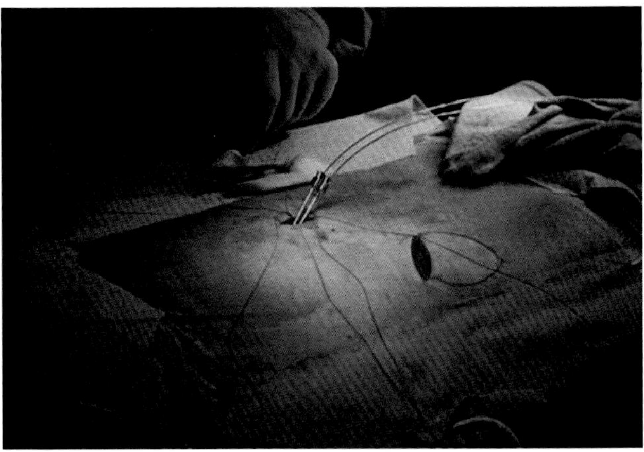

Fig. 10.5 Dual needles are seen with a pocket created prior to anchoring to allow for observation of hemostasis prior to closure

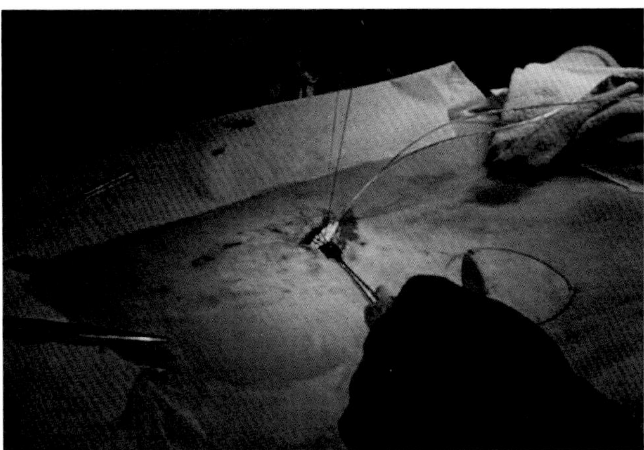

Fig. 10.6 Anchors should be abutting the fascia prior to securing them to the spine

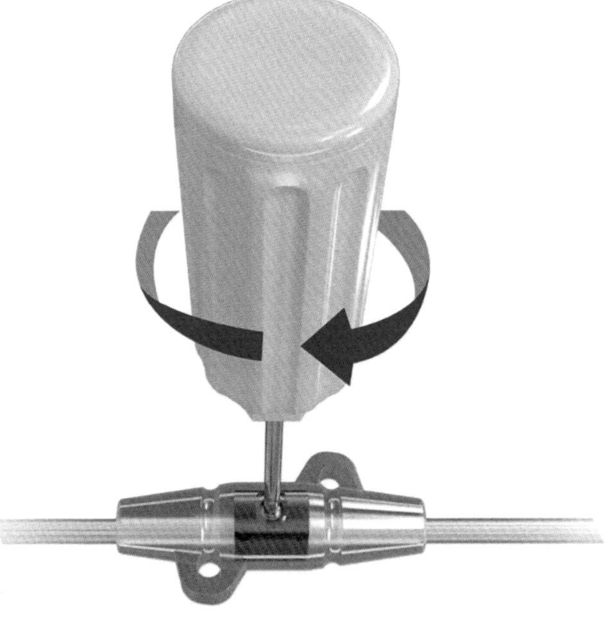

Fig. 10.7 Clik™ anchor with hex wrench

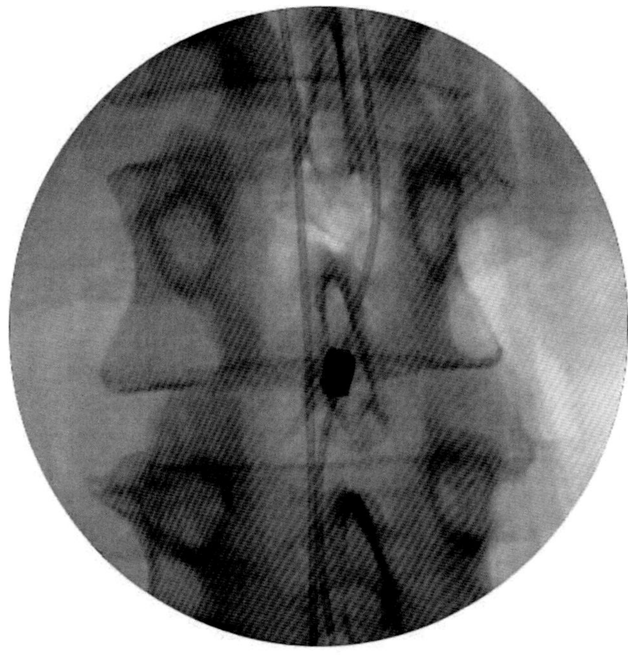

Fig. 10.8 Fluoro image of Clik™ anchor

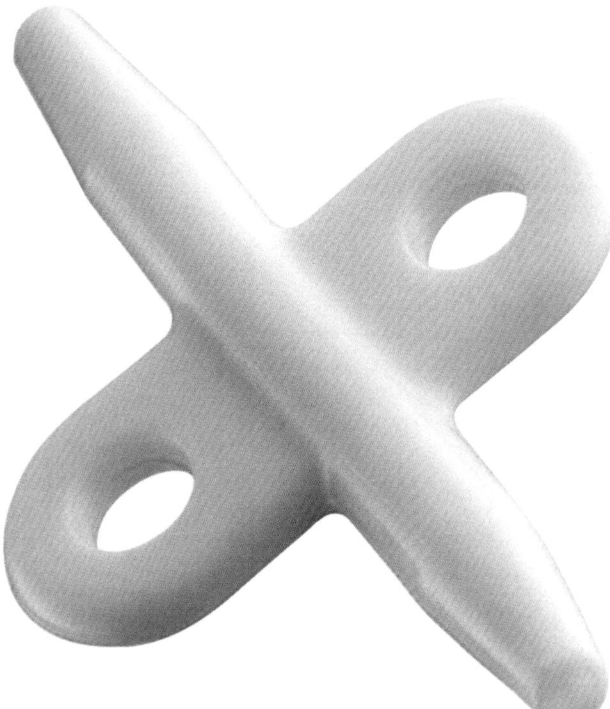

Fig. 10.9 Injex® bi-wing anchor

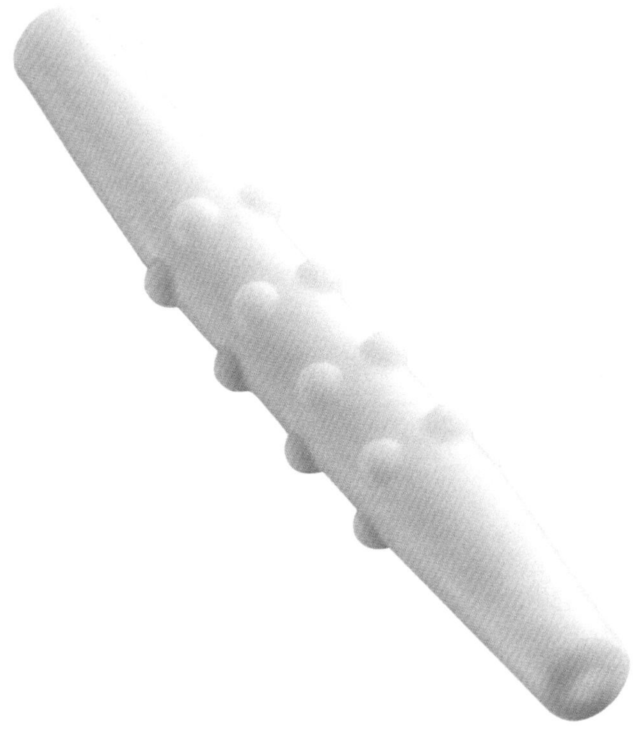

Fig. 10.10 Injex® Bumpy anchor

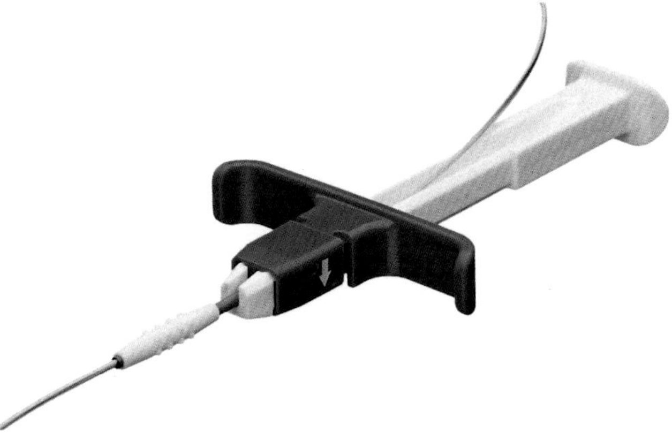

Fig. 10.11 Injex® dispenser tool

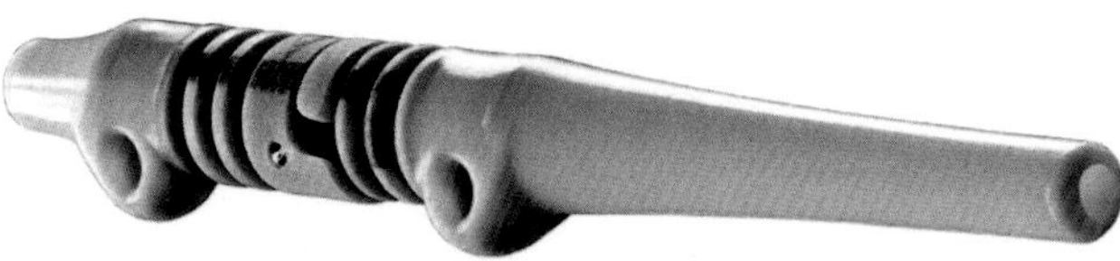

Fig. 10.12 Swift-Lock™ anchor (Reprinted with permission of St. Jude Medical)

10.3 Suturing and Anchoring Materials

The suture used to anchor the lead should be nonabsorbable and durable. In the past, many texts and articles have recommended silk as a mainstay of anchoring, but over time, the use of silk can lead to migration because the silk can degrade and eventually break down, allowing potential movement of the lead. Sturdy, nonabsorbable sutures such as Ethibond (Ethicon, Somerville, NJ) and other similar sutures will reduce the risk of long-term migration. Also, using a large cutting needle (CT-1) will allow the physician to take a bigger bite of the fascia, thus helping to more effectively secure the anchor and lead.

Boston Scientific has recently introduced the fiXate™ Tissue Band, a novel device to assist with lead anchoring. The suture comes preloaded in the device, which is placed over the lead. The button is depressed, and device delivers the suture into the tissue. Using a knot puller, the suture is then secured. The advantage of this method may be to reduce the risk of human error, and it may be particularly helpful for those who feel that suturing for anchoring is not their strong point. The disadvantages are added costs and the potential for not properly aligning the anchor and sutures.

The type of anchor the clinician chooses may not be very significant. Manufacturers often point out the advantages of their anchoring systems, and clinicians develop preferences based on individual experiences, but to date no long-term studies have been performed to compare anchors from competing companies. Regardless of the anchor chosen, it is important for the clinician to perform several safeguards to improve outcomes (Table 10.1).

Table 10.1 Physician action to safeguard against migration risk

Migration risk	Physician action
Needle angle	Needle angle of 30–45°
Needle entry	Paramedian approach
Fatty tissue at anchoring site	Débride fatty tissue around the needle entry site, exposing fascia and ligament for proper anchoring
Anchoring to muscle	When using an exaggerated paramedian approach, the physician should dissect medially until approaching ligament or fascia, avoiding anchoring to muscle, which may lead to migration with contraction
Lead anchor gap	The anchor should be as close to the lead entry into the ligament or fascia as possible, avoiding room for migration distal to the anchor
Suturing with silk	Avoid silk sutures when anchoring
Dependence on lock systems	When using anchor lock systems, the clinician should give attention to avoiding tension on the lead and to properly securing the anchor
Hematoma below anchor	Hemostasis should be obtained prior to closing the wound
Minimal migration changes	Final lead placement should result in accommodation of small migrations (<5 mm) with reprogramming rather than reoperation

10.4 The Deer-Stewart Anchoring Method

In our experience, the commitment to excellence in anchoring is worth adding a few minutes to the surgical procedure. To properly secure the lead that has been placed percutaneously, it is important to space the sutures properly. This can be achieved by using both strategically placed sutures that use the benefits of the anchor and figure-of-eight sutures that lead to tissue fibrosis around the anchor lead complex. Figure 10.1 illustrates the technique in which three sutures are placed through the fascia and ligament (prior to needle removal), and two additional figure-of-eight sutures are placed at the proximal and distal ends of the anchor. This technique can be applied to any manufacturer's lead to secure better anchor to tissue fibrosis and subsequent reduction in anchor shifting.

10.5 Risk Assessment

The ability of clinicians to anchor percutaneous leads and avoid migration appears to be improving. Nevertheless, migration still occurs and can require reprogramming the system, revising one or more leads, converting to a surgical lead, or removing the device. Because these systems are often therapies offered late in the algorithm, these occurrences are unfavorable. Several situations increase the risk:

- If the physician fails to remove adipose tissue from the fascia and ligament before anchoring, the tissue can become ischemic and the lead can migrate.
- In extreme paramedian approaches, the cut-down can be over muscle tissue. When anchoring is performed to muscle tissue, migration can occur as the patient's normal movement requires muscle contraction.
- Suture breakage can occur, making one-suture anchoring techniques extremely risky. Breakage of the suture may lead to shifting of the lead or anchor.
- The anchor can cause discomfort if it is superficial in the tissue. The new mechanical anchors have not resolved this problem.

10.6 Risk Avoidance

Applying the following precautions can greatly reduce the risk of lead migration:

- Migration can be reduced by using an angle of 45° or less for needle entry into the epidural space and by using a paramedian approach with needle placement. Needle entrance is best approached medial to the pedicle 1.5–2 levels inferior to the targeted entrance interlaminar level.

- Anchoring should occur only after all fatty tissue has been débrided from the area surrounding the needle.
- When the paramedian approach is used in an extreme manner, the amount of fascia and ligament available for anchoring is unacceptable. The paramedian approach should be used in all cases of implantation, but the needle entry point should remain in the area of the spine that allows for proper anchoring. If the paramedian approach is extreme, the tissue underlying the needle entry is muscle tissue.
- Nonabsorbable suture should be used for anchoring. When possible, silk should be avoided because its long-term stability is worrisome.
- In thin patients, it is important to use a double-layer or triple-layer closure to reduce the risk of discomfort at the anchor placement site. If the tissue layer present to cushion the anchor is unacceptable, the surgeon can make a pocket in the muscle adjacent to the anchor to place any excess wiring or strain relief loops.
- Attention to hemostasis should be given in the area of lead placement. Hematoma development in and around the lead can lead to movement of the anchor, fracture of the sutures, or movement of the leads.

Conclusions

The implanting team should consider anchoring as a critical part of the surgery. Properly anchoring the lead is an important step in the long-term success of the procedure. Many clinicians focus on the placement of the lead, the creation of the pocket, and wound closure. Equal thought, planning, and care should be given to the anchoring technique, and appropriate training should focus on this critical part of the procedure.

Suggested Reading

Alo K, Redko V, Charnov J. Four year follow-up of dual electrode spinal cord stimulation for chronic pain. Neuromodulation. 2002;5: 79–88.

Justiz 3rd R, Bentley I. A case series review of spinal cord stimulation migration rates with a novel fixation device. Neuromodulation. 2013. doi:10.1111/ner.12014.

Ohnmeiss DD. Patient satisfaction with spinal cord stimulation for predominant complaints of chronic, intractable low back pain. Spine J. 2001;1:358–63.

Raphael JH, Mutagi H, Hanu-Cernat D, Gandimani P, Kapur S. A cadaveric and in vitro controlled comparative investigation of percutaneous spinal cord lead anchoring. Neuromodulation. 2009;12:49–53.

Tunneling Spinal Cord Stimulation Systems

11

Timothy R. Deer and Jason E. Pope

11.1 Introduction

Every aspect of the surgical procedure to implant a spinal cord stimulation system demands respect. This globally encompasses: good surgical technique and knot tying, but can be broken down into its components: placement of the leads and anchoring, creation of the pocket for the internal programmable generator (IPG) and tunneling from the paraspinal incision to the pocket location. Often overlooked, the process of tunneling the lead or lead connectors from their neurostimulation target to the IPG location is critical for the device to be functional and allow communication between the electrode contacts and the desired neurological tissue. This chapter focuses on the procedure of tunneling for spinal cord stimulation.

11.2 Technical Overview

The patient is positioned, prepped, and draped in a normal fashion. Commonly, one of two approaches are employed: (1) placement of the needle(s) and lead(s) first, followed by a cut-down to expose the fascia and ligament for anchoring, or (2) performing the cut-down and surgical dissection to the fascia first, followed by placement of the needle(s), leads(s), and then anchoring. Nevertheless, anchoring should occur prior to tunneling, as the leads should be secured with a strain relief loop in the tissue to reduce the risk of migration. In addition to securing the lead, an incision is made to create a pocket for the generator. The pocket is sized to properly fit the desired device, and hemostasis is confirmed. In our center, typically both the paraspinal and pocket surgical dissection is performed prior to needle and lead placement for implantation of the device. Please refer to Chaps. 6, 7, 9, 23, and 24 for a detailed description of the various other components of the surgical implantation procedure.

Once both incisions are sufficiently created, hemostasis is achieved, the leads are deployed and anchored, and the course of planned tunneling is determined. The course of tunneling is based on landmarks, body habitus, and bony margins, avoiding acute angles and bony prominences. Once the course is determined, a sterile skin marker is used to outline this pathway of planned tunneling. Depending on the distance between the IPG location and the anchoring site, local anesthesia may be placed along the marked path. If local anesthetic is chosen, care must be taken to ensure that maximum doses are avoided. Further, if deepening the sedation or increased intravenous analgesia for tunneling proposes during the case, it is recommended that a trained anesthesia provider perform the monitored anesthesia care (MAC).

Tunneling devices are commonly a component of the implantation kit provided by the spinal cord stimulation manufacturer and may necessitate the direction of its passage. It is the author's preference to tunnel from the IPG location to the lead incision. It is recommended to use fluoroscopy and perform a "scout" image to signify any bony anatomy that needs to be avoided, along with palpation. A marking pen should be used to outline any prominences identified. Once the tract is identified potential barriers marked, a slight bend is placed in the tunneling tool to ensure ease with location identification as the tunneling is performed.

The implanter should palpate the tract as the tunneling tool is advanced to gauge the depth and course of the progress. The depth of the tunneling process should be in the subcutaneous adipose tissue. The tunneling can be painful and potentially dangerous if it occurs in the wrong tissue plain. It is always recommended to know the location of the distal end (tip) of the tunneling tool as it is passed. If the course of

T.R. Deer, MD (✉)
The Center for Pain Relief, 400 Court Street, Suite 100, Charleston, WV 25301, USA
e-mail: DocTDeer@aol.com

J.E. Pope
Summit Pain Alliance, 392 Tesconi Court, Santa Rosa, CA 95401, USA
e-mail: popeje@me.com

T.R. Deer, J.E. Pope (eds.), *Atlas of Implantable Therapies for Pain Management*, DOI 10.1007/978-1-4939-2110-2_11

tunneling is too superficial, it can be very painful and lead to skin erosion. Conversely, if the tunneling course is too deep, for example in the muscle, abdominal cavity, or pleura, this can lead to significant injury and result in potential morbidity and potential mortality.

After the tunneling device has been passed, it is removed carefully and deliberately, leaving the plastic tunnel for placement of the leads. The leads or extensions are passed into the plastic tunnel and fed through to the pocket location or counter incision. The plastic tunnel is then removed, leaving the leads in place. It is then recommended that the lead be cleaned and then placed within the IPG. See Figs. 11.1, 11.2, 11.3, 11.4, 11.5, 11.6, 11.7, 11.8, 11.9, and 11.10.

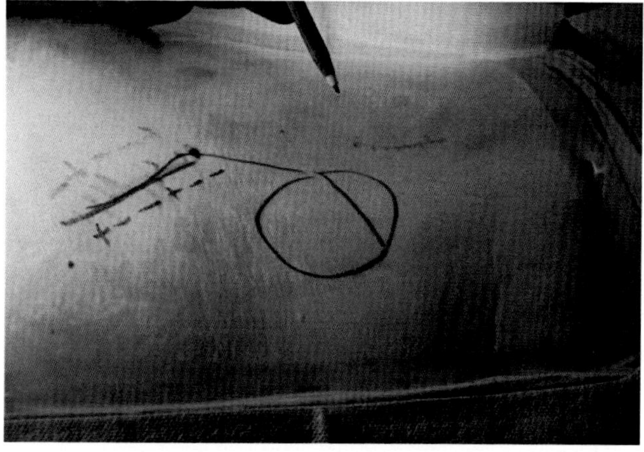

Fig. 11.1 The course of tunneling is planned based on landmarks and the best direction for placing the tunneling tool

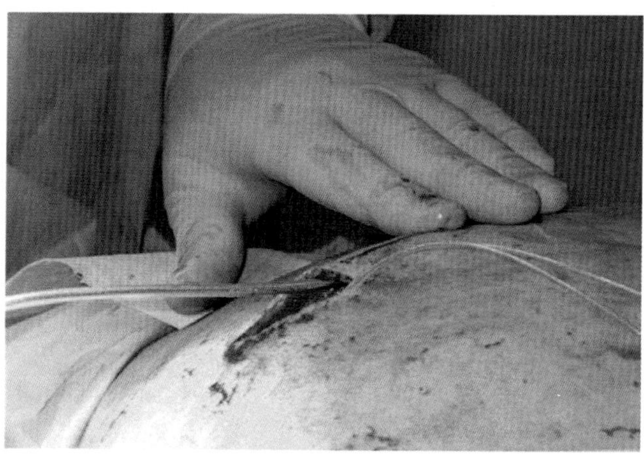

Fig. 11.3 Initiation of tunneling at lead insertion site

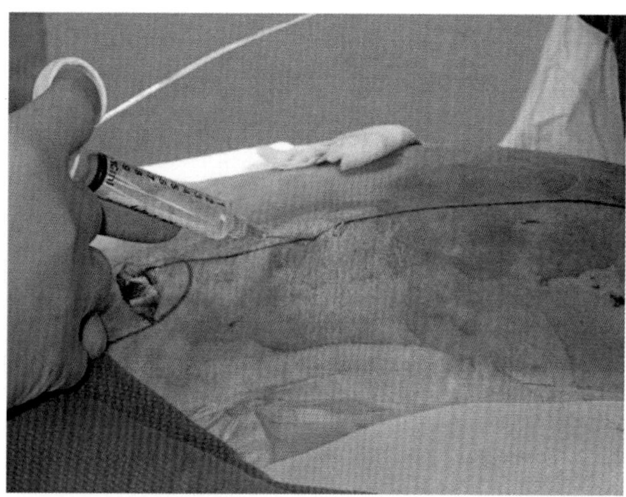

Fig. 11.2 Local anesthesia placed along the tract for tunneling

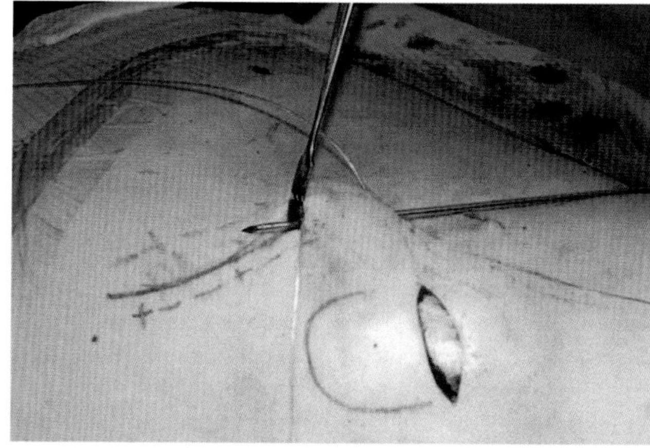

Fig. 11.4 Angle of tunneling with attention to sterile technique

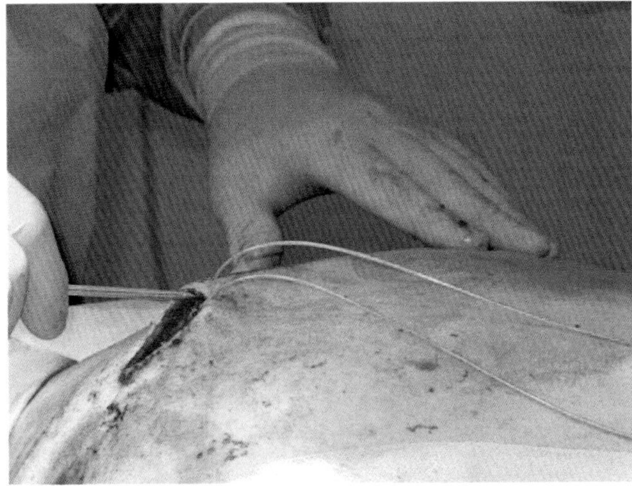

Fig. 11.5 Palpation of the course of tunneling to ensure adequate depth

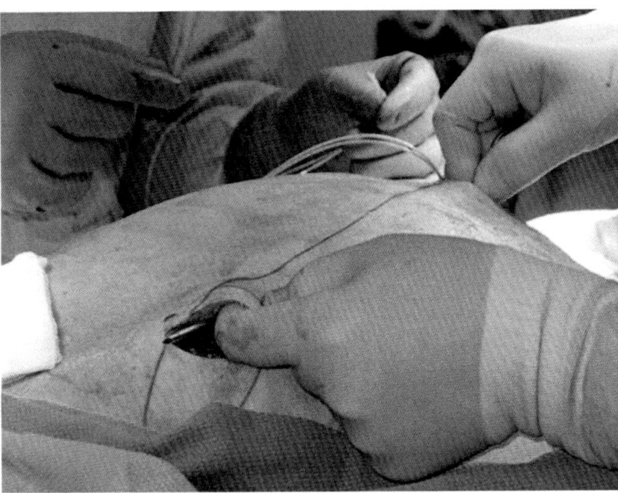

Fig. 11.6 Continued progress of tunneling toward the pocket

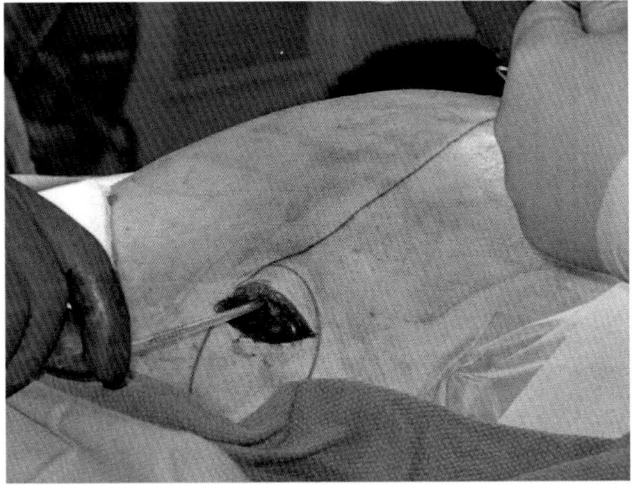

Fig. 11.7 Final passing of the device through the tissue to complete the tunneling process

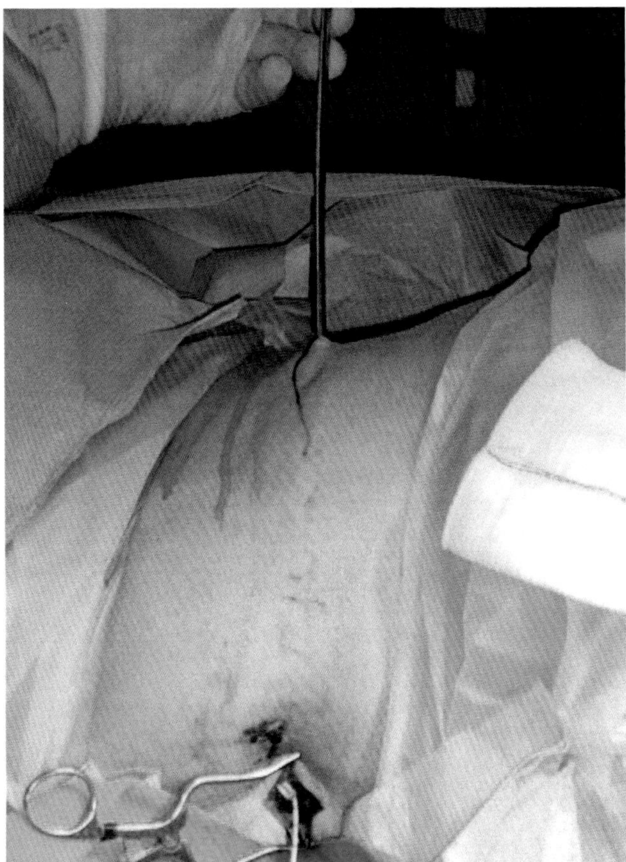

Fig. 11.8 Lateral decubitus representation of tunneling along a planned direction

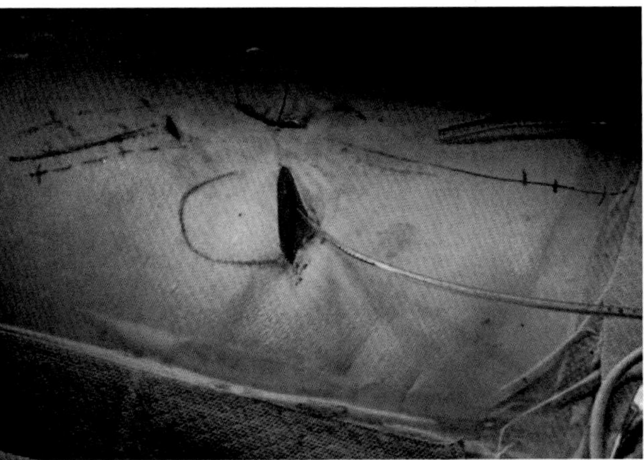

Fig. 11.9 Depiction of tunneling from the posterior lead position to the generator pocket

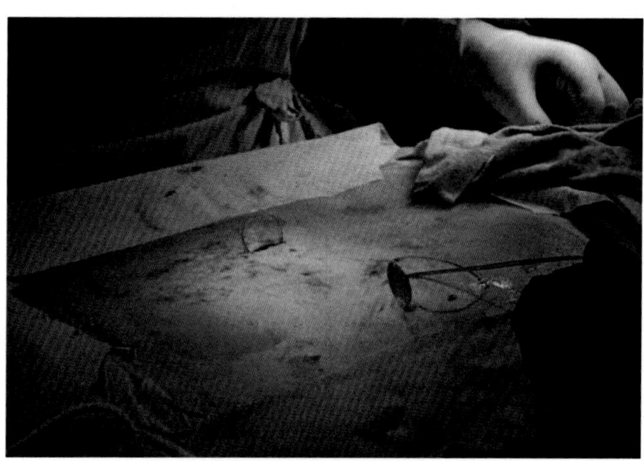

Fig. 11.10 The completed tunneling procedure in lateral decubitus position

11.3 Risk Assessment

1. The risk of tunneling depth should be considered. The physician may tunnel in a superficial plane, causing skin irritation or eventual erosion. The physician may tunnel too deeply, causing injury to muscle or more serious dilemmas such as visceral or pleural injury.
2. Tunneling can lead to hematoma formation, which can lead to pain and potential loss of the system.
3. Strict sterility of the surgical field needs to be maintained and the tunneled path should be included in the surgically prepped area. Alcohol-based prep is recommended as it is more bacteriocidal.
4. Tunneling can place the physician in physically awkward positions requiring the rod to be placed well above the patients head, or below the table when tunneling from a lateral decubitus position. This positional challenge can lead to wound contamination or field contamination.
5. Tunneling can be traumatic and may cause severe pain, making the level of comfort difficult to control for the patient, and to those providing sedation. This is a common problem when tunneling from the head and neck to the lower flank or buttocks. Care must be taken to ensure a quite operative field, by employing deepened sedation or increased analgesia.
6. Tunneling can lead to tissue infection and eventual loss of the system.
7. Tunneling can result in an injury to components of the system since a sharp metallic object is placed in proximity to the leads, anchors, and wire loops.

11.4 Risk Avoidance

1. The physician should constantly monitor the depth of the tunneling path. This is accomplished by using the non-tunneling (typically nondominant) hand to palpate the course of the tunneling tool as it is advanced toward the target incision. With adherence to this policy, the risk of injury is greatly reduced.
2. Placing a slightly contoured bend on the device aids identification of the distal (tip) end of the tunneling tool.
3. The patient should be evaluated preoperatively for bleeding disorders and medications that may affect clotting. If the area of tunneling appears to be swelling or expanding, tissue pressure should be applied until the situation has stabilized.
4. While prepping and draping for permanent stimulation implants, the physician should consider the course that will be used for tunneling and properly conduct the surgical field so that the physician's elbows, hands, and the tunneling rod itself will not come into proximity with any unsterile area.
5. Prior to tunneling the device, the physician should apply local anesthetics to the planned tract to reduce pain associated with the procedure. Additional local anesthetics can be added if tunneling is painful, with time allotted to allow the anesthetic effect to commence. In some instances, the anesthesia team will slightly increase sedation just prior to tunneling. Some clinicians advocate an epidural block prior to placing the leads to reduce the pain of tunneling. The author does not support this idea for several reasons, but the most convincing is the need to avoid high volumes of fluid in the epidural space at the time of implanting new leads.
6. The entire procedure requires vigilance to reduce the risk of infection. The skin should be prepped widely, draping should be extended to widen the surgical field, and the clinician should avoid contact with any unsterile area. The use of antibiotic solution to coat the tunneling tool, and to irrigate the tunneling tract may reduce the risk of infection.
7. When tunneling near components of the system, the physician should be able to clearly visualize the entire implant and strive to avoid any contact with the tunneling tip. The use of an Army-Navy, or rake, or similar retractor, may be helpful in protecting the system.

Conclusions

The placement of a spinal cord stimulation system is a complicated procedure requiring technical skills, good clinical judgment, and vigilance to good outcomes. Many physicians have great concern regarding proper lead placement, and creation of a pocket, but do not give the tunneling process proper consideration. This chapter summarizes potential pitfalls and need for attention to this important part of the procedure. Competence in tunneling can lead to an improved cosmetic outcome, improved patient comfort, and improvements in the overall patient experience.

Suggested Reading

Falco F, Rubbani M, Heinbaugh J. Anterograde sacral nerve root stimulation (ASNRS) via the sacral hiatus: benefits, limitations, and percutaneous implantation technique. Neuromodulation. 2003;6(4): 219–24.

Falowski S, Celii A, Sharan A. Spinal cord stimulation: an update. Neurotherapeutics. 2008;5:86–99.

Quigley DG, Arnold J, Eldridge PR, et al. Long-term outcome of spinal cord stimulation and hardware complications. Stereotact Funct Neurosurg. 2003;81:50–6.

12 Pocketing Techniques for Spinal Cord Stimulation and Peripheral Nerve Stimulation

Timothy R. Deer and C. Douglas Stewart

For too many young implanters, the creation of a pocket is a hurdle that intimidates them from offering permanent implants. Conversely, experienced implanters should be cautioned not to take this process too lightly, as optimal pocketing can greatly impact the overall device experience.

12.1 Technical Overview

The technical aspects of the spinal cord stimulation implant are often centered on lead placement and spinal interventions, but the pocket is an equally important part of the procedure that deserves special attention. The decision-making for pocketing begins prior to implantation. When choosing the pocket site, the physician should consider the patient's body habitus, the site of the lead implant, the likelihood of weight gain or loss, the risk of migration, and the impact on the sterile field (Table 12.1). The patient (especially those with very large body habitus) should be evaluated while sitting, standing, and lying down, to make sure that no significant shift in the soft tissue will adversely affect outcome. If the lead entry anchoring point is in the upper lumbar spine, placing the pocket above the beltline should resolve this issue in most cases, as significant tissue shifts have little impact in this body region.

New devices are becoming smaller, and the choice of pocketing sites may continue to evolve, providing less impact on body contours and greater comfort. One factor affecting the selection of the surgical site is the direction of Langer's lines, sometimes called cleavage lines, which correspond to the natural orientation of collagen fibers in the dermis (Fig. 12.1). Knowing the direction of Langer's lines within a specific area of the skin is important for surgical operations, particularly cosmetic surgery. Given a choice about where and in what direction to place an incision, the surgeon may choose to cut in the direction of Langer's lines. Incisions made parallel to Langer's lines may heal better and produce less scarring than those that cut across. Incisions perpendicular to Langer's lines have a tendency to scar and create an unsightly cosmetic outcome, although sometimes such incisions are unavoidable.

Another factor that can result in a poor outcome is placement of the pocketing incision across a previous surgical scar. The result can be poor healing, poor cosmesis, and sometimes chronic pain.

It is important to carefully mark the site of implant preoperatively to ensure that the physician does not become distracted by other issues in the operating room (Fig. 12.2). Once the pocket site is determined, the patient is positioned to expose the site for surgical intervention.

The incision should be made with one distinct motion to ensure an even cut to improve closure. The surgeon should retract the skin at the time of incision to allow for an even tissue plane for dissection. The incision depth varies based on the patient's body fat and adipose tissue. Routinely, the incision is made between 1.5 and 3.0 cm in depth. It should be deep enough to avoid generator erosion through the tissue, but superficial enough to allow for computer telemetry. When the proper tissue plane is achieved, the tissue is dissected by blunt dissection, cutting electrocautery dissection, or sharp dissection; clinicians differ in their preferences. The blunt dissection technique, which is associated with less tissue trauma and bleeding, is often preferred, although aggressive blunt dissection increases the likelihood of seroma formation. In some patients, fibrous tissue is present and must be dissected by sharper and more aggressive techniques. The use of sharp scissors to separate rather than cut the tissue is a common strategy to combine both the sharp and the blunt tissue dissection techniques.

The ideal pocket size should be 120–130 % of the generator volume. The extra room will allow tissue slack, to avoid

T.R. Deer, MD (✉) • C.D. Stewart
The Center for Pain Relief,
400 Court Street, Suite 100, Charleston, WV 25301, USA
e-mail: DocTDeer@aol.com;
dstewart@centerforpainrelief.com

T.R. Deer, J.E. Pope (eds.), *Atlas of Implantable Therapies for Pain Management*, DOI 10.1007/978-1-4939-2110-2_12

wound dehiscence and to decrease pain. If the pocket is larger than the recommended size, the patient may be prone to generator flipping, which can lead to a need for surgical revision.

Hemostasis is important, as bleeding can lead to hematoma, seroma, wound dehiscence, and the need to explore the wound. When making the pocket, the clinician should carefully retract the tissue and examine the pocket for bleeding. Bleeding can be controlled by cautery or, in the case of pulsatile arterial bleeds, by an absorbable ligature suture. Suture is used to ligate the bleeder when cautery is not successful. It is important to avoid cautery at the surface of the skin, where wound closure occurs. Being too aggressive with the tissue heating can lead to necrosis and poor tissue healing.

Prior to closing the wound, the pocket should be irrigated aggressively with an antibiotic such as bacitracin. The irrigation should be copious, using 500–1000 mL or more. Irrigation of the wound is a critical factor in reducing infection risks, and the clinician should strive to make this part of the routine pocketing methods.

After the pocket is completed, a tunneling procedure is performed to bring the lead wiring to the pocket (Figs. 12.3 and 12.4). This wire should be long enough to allow for a strain relief loop to reduce the risk of migration. The loop of wire should fit smoothly behind the generator. The importance of making the pocket 20–30 % larger than the generator is helpful with this step, to ensure that there is proper room for the wiring.

Wound closure should be seen as another critical point in the implant process. It is important to use a two-layer to three-layer closure technique, to ensure proper skin alignment, and to avoid tension of the tissue, which can lead to necrosis.

Table 12.1 Pocket site selection information

Location	Advantages	Disadvantages	Ideal uses
Buttock	The generator is close to the implant site for the lumbar and thoracic spine Patients with implants for back and leg pain do not require repositioning The amount of adipose tissue is adequate in normal or obese patients	The generator can cause pain from irritation by the belt or clothing In the immediate postoperative period, putting pressure on the tissue when sitting can open the wound (a greater concern for the obese patient) Bending at the waist can place pressure on the wiring and may cause concern about migration	Sacral and caudal implants Lumbar and thoracic spine implants
Abdomen	The generator is in an area with low pressure during sitting and lying The generator is easily accessible for patient programming	The amount of wiring between the spine and the pocket may increase the risk of lead migration In obese patients, the abdominal wall contour may lead to generator discomfort When the leads are implanted simultaneously with the generator, the patient must be repositioned, reprepped, and redraped, a process that can increase the risk of infection	Patients who have discomfort from implants at other sites Staged implant procedures, in which the trial leads are surgically implanted for the trial Peripheral nerve implants of the pelvis, abdomen, or chest wall
Posterior flank	The ideal implant site for most implants The location above the beltline has less stress on the tissue than the buttock The area is less contaminated, owing to its distance from the anus and pelvis Compared with the buttocks and abdomen, the stress on the leads is less when tunneling from the cervical spine and head and neck; this may reduce the risk of migration Lumbar incisions are in close proximity to the flank, which may reduce the risk of migration	Sensitivity may result in pain at the generator site	Lumbar, thoracic, and cervical spine implants Head and neck implants

Table 12.1 (continued)

Location	Advantages	Disadvantages	Ideal uses
Spine implant site, through same incision (possible for very small generator)	The distance between the spinal leads and the generator reduces the risk of migration Single incision means fewer sites to become infected	Excessive wire length of the leads may make it difficult to place the generator into the pocket Discomfort may occur with sitting or reclining	Patients with adequate tissue to support a generator in the paravertebral tissue
Chest	Chest wall position puts minimal stress on implants in the occiput, and facial nerves for peripheral implants	Area is sometimes difficult to reach by tunneling (When tunneling from the head and neck, it is important to be aware of the vessels of the neck and the lung position) Tunneling must occur over the clavicle	Implants of the head and neck, including peripheral nerve and intracranial nerve implants
Subpectoral	May avoid the risk of skin erosion in children or patients with very low body fat	Technically difficult procedure requires additional training	Children or very thin patients without enough subcutaneous fat to support the metal under the dermis
Extremity (possible for small generator)	Not necessary to tunnel the wiring over joints, which can cause migration	The subcutaneous tissue of the limb may not support the device, because of pain or erosion Site not possible with larger internal programmable generators	Peripheral nerve implants
Axillary line at T4	Reduced need for tunneling, compared with flank or buttock Brassiere can be used to secure the antenna of a radiofrequency device	The tissue may be irritated by arm movement Device may be difficult to reach with the opposite arm for programming	Cervical spine or head and neck implants

Fig. 12.1 Langer's lines on a map of the human body

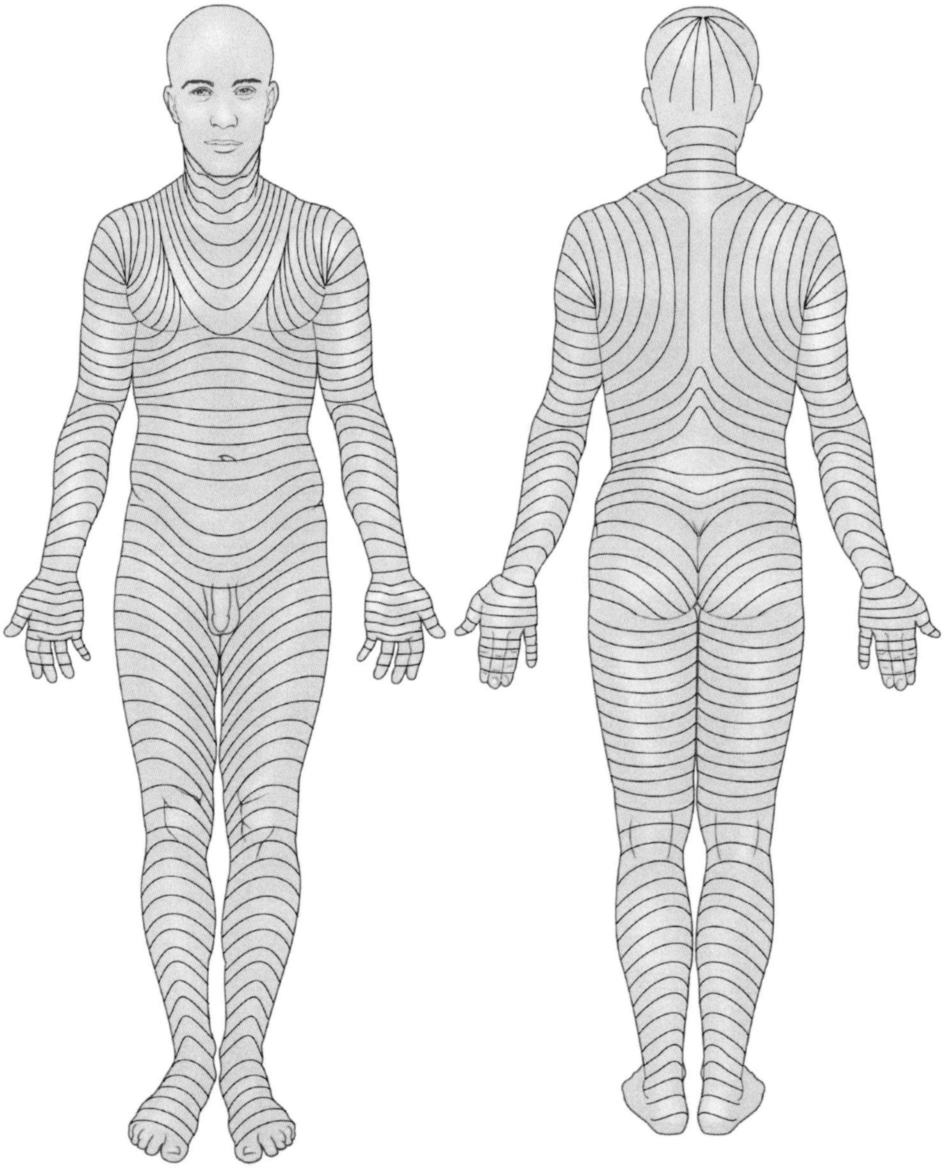

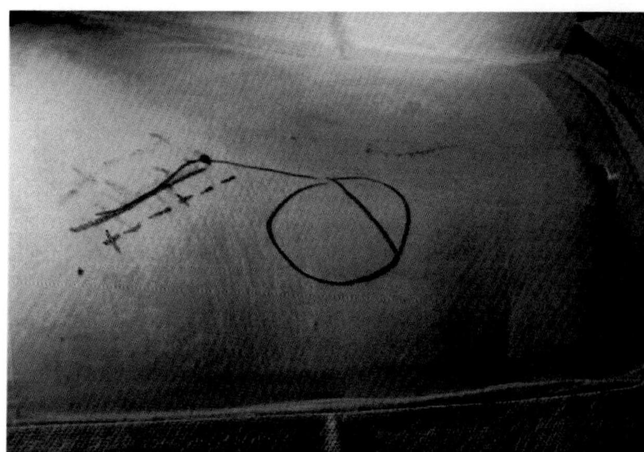

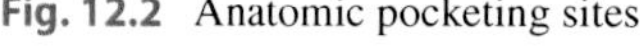

Fig. 12.2 Anatomic pocketing sites

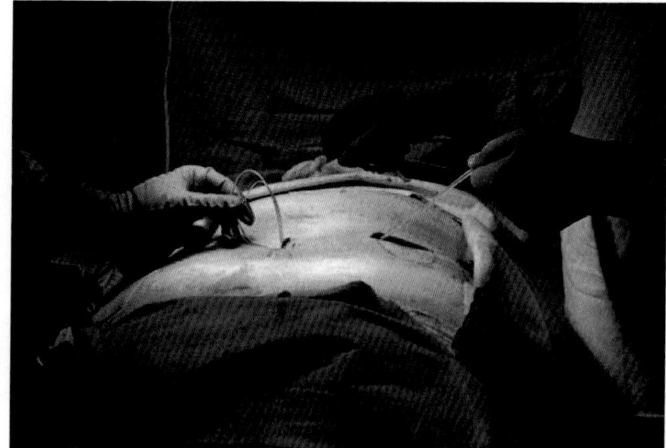

Fig. 12.3 After the pocket is completed, a tunneling procedure is performed to bring the lead wiring to the pocket

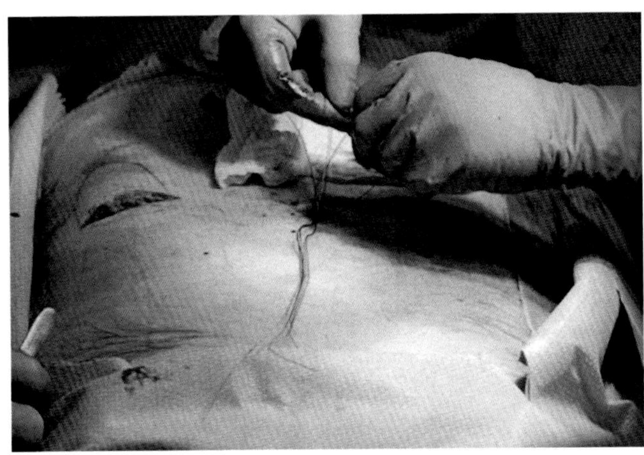

Fig. 12.4 Posterior flank incision in close proximity to the site of L3 lumbar incision.

12.2 Risk Assessment

A risk of complications can accompany the pocketing portion of the procedure:

- The generator can cause pain and irritation if placed too superficially.
- The generator may be unable to communicate with telemetry if it is placed too deeply.
- The generator can cause pain if placed close to a bony prominence.
- Seroma of the pocket can lead to wound dehiscence and pain.
- Hematoma of the wound can lead to the need for surgical evacuation, and wound dehiscence or infection.
- Cautery lesioning for hemostasis can lead to skin breakdown if done too near the surface.
- Coiling the wire above the generator can lead to pain or erosion.

12.3 Risk Avoidance

The clinician should take all possible steps to avoid risks to the patient:

- The depth of the generator must be in the subcutaneous tissue with appropriate adipose tissue for cushioning.
- The generator must be superficial enough to allow communication. Prior to leaving the operating room after permanent implantation, the clinician should test the device for impedance.
- The bony prominences of the pocket region should be examined preoperatively and at the time of implantation. The implant should avoid the rib, anterior superior iliac spine, posterior superior iliac spine, and sacrum.
- Seroma can be reduced by using blunt dissection, limiting tissue trauma, and ensuring good hemostasis of venous bleeders. Hemostasis can be improved by packing the pocket with antibiotic-soaked sponges for 5–10 min during the course of the procedure.
- Hematoma can be avoided by close attention to preoperative medications that affect clotting or change platelet function. Careful attention to identifying and resolving bleeding is critical prior to wound closure. Bleeding can be resolved by cautery, suturing, and applying pressure.
- When using cautery, the physician should avoid surface bleeders that border the skin margin.
- Wire that is in excess of that needed for spine insertion and tunneling should be carefully secured in a strain relief loop at the spinal site of lead placement and at the pocket site, with attention to placing the wire below the generator (Figs. 12.5 and 12.6).

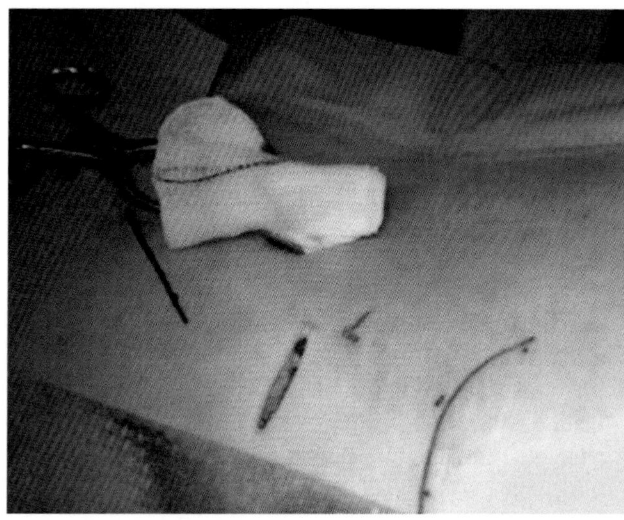

Fig. 12.5 Wire for strain relief behind the generator, which is being secured with a hex wrench

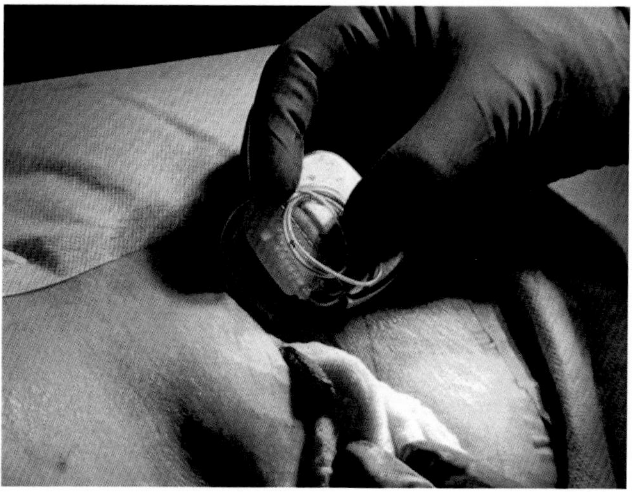

Fig. 12.6 Wire strain relief loop

Conclusions

When creating a pocket, the physician should carefully plan its location based on factors such as lead target, body habitus, and patient function. The pocket should be made with careful surgical skill, and attention should be given to avoid risks. Wound closure and postoperative follow-up should be performed with a focus on reducing tissue trauma and optimizing wound healing (Fig. 12.7).

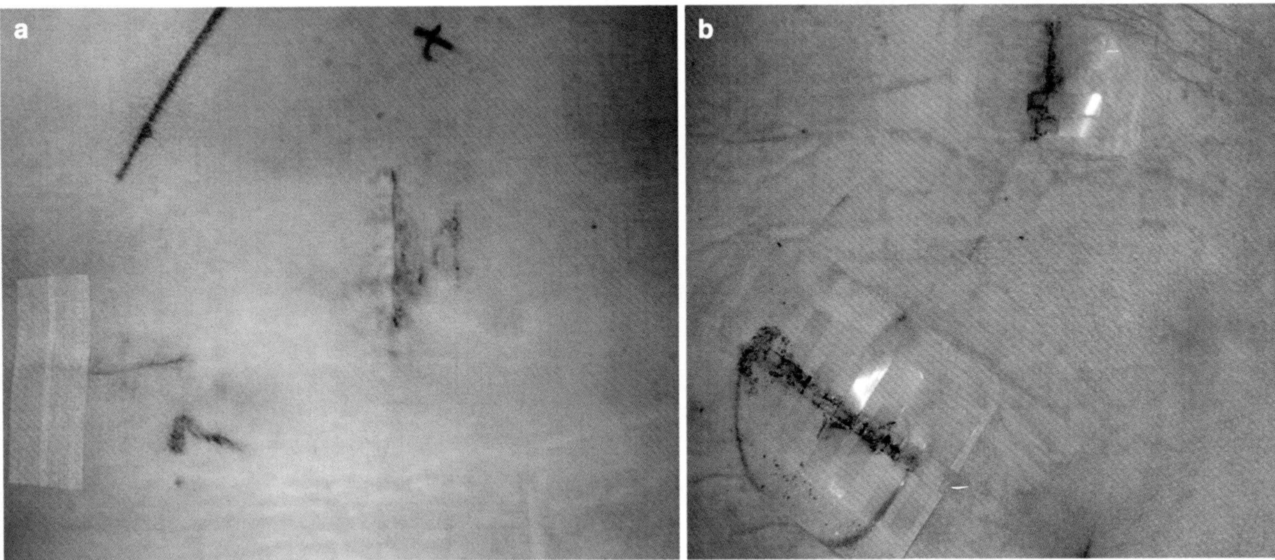

Fig. 12.7 (**a**, **b**) Examples of a well-healed pocketing site

Suggested Reading

Scheepens WA, Weil EH, van Koeveringe GA, Rohrmann D, Hedlund HE, Schurch B, et al. Buttock placement of the implantable pulse generator: a new implantation technique for sacral neuromodulation—a multicenter study. Eur Urol. 2001;40:434–8.

Townsend CM, Beauchamp RD, Evers BM, Mattox KL, editors. Sabiston textbook of surgery: the biological basis of modern surgical practice. 19th ed. Philadelphia: Saunders; 2012.

Vanhauwaert DJ, Kalala JP, Baert E, Hallaert G, Crombez E, Caemaert J, et al. Migration of pump for intrathecal drug delivery into the peritoneal cavity. Case report. Surg Neurol. 2009;71: 610–2.

Winkelmuller M, Winkelmuller W. Long-term effects of continuous intrathecal opioid treatment in chronic pain of nonmalignant etiology. J Neurosurg. 1996;85:458–67.

Wound Closure

13

Timothy R. Deer and C. Douglas Stewart

13.1 Introduction

Over the past two decades I have trained hundreds of physicians to implant devices. The excitement of learning to implant a spinal cord stimulation lead or an intrathecal catheter can be a significant professional achievement. Unfortunately the number of physicians who are students of the entire procedure is less common. Part of the total implant package includes learning the finer points of wound closure. This chapter is dedicated to that pursuit.

13.2 Overview

As a method for closing cutaneous wounds, the technique of suturing is thousands of years old. Although suture materials and aspects of the technique have changed, the goals remain the same: closing dead space, supporting and strengthening wounds until healing increases their tensile strength, approximating skin edges for an aesthetically pleasing and functional result, and minimizing the risks of bleeding and infection.

Proper suturing technique is needed to ensure good results in dermatological surgery, not only for cosmetic reasons but also for anchoring implantable therapies. The postoperative appearance of a wound can be compromised if an incorrect suture technique is chosen or if the execution is poor. Conversely meticulous suturing technique cannot fully compensate for improper surgical technique, because poor incision placement, with respect to relaxed skin tension lines, excessive removal of tissue, or inadequate undermining, may limit the surgeon's options in wound closure and suture placement. Gentle handling of the tissue is also important to optimize wound healing.

The choice of suture technique depends on the type and anatomical location of the wound, the thickness of the skin, the degree of tension, and the desired cosmetic result. The proper placement of sutures enhances the precise approximation of the wound edges, which helps minimize and redistribute skin tension. For our discussion wound placement is fairly mandated by the type of advanced implantable therapy. The location of the implantable internal pulse generator (IPG) or reservoir is commonly dictated by avoiding bony anatomy and placement overlying pressure points, accommodating the size of the device.

The IPG for either dorsal column stimulation or peripheral stimulation strategies is commonly placed within the flank, ipsilateral to the lead entry or placement, so as to avoid crossing the midline. Other sites for IPG placement include the infraclavicular area, buttock, or abdomen. For peripheral nerve stimulation, IPG location is limited by size and can be placed within the leg or arm, taking care with the leads crossing major joints. The placement for intrathecal reservoir is on-label and commonly placed within the abdomen, although some authors advocate posterior placement.

The aforementioned acknowledged, the surgical sites are fairly open and flat, thus lending themselves to a few common closure techniques. Regardless of technique chosen, wound eversion is essential to maximize the likelihood of good epidermal approximation and is desirable to minimize the risk of scar depression secondary to tissue contraction during healing. The elimination of dead space (Fig. 13.1), the restoration of natural anatomical contours, and the minimization of suture marks are also important to optimize the cosmetic and functional results.

T.R. Deer, MD (✉) • C.D. Stewart
The Center for Pain Relief,
400 Court Street, Suite 100, Charleston, WV 25301, USA
e-mail: DocTDeer@aol.com;
dstewart@centerforpainrelief.com

T.R. Deer, J.E. Pope (eds.), *Atlas of Implantable Therapies for Pain Management*, DOI 10.1007/978-1-4939-2110-2_13

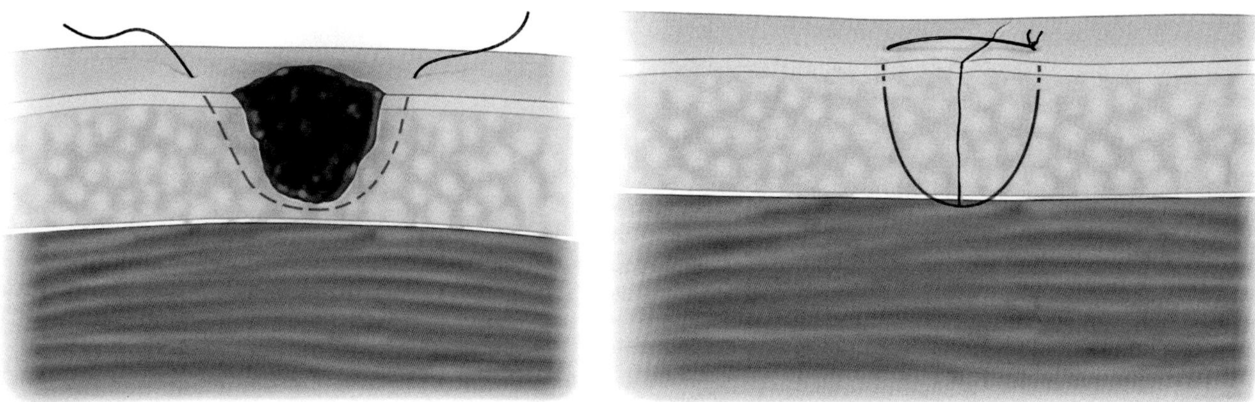

Fig. 13.1 Wound closure with elimination of dead space. Note the elimination of any dead space in the wound

13.3 Techniques

A few simple rules promote the opportunity for a success wound closure:

1. Clean and dry, well-controlled hemostasis and removal of tissue debris and clot
2. Adequate room for implanted devices
3. Elimination of dead space
4. Appropriate technique for closure of skin

There are as many closure techniques as individuals doing them. Excellent outcomes are produced by attention to detail. The authors have spent many years using these techniques; experience, empirical study, and anecdotal observation have proven their worth in the low complication rate and high degree for success. Consideration of type of stitch employed and choice of suture used (Table 13.1), along with type of needle (Fig. 13.2), improve the chance for desirable outcomes.

The choice of suture material is left to the surgeon; however in most instances absorbable material is the best choice. Most surgeons have a basic "suture routine," a preference for using the same material(s) unless circumstances dictate otherwise. A monofilament material is the material of choice. The exception would be the anchoring stiches, because synthetic nonabsorbable suture is used to anchor implanted devices.

Wound closure can be accomplished using sutures, staples, adhesives, or adhesive strips. We look at all these techniques but focus primarily on suturing.

Table 13.1 Characteristics of common absorbable and non-absorbable sources

Suture	Surgical gut	Surgical gut	Polyglycolic acid (PGA)	Rapid polyglycolic acid (RPGA)	Silk	Nylon	Polypropylene
Types	Plain	Chronic	Braided	Braided	Braided	Monofilament	Monofilament
Common material color	Yellowish tan	Blue	White	Undyed (beige)	Black	Black	Blue
Raw material	Collagen from beef and shrimp	Collagen from beef and shrimp	Lactide and glycolide co-polymer	Lactide and glycolide co-polymer	Organic protein (fibroin)	Long-chain aliphatic polymers	Long-chain polyolefin polymers
Tensile strength	Low	Low	High	High	Moderate	Moderate	High
Tensile strength (in vivo)	3–5 days	7–10 days	28–35 days	10–14 days	Progressive degradation of fiber results in gradual loss of tensile strength	Progressive hydrolysis results in gradual loss of tensile strength	No significant changes known to occur in vivo
Tissue inflammatory reaction	Moderate	Moderate	Minimal	Minimal	Mild to moderate	Minimal	Minimal
Indications/contraindications	Exhibit mild tensile strength. Used for approximating tissues with little tension Absorbable and should not be used where extended approximation of tissues under stress is required Should not be used in patients with known sensitivities or allergies to collagen	Exhibit mild tensile strength. Used for approximating tissues with little tension Absorbable and should not be used where extended approximation of tissues under stress is required Should not be used in patients with known sensitivities or allergies to collagen or chromium	Periodontal surgery, implant surgery, oral maxillofacial surgery Exhibit high tensile strength. Can be used to resist muscle pull Absorbable and should not be used where extended approximation of tissues under stress is required	Periodontal surgery, implant surgery, oral maxillofacial surgery Exhibit high tensile strength. Can be used to resist muscle pull Absorbable and should not be used where extended approximation of tissues under stress is required	Periodontal surgery, implant surgery, oral maxillofacial surgery Should not be used in patients with known sensitivities or allergies to silk	Periodontal surgery, implant surgery, oral maxillofacial surgery	Periodontal surgery, implant surgery, oral maxillofacial surgery

Fig. 13.2 Types of needles

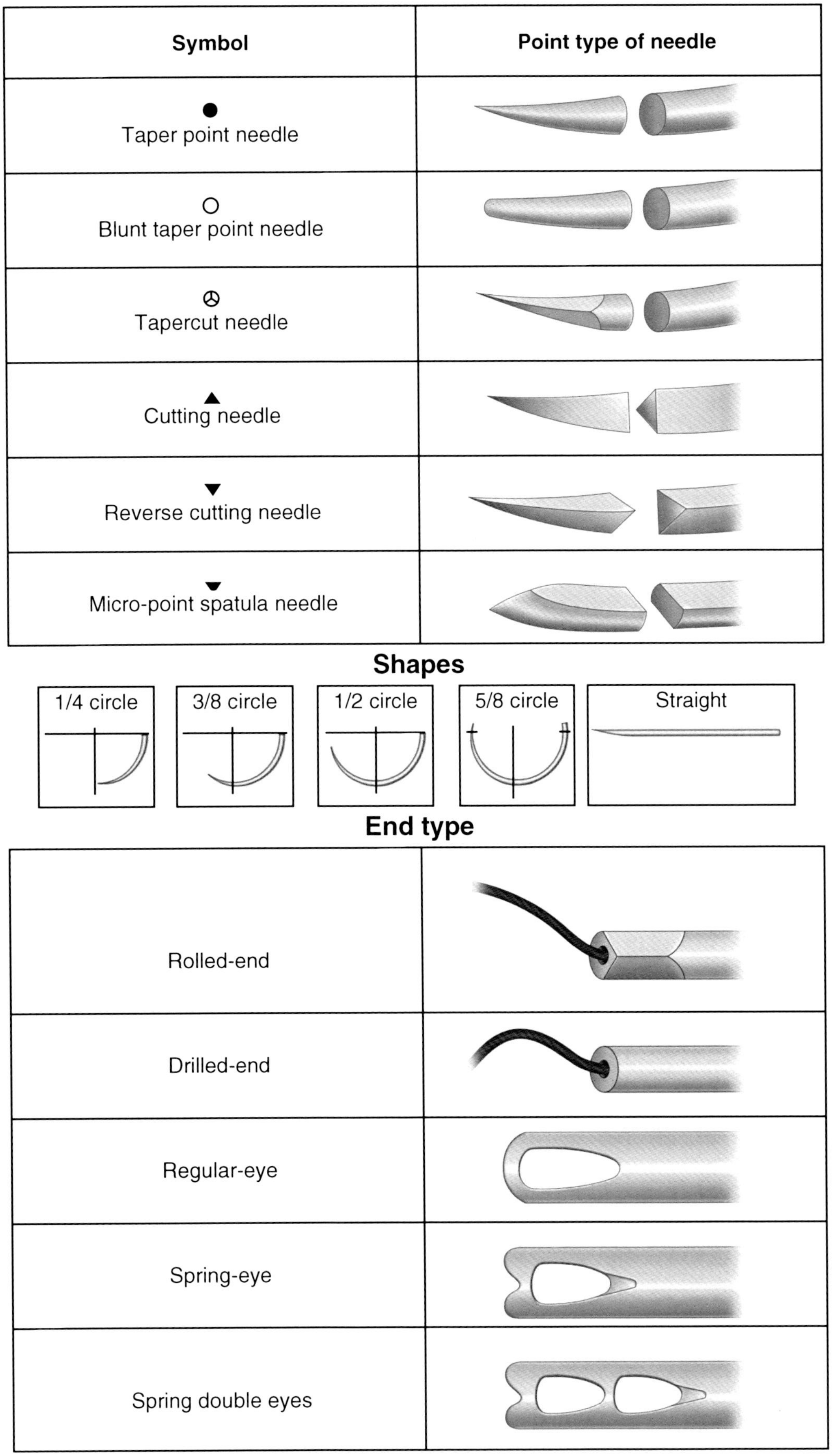

Symbol	Point type of needle
● Taper point needle	
○ Blunt taper point needle	
⊗ Tapercut needle	
▲ Cutting needle	
▼ Reverse cutting needle	
▼ Micro-point spatula needle	

Shapes

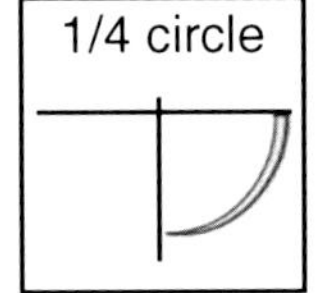

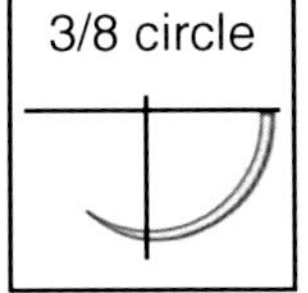

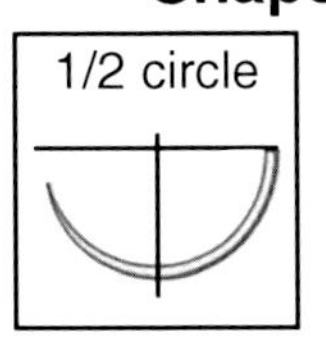

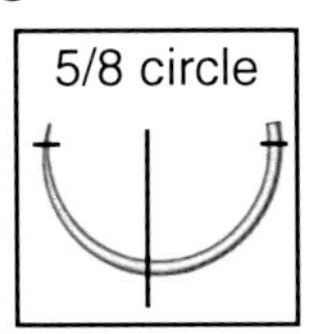

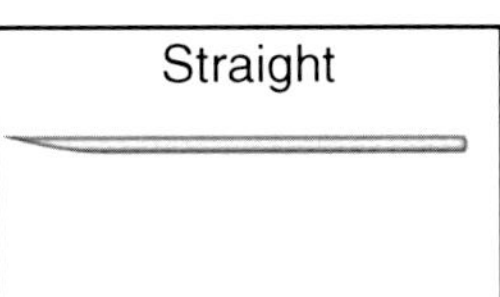

End type

Rolled-end	
Drilled-end	
Regular-eye	
Spring-eye	
Spring double eyes	

13.4 Closure Methods

13.4.1 Suturing: Knot Tying

Once the suture is satisfactorily placed, it must be secured with a knot. The instrument tie is used most commonly in cutaneous surgery. The square knot is traditionally used (Fig. 13.3). First, the tip of the needle holder is rotated clockwise around the long end of the suture material for two complete turns. The tip of the needle holder is used to grasp the short end of the suture. The short end of the suture is pulled through the loops of the long end by crossing the hands, such that the two ends of the suture material are situated on opposite sides of the suture line. The needle holder is rotated counterclockwise once around the long end of the suture. The short end is grasped with the needle holder tip, and the short end is pulled through the loop again.

The suture should be tightened sufficiently to approximate the wound edges without constricting the tissue. Sometimes leaving a small loop of suture after the second throw is helpful. This reserve loop allows the stitch to expand slightly and is helpful in preventing the strangulation of tissue because the tension exerted on the suture increases with increased wound edema. Depending on the surgeon's preference, one or two additional throws may be added.

Properly squaring successive ties is important. That is, each tie must be laid down perfectly parallel to the previous tie. This procedure is important in preventing the creation of a granny knot, which tends to slip and is inherently weaker than a properly squared knot. When the desired number of throws is completed, the suture material may be cut (if interrupted stitches are used) or the next suture may be placed (Fig. 13.3).

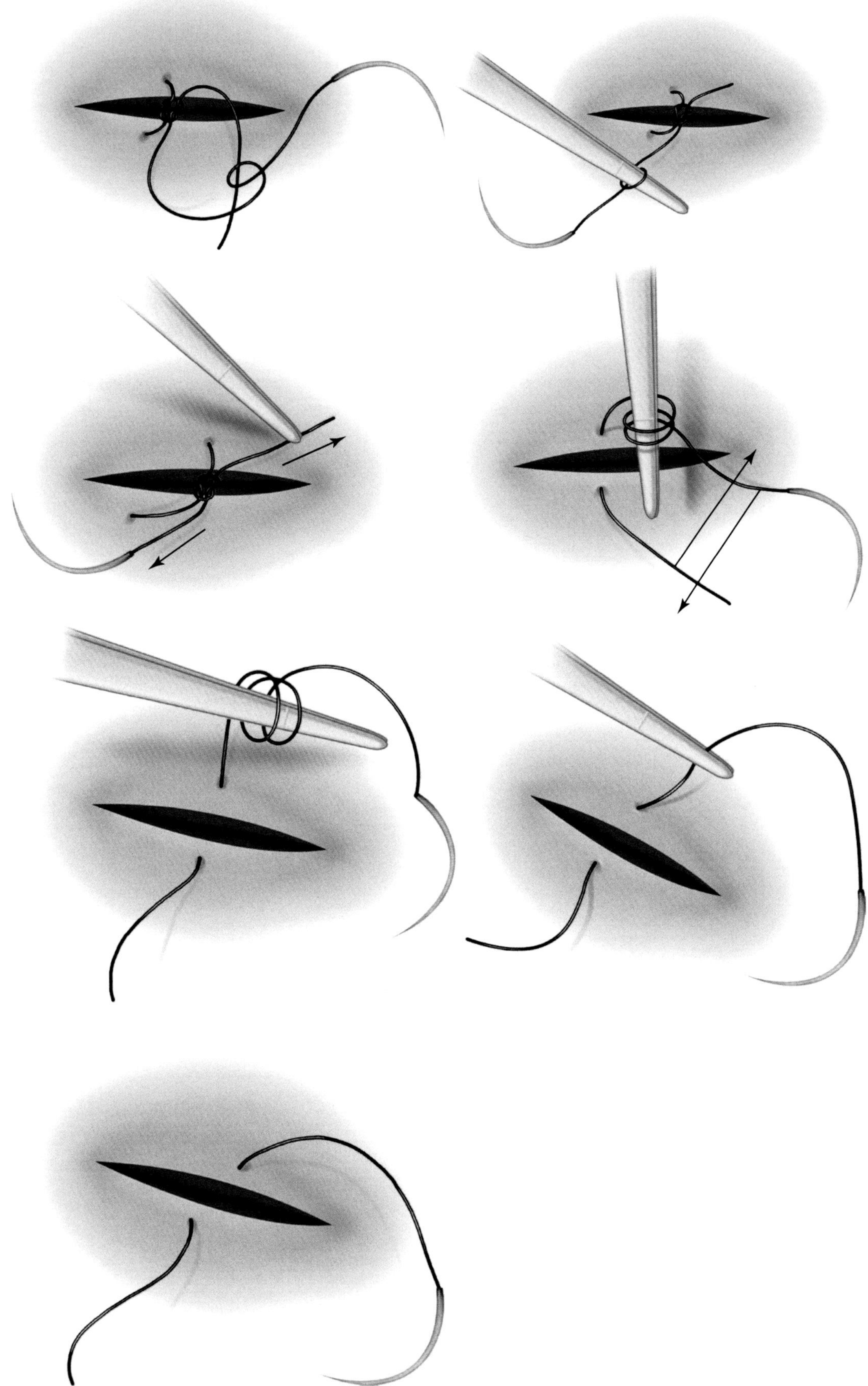

Fig. 13.3 Knot tying: square knot using instruments

13.4.2 Suturing: Stitch Techniques

13.4.2.1 Simple Interrupted Stitch (Fig. 13.4)

Compared with running sutures, interrupted sutures are easy to place, have greater tensile strength, and have less potential for causing wound edema and impaired cutaneous circulation. Interrupted sutures also allow the surgeon to make adjustments as needed to properly align wound edges as the wound is sutured.

Before the dermis is closed, all tension should be removed from the wound with subcuticular stitches. The stitches placed in the most superficial layer are only there to approximate the edges and make the wound watertight.

If there is tension on the wound, there will be deposition of excess collagen material if there is a widening of the subcutaneous layer, causing a wide unattractive scar. If the subcutaneous tissue is not closed or closed poorly then there will be excessive tension on the suture line that will interrupt microcirculation and cause poor or delayed healing, thus presenting the potential for a failure of the wound line itself.

Disadvantages of interrupted sutures include the length of time required for their placement and the greater risk of cross-hatched marks across the suture line. The risk of cross-hatching can be minimized by removing sutures early to prevent the development of suture tracks.

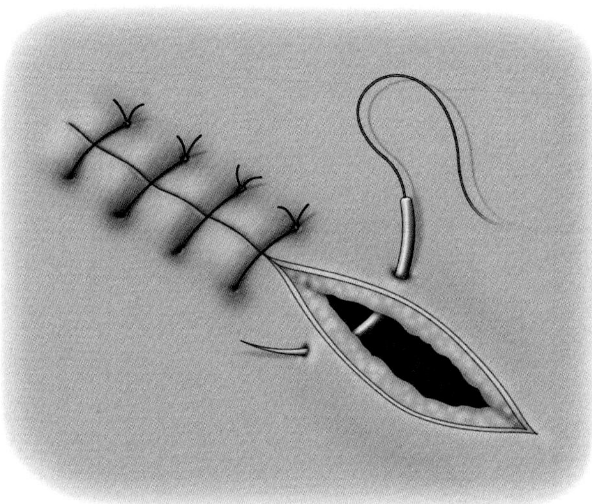

Fig. 13.4 Simple interrupted stitch

13.4.2.2 Simple Running Stitch (Fig. 13.5)

Running sutures are useful for long wounds in which wound tension has been minimized with properly placed deep sutures and in which approximation of the wound edges is good. This type of suture may also be used to secure a split- or full-thickness skin graft. Theoretically, less scarring occurs with running sutures than with interrupted sutures because fewer knots are made with simple running sutures; however, the number of needle insertions remains the same.

Advantages of the simple running suture include quicker placement and more rapid reapproximation of wound edges, compared with simple interrupted sutures.

Disadvantages include possible cross-hatching, the risk of dehiscence if the suture material ruptures, difficulty in making fine adjustments along the suture line, and puckering of the suture line when the stitches are placed in thin skin. Again this can be minimized with good subcutaneous closure. A good subcutaneous closure will align the wound and take tension off the wound.

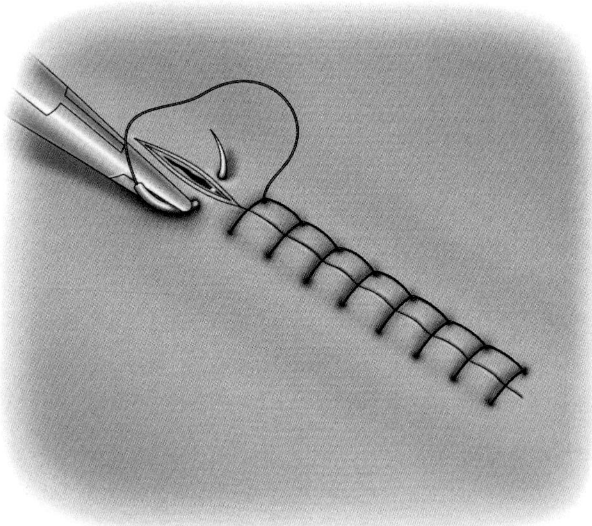

Fig. 13.5 Simple running stitch

13.4.2.3 Horizontal Mattress Stitch

The horizontal mattress suture is placed by entering the skin 5–7 mm from the wound edge. The suture is passed deep in the dermis to the opposite side of the suture line and exits the skin equidistant from the wound edge, much like placing two simple sutures using the same stich. The needle reenters the skin on the same side of the suture line 5–7 mm lateral to the exit point. The stitch is passed deep to the opposite side of the wound where it exits the skin and the knot is tied (Fig. 13.6).

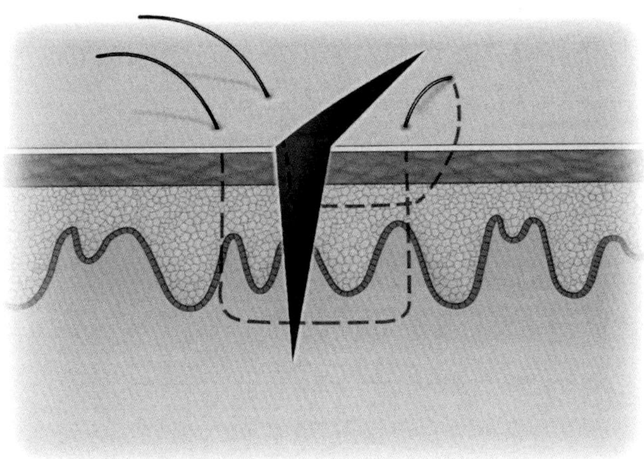

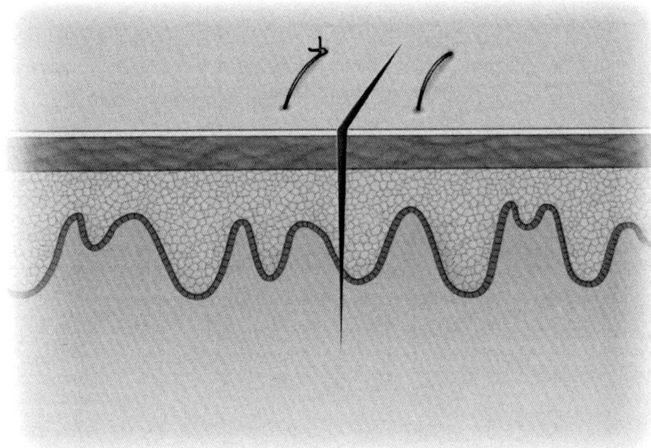

Fig. 13.6 Horizontal mattress stitch

13.4.2.4 Vertical Mattress Stitch

The vertical mattress suture is a variation of the simple interrupted suture. It consists of a simple interrupted stitch placed wide and deep into the wound edge and a second more superficial interrupted stitch placed closer to the wound edge and in the opposite direction. The width of the stitch should be increased in proportion to the amount of tension on the wound. However, remember there should be no tension on the wound. The tension should be minimized by the use of subcuticular sutures whether running or interrupted (Fig. 13.7).

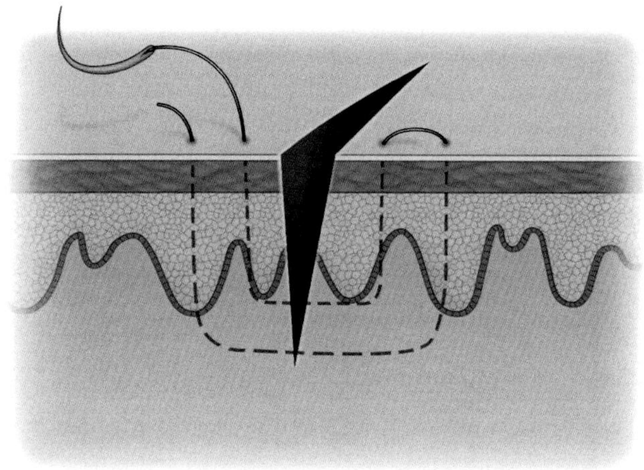

Fig. 13.7 Vertical mattress stitch

13.4.3 Non-suture Closure Techniques

Non-suture closure techniques include steri-strips (Fig. 13.8a), staples (Fig. 13.8b), and skin adhesives. These strategies impart a reduction of stress along the incision line. Staples need to be removed within 5–7 days following placement for most applications in the pain space.

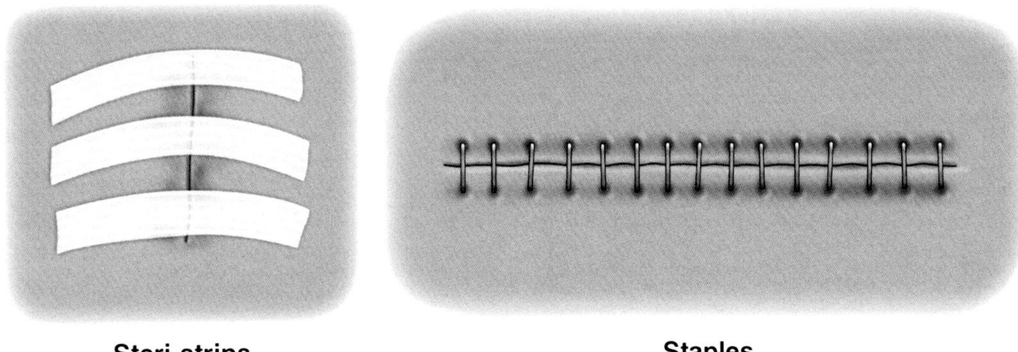

Fig. 13.8 (**a**) Steri-stripes; (**b**) Staples

Conclusions

Patient identification of implantable, advanced technologies begins the journey of securing sustained care for patients. Implementation of the advanced therapy largely hinges on the ability to place and secure the system, along with an efficacious and succinct surgical technique.

Suggested Reading

Mackay-Wiggan J. Suturing techniques. In: Elston DM, editor. Medscape. Available at http://emedicine.medscape.com/article/1824895-overview. Accessed 19 Feb 2015.

Townsend CM, Evers BM. Atlas of general surgical techniques: expert consult. Philadelphia: Saunders; 2010.

Zollinger R, Ellison E. Zollinger's atlas of surgical operations. 9th ed. New York: McGraw-Hill Companies; 2010.

Wound Healing

14

Timothy R. Deer and C. Douglas Stewart

Many neuromodulators have a background in pharmacology and physiology, but little understanding of the surgical principles that guide postoperative management. Wound healing is an intricate and spontaneous phenomenon that results in a desirable outcome when allowed to proceed in the normal fashion. When the skin is broken, the natural process of wound healing is initiated. The classic model of wound healing occurs in several ordered and overlapping phases: (1) hemostasis, (2) inflammation, (3) proliferation, and (4) remodeling. While this process takes place, the tissue must be held in apposition until the healing mechanisms provide the wound with sufficient strength to withstand stress without mechanical support. This chapter discusses the basics involved in wound healing and what it means to the implanting and managing physician.

14.1 Technical Overview

Tissue is defined as a collection of similar cells and the intercellular substances surrounding them. There are four basic tissues in the body: (1) epithelium; (2) connective tissues, including blood, bone, and cartilage; (3) muscle tissue; and (4) nerve tissue. In most instances, wounds will heal spontaneously if no distractors interfere with the process. Processes such as uncontrolled diabetes, immunosuppression, and poor skin apposition can disrupt this process. In wounds that are created in a sterile operating room environment, the process should occur in an ordered and defined fashion. The choice of wound closure materials and the techniques of using them are prime factors in the restoration of continuity and tensile strength to the surgical wound during this process.

The rate at which wounds regain strength during the wound healing process must be understood as a basis for selecting the most appropriate wound closure material. Other factors to consider include suture removal, staple removal, and wound care.

14.2 Recovery of Tensile Strength

Tensile strength is a tissue characteristic that affects the tissue's ability to withstand injury but is not related to the length of time it takes the tissue to heal. As collagen accumulates during the reparative phase, strength increases rapidly, but it may take 12–26 weeks before a plateau is reached. In the initial days after wound creation, optimal healing requires extrinsic support of the wound from the method used to bring it together—usually sutures. Although skin and fascia (the layer of firm connective tissue covering muscle) are comparatively strong tissues, they regain tensile strength slowly during the healing process. Variations in tissue strength also may be found within the same organ. Factors that determine tissue strength include the general health, age, and weight of the patient, the thickness of tissue, the presence of edema, and the duration of tissue injury, which can be affected by pressure, ongoing tissue trauma, and blood flow. Table 14.1 highlights major factors that can adversely affect wound healing:

- **Age**—With the aging process, both skin and muscle tissue lose their tone and elasticity. Metabolism also slows, and circulation may be impaired. Aging alone is not a major factor in wound healing, but aging and chronic disease states often go together, and both delay repair processes through delayed cellular response to the stimulus of injury, delayed collagen deposition, and decreased tensile strength in the remodeled tissue. All of these factors lengthen healing time and may lead to wound breakdown.
- **Weight**—Obesity results in adipose deposition at the wound site that may prevent a good closure. Fatty tissue

T.R. Deer, MD (✉) • C.D. Stewart
The Center for Pain Relief,
400 Court Street, Suite 100, Charleston, WV 25301, USA
e-mail: DocTDeer@aol.com;
dstewart@centerforpainrelief.com

T.R. Deer, J.E. Pope (eds.), *Atlas of Implantable Therapies for Pain Management*, DOI 10.1007/978-1-4939-2110-2_14

does not have a rich blood supply, making it very susceptible to infection. In addition, suturing to adipose can result in poor tissue closure and wound breakdown.

- **Nutritional status**—Specific deficiencies or overall malnutrition associated with chronic disease or cancer can impair the healing process. Dietary inadequacies and poor absorption can lead to poor overall health and deficiencies of vitamins and minerals that are important in tissue recovery. Recent analyses suggest that zinc, magnesium, and vitamins A, B, and C are essential to support cellular activity and collagen synthesis in the healing process. In many cases, supplementing these substances is not helpful because they are discharged in the urine, so it is essential to eat a healthy and balanced diet.
- **Dehydration**—If the patient's system has been depleted of fluids, the resulting electrolyte imbalance can affect cardiac function, kidney function, cellular metabolism, oxygenation of the blood, and hormonal function.
- **Inadequate blood supply to the wound site**—Oxygen is necessary for cell survival, and thus for healing. Skin healing takes place most rapidly in the face and neck (which receive the greatest blood supply) and most slowly in the extremities. The presence of any condition that compromises the supply of blood to the wound, such as poor circulation to the limbs in a diabetic patient or arteriosclerosis with vascular compromise, will slow and can even arrest the healing process.
- **Immune responses**—Because the immune response protects the patient from infection, immunodeficiency may seriously compromise the outcome of a surgical procedure. Factors related to immunodeficiency that impact healing include recent chemotherapy, malignancy, prolonged doses of catabolic steroids, and (in some settings) infection with hepatitis or HIV. With new drugs for the latter two illnesses, the degree of immunosuppression varies. On the other hand, an overactive immune response also can interfere with the healing process through an exaggerated immune response to specific suturing materials or implanted devices that will have an impact on the healing of the wound.
- **Chronic disease**—A patient whose system has already been stressed by chronic illness—especially endocrine disorders, diabetes, malignancies, localized infection, or debilitating injuries—will heal more slowly and will be more vulnerable to postsurgical wound complications. All of these conditions merit concern, and the surgeon must consider their effects upon the tissues at the wound site, as well as their potential impact upon the patient's overall recovery from the procedure. Collaboration with a physician well versed in management of the disease(s) specific to the patient can be helpful.
- **Radiation therapy**—Radiation therapy to the surgical site prior to or shortly after surgery can produce considerable impairment of healing and lead to substantial wound complications. Surgical procedures in patients who have had radiation for malignancies in the area of the planned surgery must be carefully considered to help avoid potential healing problems. In some of these settings, the generator for the stimulation device or intrathecal pump pocket must be adapted to the area of the radiation field.
- **Old scar**—If an implant is planned in an area of previous surgical intervention, problems due to fibrosis and decreased vascularization can arise. This concern can be compounded if an incision must cross an old surgical wound. This practice can be limited by careful preoperative planning.

Table 14.1 Factors that can adversely affect wound healing

Patient factor	Adverse impact on healing
Age	Extremes of aged and youth
Weight	Extremes of obesity and cachexia
Nutrition	Negative protein balance
Blood supply	Ischemia and edema
Immune function	Immunosuppression
Chronic disease	Overall poor response to tissue trauma
Radiation therapy	Negative tissue response
Chemotherapy	Negative tissue response
Previous surgical scar at wound site	Negative impact on healing

14.3 Phases of Wound Healing

Once a surgical wound is created, a cascade of events is set into motion. In the time immediately after the incision, platelets aggregate at the injury site to form a fibrin clot, which reduces active bleeding and creates the initial phases of hemostasis. This process is dependent upon the platelet level and function, fibrin, and the overall hormonal response.

The inflammation phase is next. This phase is important for wound healing and tissue sterilization. In this part of wound healing, bacteria and cell debris are phagocytosed and removed from the wound by white blood cells. Immunosuppression can have its biggest negative impact during this phase. The body also releases tissue factors in blood that cause the migration and division of cells during the proliferation phase.

The proliferation phase consists of several complex processes. Angiogenesis is the process where vascular endothelial cells form new vascular structures. Collagen deposition occurs simultaneously, and is followed by the deposition of collagen and the eventual formation of granulation tissue. As the wound undergoes epithelial cell molding, the wound contracts. Fibroblasts grow and develop an important new provisional extracellular matrix, as the cells deposit collagen and fibronectin. As this progress occurs, epithelial cells simultaneously gather and cover the new tissue.

After the epithelial matrix is deposited, wound contraction occurs. This process occurs when myofibroblasts function to grip the wound edges and pull the tissue together. At the end of the process, the body uses phagocytosis to destroy unwanted or unnecessary cells.

In the end process, collagen deposition results in the permanent scar and tissue restructuring that is a completely healed wound (Fig. 14.1).

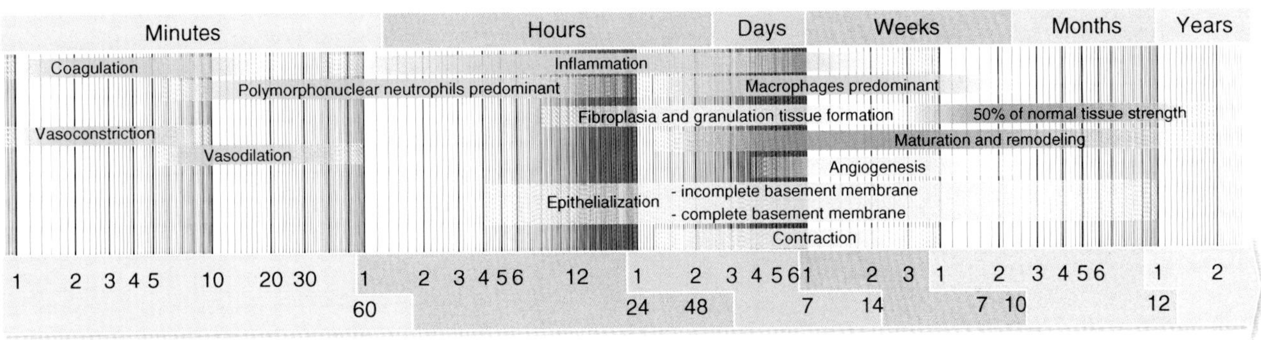

Fig. 14.1 The process of wound healing

Conclusion

The wound healing experience is a perfect example of the body's "fixing itself." The surgeon's job is to see that the process takes place without interruption and as seamlessly as possible, to afford the patient the best possible surgical and cosmetic result.

Suggested Reading

Martin P. Wound healing–aiming for perfect skin regeneration. Science. 1997;276:75–81.

Midwood KS, Williams LV, Schwarzbauer JE. Tissue repair and the dynamics of the extracellular matrix. Int J Biochem Cell Biol. 2004;36:1031–7.

Singer AJ, Clark RA. Cutaneous wound healing. N Engl J Med. 1999;341:738–46.

15 Complications of Spinal Cord Stimulation

Timothy R. Deer and Jason E. Pope

Spinal cord stimulation (SCS) is a therapy that offers hope to thousands of patients who suffer from chronic pain. The therapy has undergone significant advancements in recent years, including improved leads, more complex programmable generators, different arrays for achieving nerve activation, innovations in software, and novel waveform applications. But the implementation of SCS requires violation of our natural barrier, the skin, which innately can create adverse effects. Further, placement requires reliable identification of the epidural space and basic surgical skills, including sterile technique, anchoring, and incision closure. The assessment of the complications associated with SCS is difficult. Complications commonly are considered to be either biological or device-related. Systematic analyses have shown device complications to be 14–43 %. Nearly 80 % of these may require a surgical revision, and 11 % of patients in chronic therapy have a complication that requires removal of the device. The risk of life-threatening complications appears to be less than 1 %. The purpose of this chapter is to give an overview of important complications and to evaluate strategies to reduce the risk to the patient.

The physician must be vigilant to prevent, identify, and resolve complications (Table 15.1). Even in the most talented hands, complications will occur. By optimizing patient comorbidities and anticipating potential challenges, your complication rate can be mitigated (but not eliminated), and the overall safety and satisfaction of your neuromodulation practice will be far-reaching.

T.R. Deer, MD (✉)
The Center for Pain Relief,
400 Court Street, Suite 100, Charleston, WV, 25301, USA
e-mail: DocTDeer@aol.com

J.E. Pope
Summit Pain Alliance, 392 Tesconi Court,
Santa Rosa, CA 95401, USA
e-mail: popeje@me.com

T.R. Deer, J.E. Pope (eds.), *Atlas of Implantable Therapies for Pain Management*, DOI 10.1007/978-1-4939-2110-2_15

Table 15.1 Complications of stimulation

Complication	Diagnosis of problem	Treatment of problem
Neuraxis complications		
Nerve injury	CT or MRI, EMG/NCS/physical exam	Steroid protocol, anticonvulsants, neurosurgery consult
Epidural fibrosis	Increased stimulation amplitude	Lead reprogramming, lead revision
Epidural hematoma	Physical exam, CT or MRI	Surgical evacuation, steroid protocol
Epidural abscess	Physical exam, CT or MRI, CBC, blood work	Surgical evacuation, IV antibiotics, Infectious Disease consult
Post–dural puncture headache	Positional headache, blurred vision, nausea	IV fluids, rest, blood patch if required
Device complications		
Unacceptable programming	Lack of stimulation in area of pain	Reprogramming of device, revision of leads
Lead migration	Inability to program, x-rays	Reprogramming, surgical revision
Current leak	High impedance, pain at leak site	Revision of connectors, generator, or leads
Generator failure	Inability to read device	Replacement of generator
Nonneurological tissue complications		
Seroma	Serosanguinous fluid in pocket	Aspiration; if no response, surgical drainage
Hematoma	Blood in pocket	Pressure and aspiration; surgical revision
Pain at generator	Pain on palpation	Lidoderm patches, injection, revision
Wound infection	Fever, rubor, drainage	Antibiotics, incision and drainage, removal

CBC complete blood count, *EMG* electromyography, *NCS* nerve conduction study

15.1 Complications of the Neuraxis

15.1.1 Epidural Hematoma

Bleeding in the epidural space is common when needles and leads are introduced. In most patients, this bleeding is unnoticed and causes no sequelae. In rare patients, the bleeding progresses to the development of an epidural hematoma. If a developing epidural hematoma progresses, it can lead to numbness, back and leg pain, weakness, and eventual paraplegia. The treatment for clinically significant epidural hematoma is surgical evacuation. It is critical that this problem be identified early and treated within 24 h of the development of symptoms. Weakness in the postoperative period after device implantation is a red flag warning that should raise the suspicion of this tragic complication.

Risk factors for developing an epidural hematoma include the use of anticoagulants, platelet-acting drugs, aspirin, or NSAIDs. Independent risk factors for epidural hematoma following spinal surgery include male sex (4:1) and age in the 5th or 6th decade of life. Other factors may include difficult percutaneous lead placement, laminotomy approach to lead placement, and revision of previously placed leads. The need to perform surgical instrumentation and to create a bony insult dramatically increases the risk of a significant bleed.

The diagnosis of epidural hematoma is assisted by clinical suspicion, physical examination, and history, but the confirmatory diagnosis is made by CT scan. MRI can be obtained once the leads are removed. Early neurosurgical consultation is suggested if epidural hematoma is on the differential.

15.1.2 Epidural Abscess

Another major complication of the neuraxis associated with SCS is epidural abscess, one of the infectious risks of implanting devices in the body. (Other risks include incisional infection, cellulitis, meningitis, and discitis.) The risks of a serious infection appear to be less than 1 in 1000. Epidural abscess may present with severe pain in the area of the lead implant. This pain may be associated with fever, usually over 101 °F. Radicular pain may develop if the abscess extends to the canal or compresses the cord. Risk factors for abscess include immunocompromised state, history of chronic skin infections, history of methicillin-resistant *Staphylococcus aureus* (MRSA) infection or colonization, chronic diseases such as poorly controlled diabetes mellitus, or local infection at the surgery site. Abscess is diagnosed by clinical suspicion, history, and physical examination, and is confirmed by CT scan. MRI may be performed once the device is explanted.

15.1.3 Other Neurologic Injury

Neurologic injuries of the spinal cord or nerve roots are other potential risks of SCS. Injury may occur by needle trauma, lead placement or removal, or surgical manipulation during paddle lead placement. Neurologic injury is more common with paddle placement than with percutaneous cylindrical lead placement.

In many patients, the injury is associated with deep sedation or general anesthesia. In the immediate postprocedure period, the injury may be difficult to diagnose. CT scans may not show an abnormality, and MRI cannot be performed until the device is surgically removed. An electromyogram and nerve conduction study may be helpful in determining the injury, but findings may not become abnormal for several days after the insult.

Less worrisome complications include inadvertent dural puncture with post–dural puncture headache, which has been reported in up to 11 % of cases, although that number appears much higher than clinical practice would suggest. This risk is increased by obesity, calcific ligaments, patient movement, and previous surgery at the level of needle entry. A paramedian approach with an angle of less than 40° appears to lower the risk of complications.

Spinal cord stenosis can develop over time in the vicinity of an implanted lead; it may result in new radicular symptoms and can progress to myelopathy over time. This problem requires revision, decompression, or lead removal.

15.2 Complications Outside the Neuraxis

Reported incidences of wound infections involving the generator, tunneled area, or lead incision site have ranged from 0 to 4.5 % of patients. This problem is diagnosed by pain, swelling, rubor, and drainage of purulent material (Figs. 15.1 and 15.2). An elevated white blood cell count, sedimentation rate, or C-reactive protein should create concern regarding the infectious status of the implant. Other causes of infection should also be considered.

Some patients may develop a swollen, irritated wound that is not associated with infection. This complication, termed a seroma, is caused by a buildup of serosanguinous fluid, and occurs with a frequency of 0.9–5.8 %. Seroma is diagnosed by lack of fever and a normal white blood count. If the diagnosis cannot be determined, incision and drainage with cultures may be required to make a conclusive diagnosis. In most cases, seroma can be treated without device removal. Careful dissection and attention to minimizing tissue trauma may reduce the risk of this complication. Compression with an abdominal binder, if appropriate, reduces the chance of seroma development.

Bleeding can occur at the generator site or lead incision. The result can be hematoma requiring drainage, or wound dehiscence.

The best treatment is prevention, which consists of thoughtful tissue dissection, pressure to the area of bleeding, suturing of arterial bleeding, coagulation of ongoing small vessel hemorrhage, and careful inspection of the wound prior to closure.

Pain at the generator site may occur secondary to neuroma, tissue irritation, or bony contact with a rib or pelvic bones. Treatment can include topical local anesthetic patches, wound injection, or surgical revision.

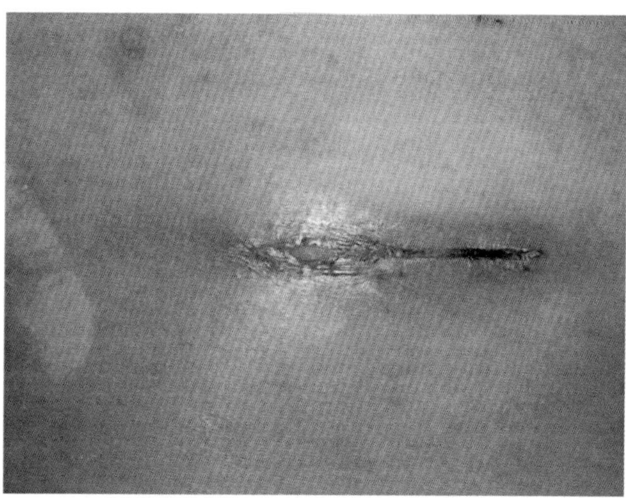

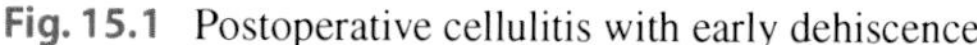

Fig. 15.1 Postoperative cellulitis with early dehiscence

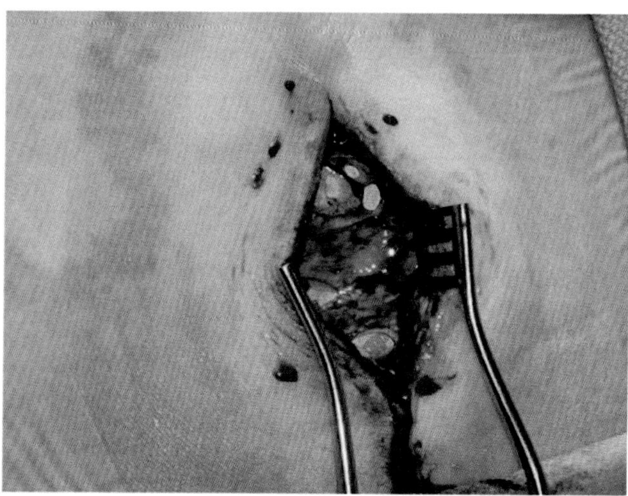

Fig. 15.2 Gross infection present at generator site

15.3 Device-Related Complications

The most commonly reported complication of SCS devices is loss of paresthesia capture over time, which can result from lead migration, the patient's development of tolerance to stimulation, or fibrosis below the lead, which increases impedance. Many of these problems can now be overcome by changes to the device. If reprogramming the system does not resolve the situation, plain films of the leads may be helpful in diagnosing migration. Eventual treatment may require lead revision or conversion to a percutaneous or traditional surgical paddle lead.

Lead migration is another complication that can lead to system failure (Fig. 15.3). This problem plagues both percutaneous and paddle systems. The authors have experienced less than 1 % migration based on x-ray evaluation, and recent studies have shown the number to be less than 11–13 % in most evaluations. The problem is diagnosed with loss of therapeutic stimulation not overcome by reprogramming, dramatic change in location or characteristics of the stimulation, and by comparison of anterior-posterior and lateral films with the original implant films. Treatment commonly requires surgical lead revision. Careful attention to anchoring to the lumbodorsal fascia may reduce the risk of this complication but cannot prevent it entirely.

Painful stimulation or loss of stimulation can occur secondary to current leakage or loss of system integrity. This problem is often diagnosed by computer analysis showing high impedance compared with baseline. Possible causes include lead migration, poor conduction secondary to fluid in or around the contacts, or partial or total lead fracture.

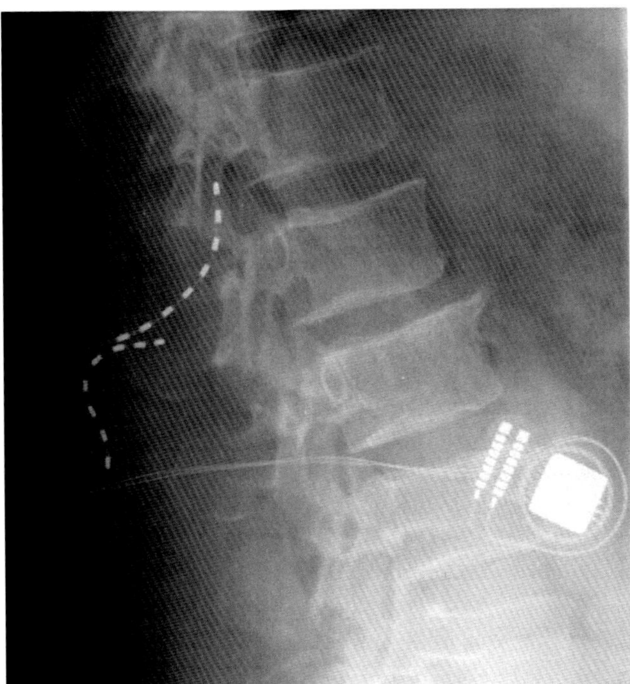

Fig. 15.3 Migration of the lead

Device flipping and generator pain may occur secondary to difficulties at the pocket. These complications can be reduced by anchoring the generator and securing the device in a pocket that is adequate to allow room for the device. If the pocket is too small, it may lead to poor wound closure, pressure on the tissue, and even erosion over time. Further, placing the incision line over the device may interfere with wound healing. A pocket that is too large may lead to flipping of the device, pain secondary to device tissue irritation, or a seroma in the area of the pocket that is not involved in the implant. The physician should be careful to measure the pocket size intermittently as it is created. Some manufacturers are now supplying spacers that can be used to check pocket size without having to place the actual device into the pocket as it is created.

Erosion of device components through the skin can lead to loss of the system. This erosion can occur secondary to poor tissue health from chronic disease, weight loss, and placement of anchors in the superficial tissues. When erythema occurs around a generator, the physician should consider surgical revision prior to the complete loss of tissue integrity, which requires removal of the system. In the placement of peripheral leads, the device should be placed below the dermis. In general, the physician should determine this depth by palpation, needle placement, and observation when making an incision to secure the lead. The use of suture for securing the peripheral lead without the use of a formal anchor should be considered, as many cases of device erosion occur at the Silastic anchor site. New anchors containing harder substances such as titanium may worsen this problem.

15.4 Risk Assessment

- The patient should be assessed for bleeding risks prior to moving forward for an implant. A careful review of medications that affect bleeding, an evaluation of coexisting diseases, and an evaluation of the spinal anatomy and challenges should be undertaken prior to moving forward.
- Perioperative comorbidities need to be optimized. Infection risk assessment includes a review of coexisting diseases, inspection of the patient's skin, and a review of preoperative laboratory studies. In patients with a history of problems such as advanced HIV disease, brittle diabetes mellitus, chronic systemic steroid use, and malignancy, caution should be exercised and implantable devices should be moved further down the treatment algorithm.
- Patients who are at risk for neural injury during implantation are hard to identify because of the low incidence of this problem. The incidence of neurologic injury is higher with paddle leads than with percutaneous leads. The patient with multiple spinal instrumentation procedures, the morbidly obese, the extremely anxious, and the patient with extensive spinal disease such as significant scoliosis should be approached with caution.
- Inadvertent dural puncture can lead to a headache that may impair the ability to assess the success of a stimulation trial or may complicate the postoperative period after permanent implantation. The risk of this complication is increased with obesity, scoliosis, significant stenosis, ligament calcification, and previous surgery at the site of the planned implant. The risks are also increased in a patient with extensive movement and inability to cooperate with the implant approach.
- The development of stenosis in the vicinity of a previously implanted lead can produce symptoms and lead to the ultimate removal of the device. Before placing a device in the cervical spine, the doctor should consider an imaging study to assess preimplant spinal diameter. In cases of preexisting stenosis, the implant should be approached with caution.
- Wound infections can vary from mild erythema to frank dehiscence. The implanter should use great care in wound closure to ensure that tissue alignment is ideal. It is important to evaluate the patient preoperatively for local skin abnormalities and evaluate disease states for possible increased risks of systemic infections. A history of previous MRSA infections should alert the physician to potential difficulties. Preoperative infection risk assessment is mandatory.
- Seroma can develop in the wound surrounding the generator and can lead to loss of the device because of wound breakdown. History of seroma development with other surgical procedures may alert the physician to potential risks of this complication. Patients with connective tissue disorders such as lupus, rheumatoid arthritis, and scleroderma may have a greater propensity to develop these problems.
- Pain at the generator site is most common in patients with a history of complex regional pain syndrome or fibromyalgia. It is difficult to predict which patients will have problems of this kind.
- Loss of proper stimulation paresthesia can occur, leading to reduced relief or a complete loss of relief. This loss can be due to epidural fibrosis, migration, positional change, or other electrical stimulation factors. The physician should carry out a troubleshooting evaluation when loss of coverage occurs, including a physical examination, plain film evaluation, and computer analysis of the system.
- Lead migration can lead to an adverse outcome. The risk of migration is increased by movement in the early preoperative period, including bending at the waist, lifting above the head, and carrying heavy objects. The techniques used for anchoring and suturing can reduce the risk of migration, but cannot eliminate the problem.
- Lead fracture is more common with surgically placed paddle electrodes. The presence of tension on the wiring can increase this risk, as can trauma to the area of the spine where the implant is placed.
- Device flipping leads to the inability to program or use the SCS system.
- Erosion of the leads, anchors, or generators through the skin can lead to loss of the system or the need for an extensive revision.
- Loss of pain relief can occur even though paresthesias are still felt in the proper region, impedance numbers are appropriate, and the leads and generator are functioning properly.

15.5 Risk Avoidance

- Patients taking clopidogrel, warfarin, and other anticoagulants should be taken off these drugs prior to implantation. This decision should be made by the physician prescribing the medications. If the patient cannot be taken off of these agents, the procedure must be canceled. If the physician feels the procedure is critical, admitting the patient for an infusion of heparin to allow for discontinuation of oral medications can be considered.
- Preoperative antibiotics should be given prior to moving into the procedure area. The use of preoperative antibiotics is sometimes considered controversial, but it now has become standard of care for most implanters. Other risk avoidance techniques include extensive prepping and wide draping, with careful attention to sterile technique.

Vigorous irrigation should be used to create tissue dilution of any potential infectious agents. Wound closure should be considered critical to reducing complications and should be taken very seriously. Postoperative followup is needed to detect any early signs of infection such as rubor, drainage, or painful incisions. In these cases, an early intervention such as incision and drainage should be considered.

- The risk of neural injury can be reduced by proper patient education, including the need for patient cooperation with maintaining minimal movement during the procedure. The physician should focus on proper patient positioning prior to moving forward. The use of fluoroscopy should be approached carefully, with attention to aligning the spine to allow for a good approach. In difficult cases, the patient should remain alert during the implantation to provide early warning to the implanting doctor of impending nerve injury.
- Post–dural puncture headache is a known complication that is unavoidable in some patients. Several actions can reduce the risk:
  - Using a needle angle of 45° or less
  - Using a paramedian approach
  - Using both a hanging drop and loss of resistance technique
  - Using contrast and lateral views if the depth of the needle is not clear
  - Being patient and using a careful and thoughtful approach to the space
- In patients with preimplant imaging that suggests moderate to severe stenosis, the doctor should be cautious with percutaneous implants. The alternative of decompression with placement of a paddle lead is an another option when there is any doubt about a risk of disease progression causing nerve impingement. The use of small-profile leads for trialing should be considered in these patients. When this approach is taken, the patient should be alert and responsive during lead and needle manipulation.
- Wound infections are best avoided by careful preoperative screening, optimization of coexisting diseases, and evaluation of skin condition prior to making an incision. The patient should be prepped and draped widely, and careful attention should be given to wound closure. The physician should be vigilant regarding tissue approximation and the reduction of tension on the wound. The patient should be followed in the postoperative period with inspection of the wound. If a superficial infection develops, the authors recommend an aggressive approach of excising the wound tissue with an elliptical incision for incision and drainage of the wound before the infection is extended. If the infection involves the pocket or the posterior spinal incision, it is important to remove the device in its entirety and consult an infectious disease specialist when appropriate.
- Seroma formation can lead to devastating results, including failure of the system. Some clinicians recommend aspiration of the fluid with analysis. This is reasonable, but careful attention must be paid to avoid contaminating a noninfected pocket. Preventing the initial problem of a seroma is the best approach. The risk can be reduced with careful and gentle handling of the tissue, judicious use of cautery, and sharp dissection rather than vigorous blunt dissection. Some clinicians have reduced seroma by making the generator pocket prior to placing the leads, and packing the wound with antibiotic-soaked sponges to tamponade venous and small arterial bleeders.
- Hematoma can form both subcutaneously and epidurally. Epidural hematoma needs to be identified and acted upon quickly. Subcutaneous hematoma can result from poor intraoperative hemostasis or postoperative trauma. Treatment commonly requires vigilance and, in rare circumstances, evacuation.
- Pain at the generator site can lead to a bad outcome even in patients who have excellent stimulation and reduction of their primary problem. The device should be placed 1–2 cm below the dermis, with attention to avoid placing the generator too superficially. Placing the generator near the pubic bones or the rib margin can also cause pain with movement. Another important factor is the distribution of adipose tissue in the patient's body habitus. In some patients, placement of the device in the buttock leads to pain secondary to lack of adipose tissue in the region. The development of smaller implantable generators has allowed the pocket to be created closer to the spinal incision site, which may mitigate this risk.
- Loss of paresthesia can be devastating to the patient who has experienced pain relief with SCS. The physician may find that this problem can be overcome by complex computer reprogramming, with a change in lead arrays, pulse width, or amplitudes. If reprogramming fails to resolve the issue, the physician should review the impedance numbers at each contact. High impedance of the system or individual contacts may lead to the need to revise the leads, open the system and check the contacts, or revise the system to a surgical paddle lead system. A plain film showing lead migration can sometimes give insight into a reprogramming strategy that may help to avoid the need for more surgery, but if this is not possible, the treatment of this problem is with revision.
- Lead migration can be reduced by using a paramedian approach, using a shallow needle angle of 45° or less, and dissecting the tissue to anchor to fascia and ligament rather than adipose tissue (Table 15.2). Anchoring techniques vary; this atlas reviews some options in detail, but the primary construct is to anchor the lead to the device and the device to the fascia and ligament. New anchors help the physician to more easily secure the lead to

material, but even with these advances it is very important to secure the anchoring device to the body tissue. Bracing, limitation of activity, and restrictions on motion may help in avoiding this complication, but these recommendations have never been proven effective in a prospective fashion.

- Lead fracture can be reduced by using a shallow angle to insert the device, by adding a strain relief loop to the spinal incision, and by adding a strain relief loop underneath the generator.
- Device flipping can be reduced by using a nonabsorbable suture to anchor the device to the fascia in the pocket and by properly sizing the pocket to avoid excessive unoccupied volume surrounding the device.
- Erosion cannot be avoided in some patients, but it may be possible to reduce the risk. Change in body habitus over time due to weight loss or weight gain may lead to new tissue pressures on the metal or Silastic devices. In other settings, erosion may occur in patients with poor skin integrity due to chronic diseases or medications. The physician should place the initial generator in the fatty tissue below the dermis, with adequate tissue to cushion the materials. If the patient starts to experience redness or pain over the device, the physician may consider device revision. Many physicians have begun to use nonabsorbable sutures to secure peripheral leads for nerve or nerve field stimulation. The risk of erosion around Silastic anchors in the periphery appears to be substantial, requiring chronic monitoring when anchors are used.
- The loss of pain relief in an area despite adequate stimulation patterns can be very frustrating to both the patient and the physician. In some settings, there is no option to resolve this problem and treatment may require device removal.

Table 15.2 Migration risk avoidance

Migration risk	Physician action
Needle angle	Needle angle of 30–45°
Needle entry	Paramedian approach
Fatty tissue at anchoring site	Dissect fatty tissue around the needle entry site, exposing fascia and ligament for proper anchoring
Anchoring to muscle	When using an exaggerated paramedian approach, the physician should dissect medially until approaching ligament or fascia; avoid anchoring to muscle, which may lead to migration with contraction
Lead anchor gap	The anchor should be as close to the lead entry into the ligament or fascia as possible, avoiding room for migration distal to the anchor
Suturing with silk	Avoid silk sutures when anchoring
Dependence on the anchor	The anchor should be seen as one component of securing the system; total dependence on the anchor can lead to poor outcomes
Hematoma below anchor	Hemostasis should be obtained prior to closing the wound, as bleeding can lead to catheter movement owing to pressure on the anchor from hematoma compression

Conclusions

SCS is a great option for many patients who suffer from chronic pain. Although the success of these devices continues to improve in the areas of pain reduction, functional improvement, and quality of life, they are not without risks. It is critical for the physician to identify risks, reduce their occurrence, and treat them appropriately to reduce the numbers of permanent complications.

15.6 Supplemental Images

See Figs. 15.4, 15.5, 15.6, 15.7, 15.8, 15.9, and 15.10.

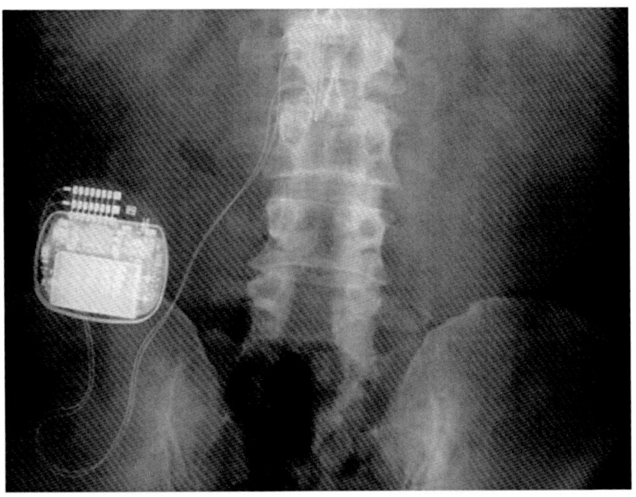

Fig. 15.4 Lead fracture, anterior view

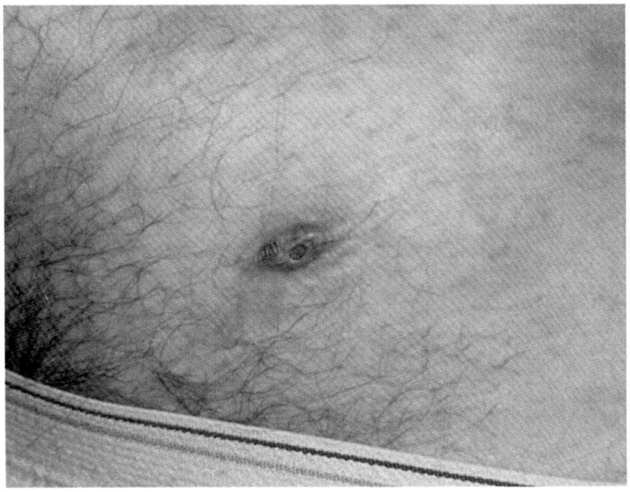

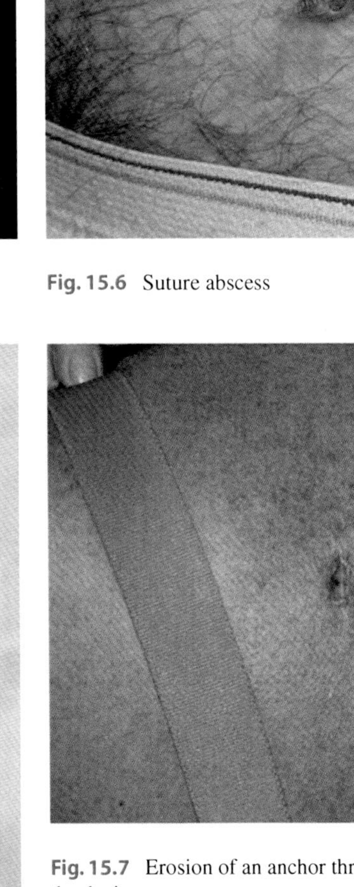

Fig. 15.6 Suture abscess

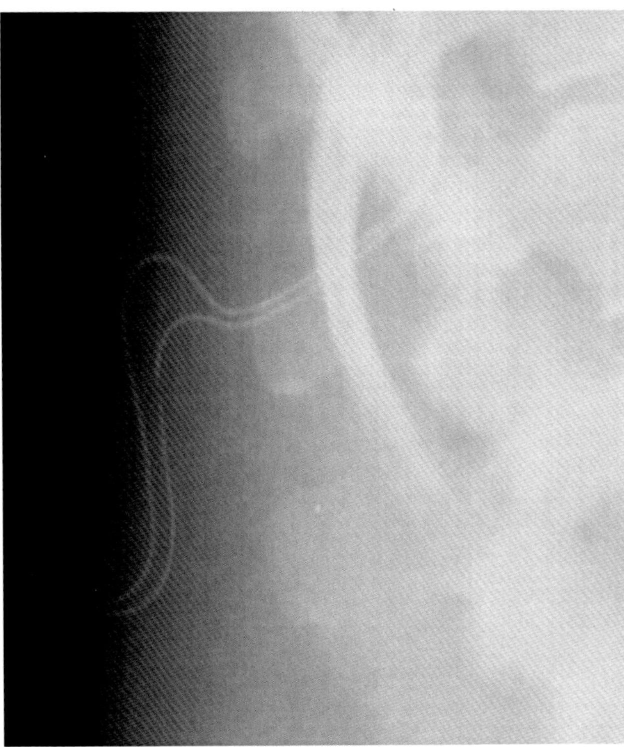

Fig. 15.5 Lead fracture, lateral view

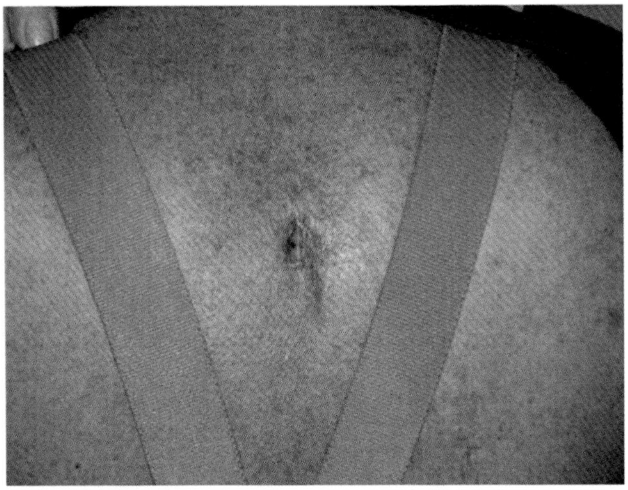

Fig. 15.7 Erosion of an anchor through the tissue, causing exposure of the device

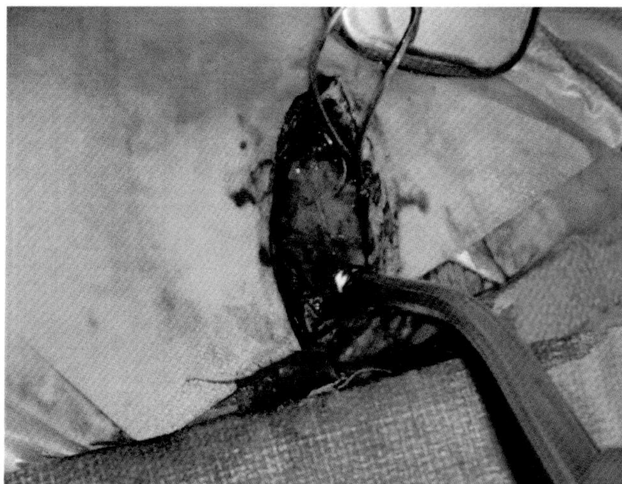

Fig. 15.8 Infected pocket requiring removal of the spinal cord stimulation device

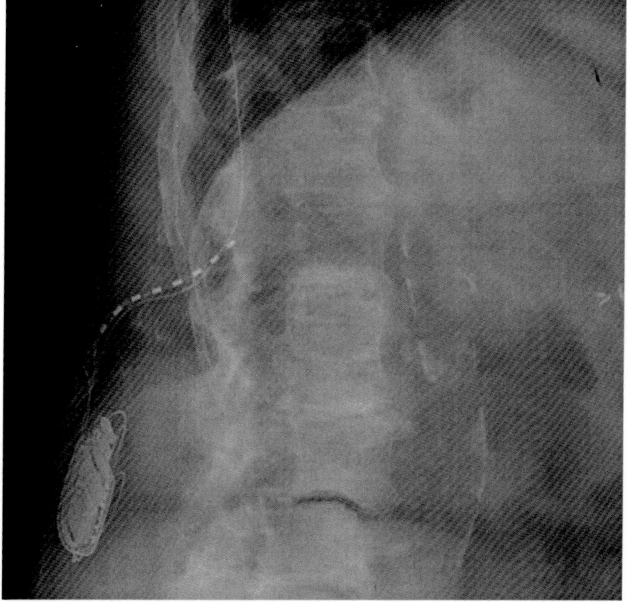

Fig. 15.9 Caudad lead migration

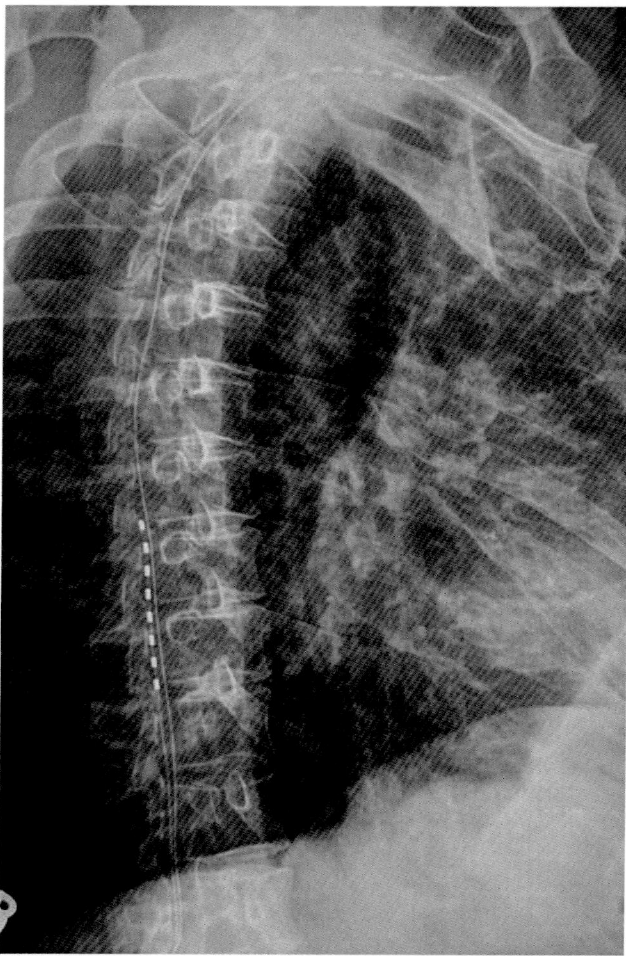

Fig. 15.10 Cephalad lead migration into the cervical nerve root

Suggested Reading

Cameron T. Safety and efficacy of spinal cord stimulation for the treatment of chronic pain: a 20-year literature review. J Neurosurg. 2004;100: 254–67.

Darouiche R. Spinal epidural abscess. N Engl J Med. 2006;355:2012–20.

Eldrige J, Weingarten T, Rho R. Management of cerebral spinal fluid leak complicating spinal cord stimulator implantation. Pain Pract. 2006;6:285–8.

Meyer SC, Swartz K, Johnson JP. Quadriparesis and spinal cord stimulation: case report. Spine. 2007;32:E565–8.

Raj PP, Shah RV, Kaye AD, Denaro S, Hoover JM. Bleeding risk in interventional pain practice: assessment, management, and review of the literature. Pain Physician. 2004;7:3–51.

Rathmell JP, Neal JM. Complications in regional anesthesia and pain medicine. New York: Elsevier Saunders; 2007.

Stimulation of the Nervous System to Treat Neuropathic Pain of the Foot

16

Timothy R. Deer and Giancarlo Barolat

16.1 Introduction

Neuropathic foot pain is a common disease state that affects more than 200 million people globally. The pain may vary from a mild tingling to an excruciating, constant burning pain, often exacerbated in the evening hours. Neuropathic pain is often difficult to treat with conservative measures, and more advanced techniques are required. This problem comes to light in those suffering from primary peripheral nerve problems, neuropathies, nerve entrapment, spinal nerve root injury or scar entrapment, and complex regional pain syndrome (Table 16.1).

Spinal cord stimulation (SCS) can be successful in treating this troubling problem. Conventional methods involve routine placement at the common locations in the spinal canal (T8 through T12), but in some cases, stimulation is required at the level of the nerve root or peripheral nerve. This chapter discusses possible strategies to successfully control neuropathic foot pain.

Table 16.1 Common disease states causing neuropathic foot pain

Neuropathies: diabetic, alcohol-induced, metabolic, nutritional deficiency, heavy metal, chemotherapy-induced, idiopathic, infectious (HIV, syphilis)
Spine-induced pain: disc impingement of the nerve, foraminal narrowing, central stenosis, epidural fibrosis, arachnoiditis, mechanical entrapment of the nerve, nerve trauma, iatrogenic, bone impingement on the nerve, failed back surgery syndrome
Complex regional pain syndromes types I and II, Raynaud's syndrome, vasculitis, ischemic pain secondary to peripheral vascular disease, vasospasm
Peripheral nerve pain: nerve injury, nerve entrapment, tarsal tunnel syndrome, postsurgical scarring, neuroma, bony deformity causing nerve pain

T.R. Deer, MD (✉)
The Center for Pain Relief,
400 Court Street, Suite 100, Charleston, WV 25301, USA
e-mail: DocTDeer@aol.com

G. Barolat, MD
Barolat Neuroscience, Presbyterian St. Lukes Medical Center,
1721 East 19th Avenue, Denver, CO 80218, USA
e-mail: gbarolat@verizon.net

T.R. Deer, J.E. Pope (eds.), *Atlas of Implantable Therapies for Pain Management*, DOI 10.1007/978-1-4939-2110-2_16

16.2 Technical Overview

Other sections of this Atlas have covered many of the pearls of this section. Needle placement, lead placement, and techniques such as anchoring and pocketing are consistent with descriptions in other sections of this text. Nerve root stimulation, paddle lead placement, and peripheral nerve placement are also covered elsewhere. The primary technical decision in treating this pain disorder is a cerebral exercise. The decision of where to target the nervous system to achieve the desired result is the most critical decision in this process (Table 16.2).

Table 16.2 Lead placement options

Approach	Location
Traditional approach	T8–T12
Modified approach	Crossing midline at T10–T11
Conus approach	Crossing midline at T12–L1
Nerve root approach	Lead capturing the nerve root in lower lumbar spine
Nerve root approach	Lead capturing the nerve root at foramen L4–5 or S1
Peripheral nerve approach	Lead placed at the peripheral nerve pain site
Dorsal root ganglion stimulation	Dermatomal placement ipsilateral to foot pain

16.2.1 The Method of Epidural Stimulation

Whether a percutaneous lead or a paddle lead is utilized, to achieve focally consistent and lasting stimulation of the foot, the active part of the lead should be at the T11–L1 level. This placement most likely entails stimulation of the cauda equina as it overlaps the tail end of the spinal cord, rather than the dorsal columns. The placement is often done in parallel or a staggered array (Fig. 16.1). If these lead arrays are successful, no further adaptations are needed, and in some cases, both foot pain and other dermatomal patterns are treated. Some physicians prefer to cross the midline with the leads used in a guarded array, with two cathodes in the center of the lead to drive the current deeper (Fig. 16.2). This pattern often leads to total coverage of the entire leg, including the feet. In selected patients, the paresthesia in the foot is troubling and not desired. The epidural approach is not the ideal treatment option for these patients.

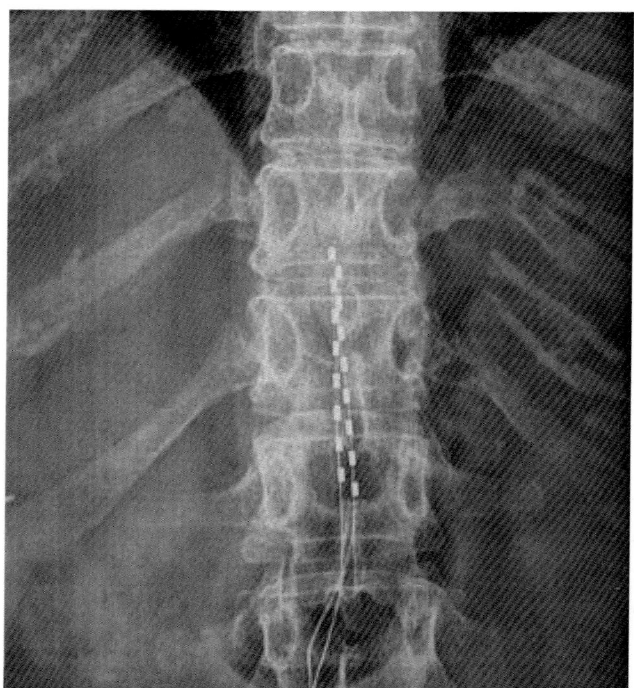

Fig. 16.1 Traditional lead placement

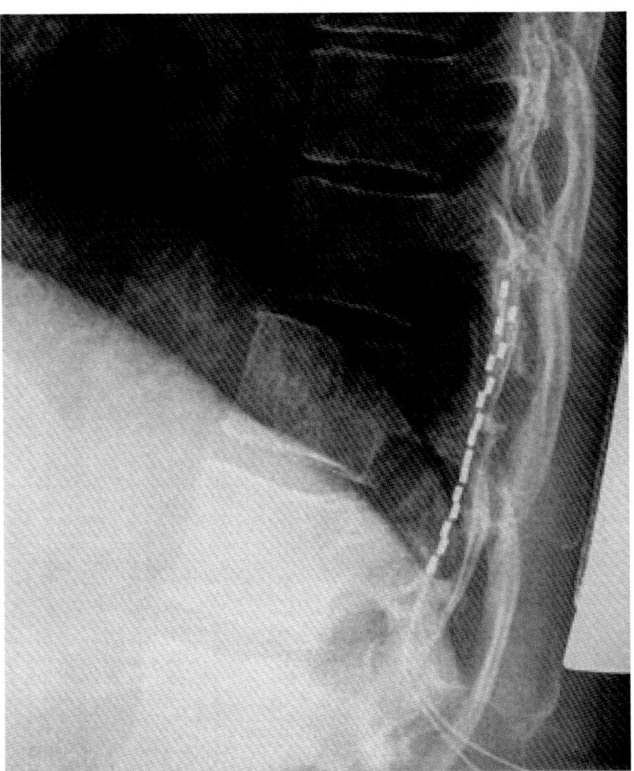

Fig. 16.2 Guarded array placement. If the foot is not stimulated by the epidural approach, a nerve root approach is an option. Either a percutaneous or paddle approach can be used

16.2.2 The Nerve Root Method of Stimulation

The lead can be placed in the area of the L5 or S1 nerve root by the percutaneous approach, using the retrograde approach or the sacral hiatus route. The retrograde approach involves entering the epidural space in a caudad approach via the intralaminar space two to three levels above the target nerve. Once the epidural needle has been successfully placed with fluoroscopic guidance, the lead is driven down the middle of the epidural space until it is one level above the desired level. Using an appropriate stylet, the lead is then directed under x-ray guidance to the nerve target. The alternative method is to use a percutaneous approach to enter the sacral hiatus with an epidural Tuohy needle and then place the lead antegrade to the desired nerve foramen. The lead is placed at the foramen or adjacent to the foramen for stimulation (Figs. 16.3 and 16.4). This approach can be very helpful, but the size of conventional leads makes it difficult to stabilize this lead placement. Current research is working on developing new technology to address these issues, but currently there are no approved leads specific to the foramen or these neurological structures.

In some patients, it is not possible or desirable to place the nerve root leads via the percutaneous approach. A paddle approach is a possible solution. The lead can capture the nerve at the foramen or in the spinal canal as it travels to the foramen. These two lead placements are depicted in Figs. 16.5, 16.6, and 16.7.

The chapter on peripheral nerve stimulation covered the possibility of placing a lead on the peripheral nerve. The target for this nerve stimulation is based on examination, pain pattern, and (when available) an electromyogram or nerve conduction study. The technique can be performed using either a percutaneous approach or a paddle lead approach, based on surgeon preference and patient characteristics. Depending on the exact topography of the pain, electrodes can be implanted on the sciatic, posterior tibial, peroneal, or saphenous nerve. In the hands of one of the authors (GB), peripheral nerve stimulation is actually the preferred initial neurostimulation approach. If the pain involves areas larger than the foot, an intraspinal stimulation target is preferable. As discussed below, the dorsal root ganglion is a possible location for stimulation for a patient with isolated foot pain.

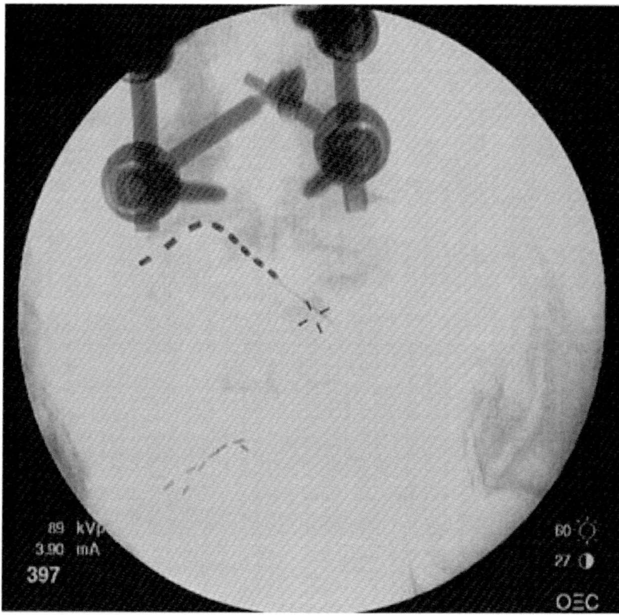

Fig. 16.3 Nerve root placement

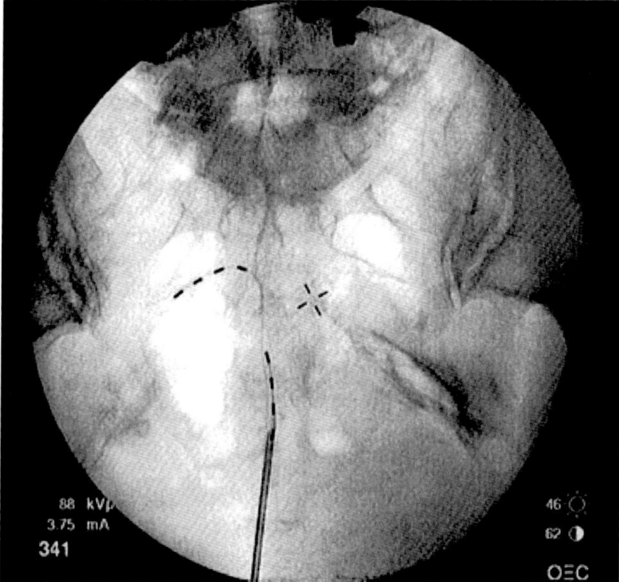

Fig. 16.4 Nerve root placement via caudal approach

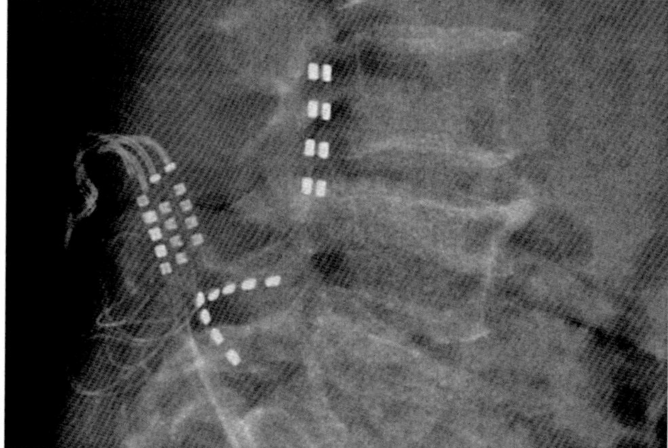

Fig. 16.5 Mixed paddle approach (Courtesy of Giancarlo Barolat, MD)

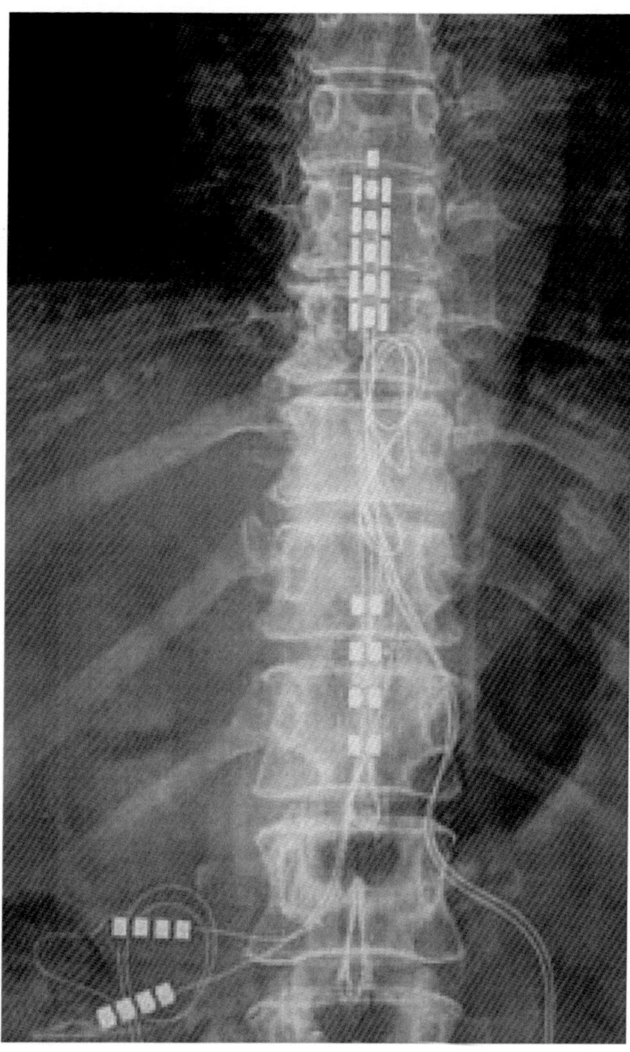

Fig. 16.6 Epidural paddle approach (Courtesy of Giancarlo Barolat, MD)

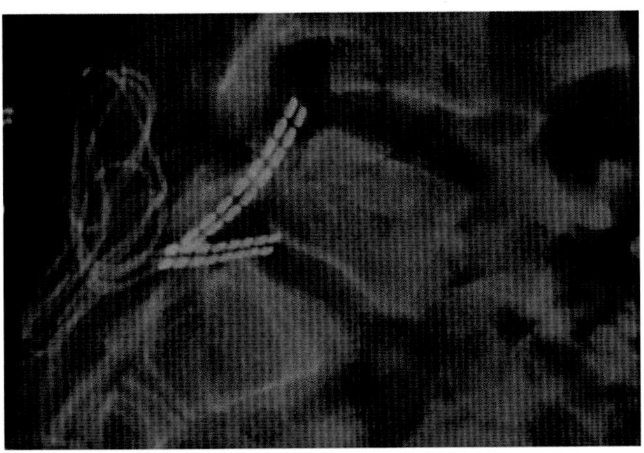

Fig. 16.7 Lateral view of paddle approach (Courtesy of Giancarlo Barolat, MD)

16.2.3 Dorsal Root Ganglion Stimulation

Novel treatment targets have emerged that may remedy the traditionally challenges of dorsal column stimulation. The dorsal root ganglion (DRG) is located bilaterally caudal to the pedicle. It is composed of the cell body of the primary afferent nociceptor and can be accessed via the epidural space. Specifically designed equipment, similar to that employed in SCS, is used to deliver a specifically designed lead to the DRG ipsilateral to the affected foot (Fig. 16.8). Because of the redundancy of afferent nociception and cross-dermatomal innervation, the lead can be placed above or below the dermatomally identified DRG. This exciting technology may remedy many challenges with foot coverage that can occur with traditional SCS, including durability and positionality. The technology is available in Europe and the pivotal Food and Drug Administration (FDA) study in the United States is currently under way.

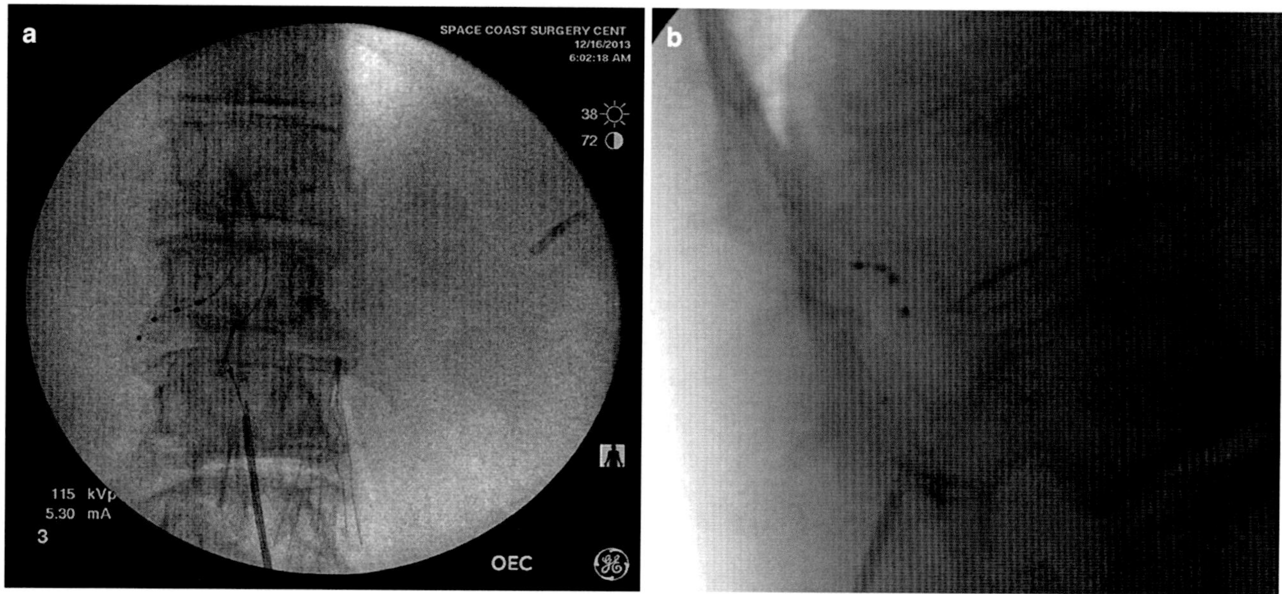

Fig. 16.8 AP (**a**) and lateral (**b**) view of left DRG placement 12

16.3 Risk Assessment

The various types of nervous system stimulation used to treat foot pain carry risks of failure or complications:

- The foot innervation can lead to a challenging problem with SCS. If the lead is placed too high in the spine, the result is a failure to achieve proper target stimulation.
- Stimulation in the upper lumbar spine, such as at the level of the conus, can lead to an unstable lead location and a varying degree of stimulation, which may be unpleasant.
- Nerve root stimulation may be felt as an intense paresthesia that is so powerful the patient gets motor recruitment.
- Stimulation of the peripheral nerve can lead to the development of scar tissue, reducing the long-term success of the device.

16.4 Risk Avoidance

The risks noted above may be avoided by following some helpful procedures:

- Crossing the midline in the thoracic spine may result in a more uniform stimulation pattern leading to coverage of the back down to the feet. This pattern is often achieved by using a "double guarded" cathode array. That involves a (+ − − +) programming of the portion of the lead crossing the midline; two leads in a staggered orientation may be required.
- Placement of the lead over the conus can be very helpful in achieving stimulation of the foot, but unfortunately lateral movement of the lead is an issue, along with movement of the conus with positional changes. This problem can be reduced by crossing the midline with the center of the configuration of programming at the conus, using a single lead or dual leads.
- When placing a stimulation lead in the vicinity of the nerve root, the programming should be started initially to capture the threshold and then backed off to a subthreshold level. The patient should be offered several programs that cover different contacts on the lead and should have a variety of pulse width options.
- Peripheral nerve stimulation leads can be placed percutaneously in the vicinity of the nerve to avoid direct nerve contact, reducing the impact of scar in some patients. If the lead must be placed directly on the nerve, a fascial graft may be helpful in stabilizing the stimulation pattern, although this technique is difficult to perform and has questionable long-term outcomes.

Conclusions

A successful outcome for patients suffering from neuropathic foot pain can be achieved with SCS. The method of lead placement, the neuropathic pain target, and lead programming may all play a critical role in the long-term efficacy of the device (Fig. 16.9). The clinician must be an active problem solver in these situations and must adapt to the patient's response.

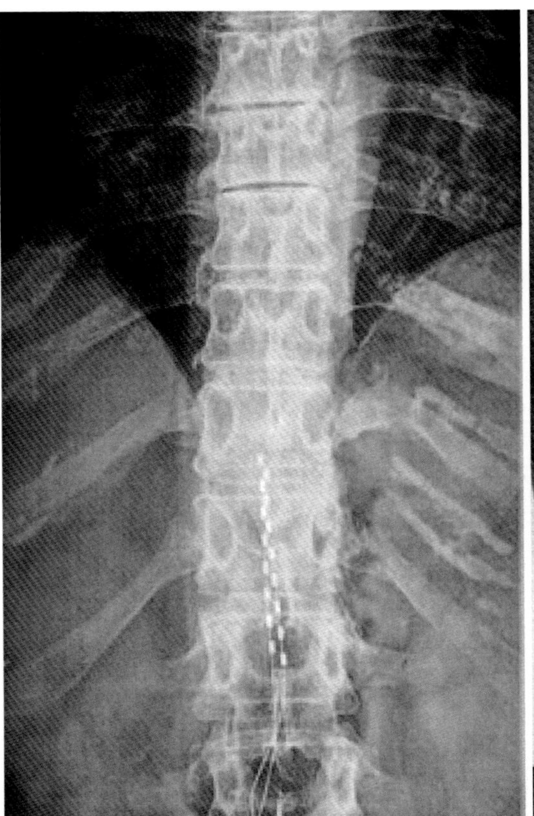
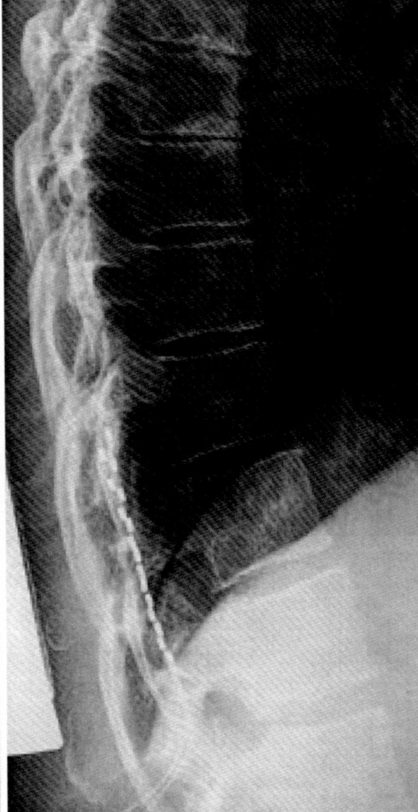

Fig. 16.9 Percutaneous lead placement for foot pain

Suggested Reading

Alo KM, Yland MJ, Redko V, Feler C, Naumann C. Lumbar and sacral nerve root stimulation (NRS) in the treatment of chronic pain: a novel anatomic approach and neuro stimulation technique. Neuromodulation. 1999;2:23–31.

Kumar K, North R, Taylor R, Sculpher M, Van den Abeele C, Gehring M, et al. Spinal cord stimulation vs. conventional medical management: a prospective, randomized, controlled, multicenter study of patients with failed back surgery syndrome (PROCESS Study). Neuromodulation. 2005;8:213–8.

Liem L, Russo M, Huygen FJ, Van Buyten JP, Smet I, Verrills P, et al. A multicenter, prospective trial to assess the safety and performance of the spinal modulation dorsal root ganglion neurostimulator system in the treatment of chronic pain. Neuromodulation. 2013. doi:10.1111/ner.12072.

Mobbs R, Nair S, Blum P. Peripheral nerve stimulation for the treatment of chronic pain. J Clin Neurosci. 2007;14:216–21.

Vinik AL, Pittenger GL, McNitt P, Stansberry G. Diabetic neuropathies: an overview of clinical aspects, pathogenesis, and treatment. In: LeRoith D, Taylor SL, Olefsky JM, editors. Diabetes mellitus. Philadelphia: Lippincott Williams & Wilkins; 2000. p. 911–34.

Yeun KC, Baker NR, Rayman G. Treatment of chronic painful diabetic neuropathy with isosorbide dinitrate spray: a double blind placebo-controlled cross-over study. Diabetes Care. 2002;25:1699–703.

Sacral Nerve Root Stimulation for the Treatment of Pelvic and Rectal Pain

17

Kenneth M. Alò, Nameer R. Haider, and Timothy R. Deer

17.1 Introduction

Pelvic, ilioinguinal, testicular, and sacral pain may have both visceral and somatic causes, lending themselves to stimulation techniques. Sacral nerve root stimulation has been recognized as a treatment of pain of the pelvis, rectum, and perineum, and serves to manage intractable pain of the bladder from interstitial cystitis, post-radiation and nerve entrapment pathologies. Further, functional improvements of bladder dynamics can be performed with sacral stimulation and intersem techniques. The sacral nerve targets are normally at S2, S3, and S4.

Ilioinguinal nerve stimulation has been utilized to treat chronic intractable pain of the groin often after herniorrhaphy-induced nerve entrapment, pelvic surgery, hysterectomy, and appendectomy (Fig. 17.1).

Chronic orchialgia may be caused by structural abnormalities including wallerian degeneration of the spermatic cord or vasal nerves. This may explain how neurostimulation of the spermatic nerves provides pain relief in patients with chronic testicular pain. Other causes of orchialgia include postoperative scarring, trauma, and chronic infection leading to nerve damage (Fig. 17.2).

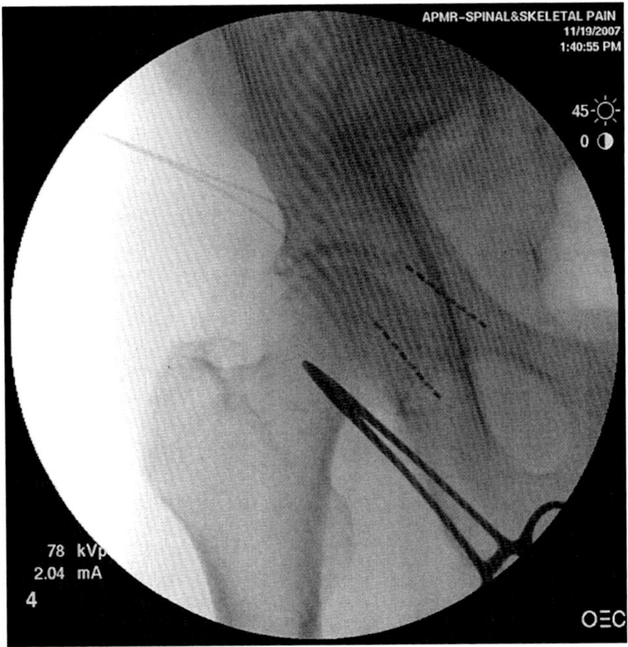

Fig. 17.1 Ilioinguinal nerve stimulation

K.M. Alò
The Methodist Hospital Research Institute,
5318 Weslayan #182, Houston, TX 77005, USA
e-mail: aglioolio@gmail.com

N.R. Haider, MD
Minimally Invasive Pain Institute, Washington, DC, USA
e-mail: drhaider@killpain.com

T.R. Deer, MD (✉)
The Center for Pain Relief, 400 Court Street, Suite 100,
Charleston, WV 25301, USA
e-mail: DocTDeer@aol.com

T.R. Deer, J.E. Pope (eds.), *Atlas of Implantable Therapies for Pain Management*, DOI 10.1007/978-1-4939-2110-2_17

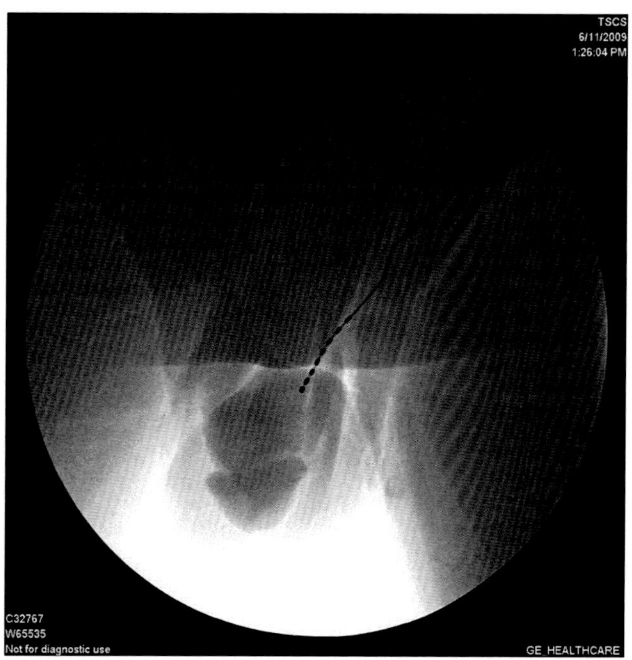

Fig. 17.2 Spermatic nerve stimulation

17.2 Selection of Candidates

Pelvic, sacral, rectal, and groin pain are complicated patient complaints that can be experienced by an eclectic group of individuals. Some of these patients are excellent candidates for stimulation whereas other patient populations have a poor prognosis. Table 17.1 identifies the important factors to consider when selecting patients for this procedure and their predictive impact on outcome.

Table 17.1 Important factors to consider when selecting patients

Factor	Consideration	Predictor
Pain generator is understood	Diagnostic workup has shown an objective abnormality	Positive
History of sexual or mental abuse	Psychological evaluation and workup	Negative
Disease is stable	No progressive condition is present	Positive
Previous treatment	History suggests some relief from other treatments	Positive
Coexisting disease	History of fibromyalgia, irritable bowel, fatigue	Negative
Pain character	Pain is burning or stabbing in nature	Positive
Drug abuse	Active drug abuse behavior	Negative
Bleeding disorders	History of active coagulopathy	Negative

17.3 Technical Overview

Traditionally four methods are used for percutaneous access to stimulate the sacral nerve roots. One surgical method to stimulate the nerves has been described.

17.3.1 Sacral Nerve Stimulation

17.3.1.1 The Retrograde Technique

The retrograde approach became very popular over the past 10 years. This method involves the placement of the epidural needle into the spinal canal, directing the bevel from a cephalad to a caudad position. The needle is placed under fluoroscopic guidance and thereafter the lead is directed from the epidural entry zone downward until it is secured in the area of the S2, S3, and S4 nerve roots unilaterally or bilaterally. The leads are then secured to the fascia and ligament at the needle entry site. This approach is usually attempted with a needle entry at L2–3 or L3–4. Entry at the L5–S1 level is difficult owing to spinal angulation and may lead to difficulty in advancing the lead into the dorsal epidural space. The disadvantage of the technique is the risk of wet tap, nerve irritation with lead placement, and potential inability to pass the lead distally (Fig. 17.3).

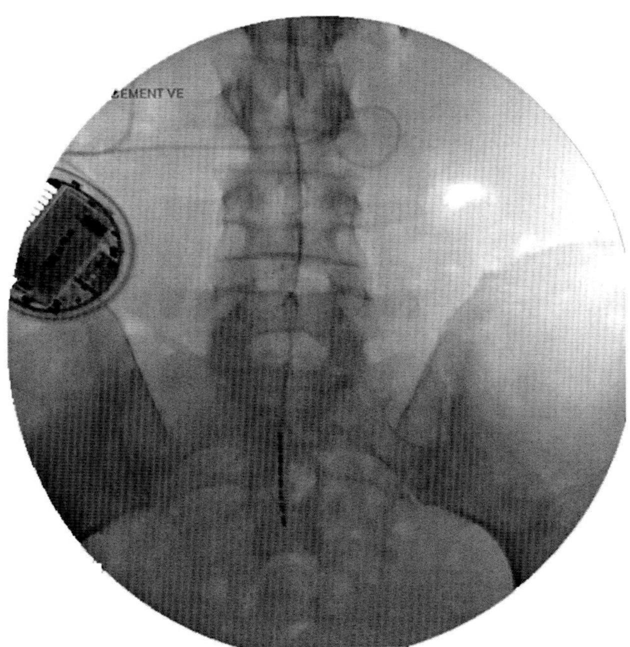

Fig. 17.3 Sacral stimulation with retrograde lead

17.3.1.2 The Lumbar Transforaminal Technique

The lumbar transforaminal approach involves placing a needle in the superior aspect of the lumbar nerve root foramen and then passing the lead inferiorly until the lead is satisfactorily placed over the sacral targets. This approach is technically difficult, may result in dorsal root entry zone injury, and may lead to difficulty in directing the lead inferiorly owing to an unsatisfactory entry angle of the lead at the foraminal entry zone. This method is covered in detail elsewhere in this Atlas.

17.3.1.3 The Sacral Transforaminal Technique

The sacral transforaminal approach involves placing the lead directly through the sacral foramen to the target nerve. This approach has been used to treat incontinence by direct nerve stimulation and to treat chronic pain. This approach is simple but has complication risks. The approach may lead to nerve injury and is difficult to anchor once the device is in place (Fig. 17.4).

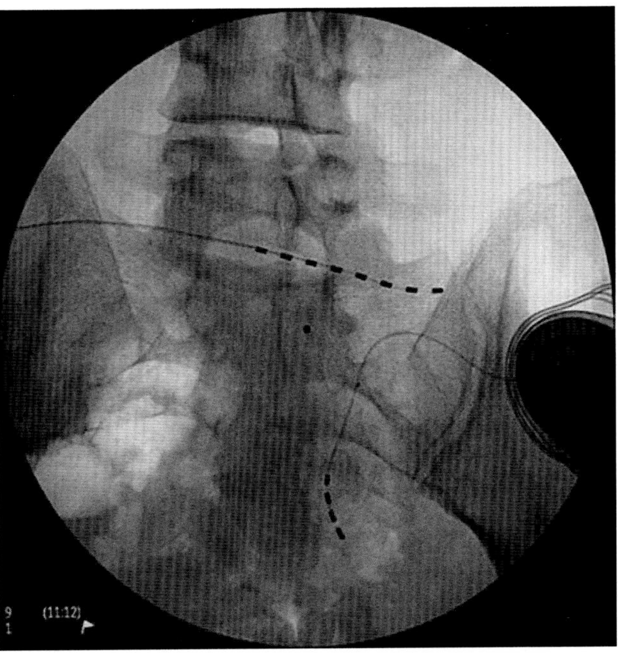

Fig. 17.4 Sacral transforaminal lead placement (lower lead)

17.3.1.4 The Sacral Hiatus or Caudal Approach Technique

The sacral hiatus can be entered by placing an epidural introducer needle into the caudal space and then driving the lead laterally to stimulate the sacral nerve targets. The target may be in the midline if the pain is in the rectum or coccyx. The advantage of this technique is the simple approach and ease of driving the lead. The disadvantage of the technique is the difficulty of anchoring the lead as it exits the sacral hiatus, especially if the body fat is not appropriate to give adequate coverage over the lead or anchor. If erosion is a risk, the permanent lead must be placed using the neurosurgical technique (Fig. 17.5).

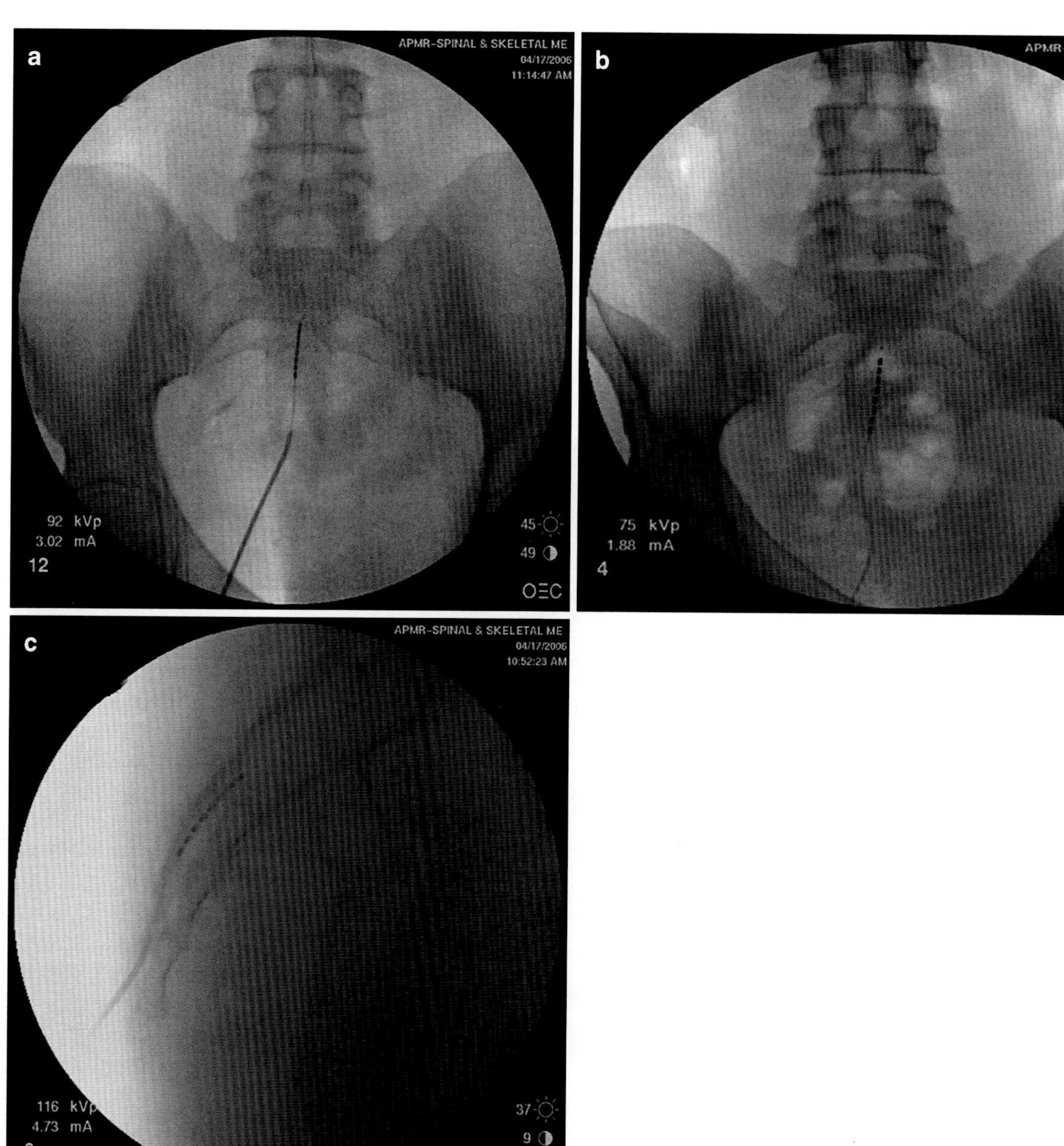

Fig. 17.5 (**a**–**c**) Placement of leads via sacral the hiatus

17.3.1.5 The Neurosurgical Laminotomy Approach

In some cases the lead cannot be placed via one of the percutaneous methods because of anatomical challenges. This approach is also used for patients who have inadequate tissue to place a permanent lead at the sacral hiatus. The approach requires the creation of a small laminotomy on the involved side or sides to place a lead over the target nerve roots.

17.3.2 Ilioinguinal Nerve Stimulation

17.3.2.1 Percutaneously Access the Ilioinguinal Nerve

The lead is placed in the tissue parallel to the inferior course of the ilioinguinal nerve. If the trial gives successful pain relief, a permanent device is placed in the nerve distribution. In the past we often dissected down to the actual nerve to place the lead under direct vision, but the use of a percutaneous nerve approach appears to be equally successful for the patient with reduced trauma overall. The generator may be placed in the lower abdominal wall near the area of the leads to reduce the risk of migration. Care should be taken to dissect down to the level of the nerve before needle/lead insertion during permanent placement to ensure that both the distal and the proximal electrode contacts of the lead are in the same plane as the nerve to ensure optimal stimulation (Fig. 17.6).

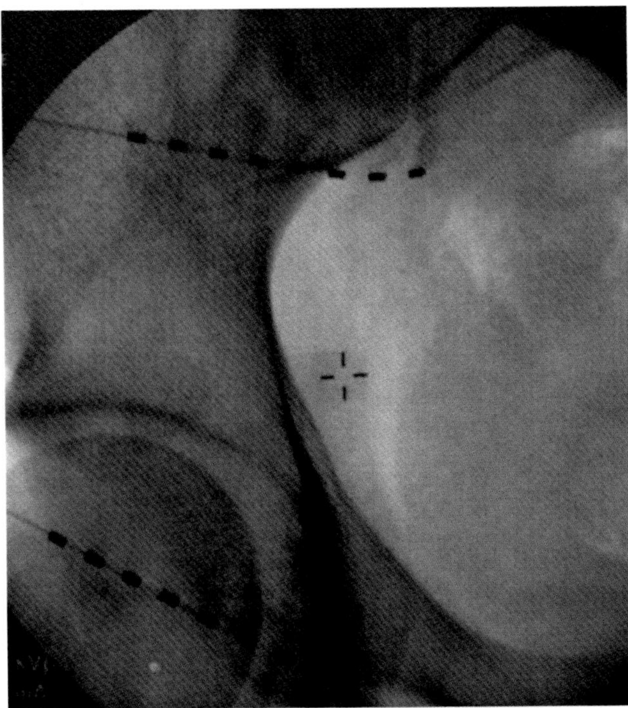

Fig. 17.6 Placement of leads for treatment of the ilioinguinal nerve

17.3.3 Spermatic or Vasal Nerves in the Vas Deferens Stimulation

17.3.3.1 Percutaneously Access the Spermatic or Vasal Nerves in Vas Deferens

The lead is placed in the tissue adjacent to the spermatic cord and vas deferens (Fig. 17.7).

The generator may be placed in the lower abdominal wall near the area of the lead to reduce the risk of migration. Ultrasound guidance may be employed to provide optimal lead placement and to mitigate risk of complications. The patient should be made aware of this risk.

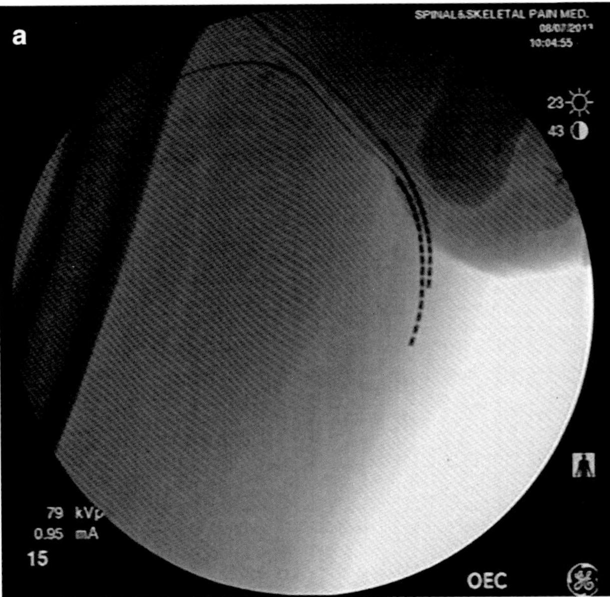

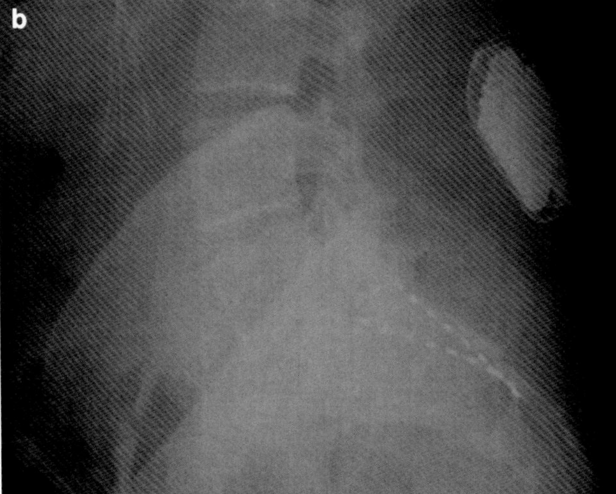

Fig. 17.7 (a, b) Spermatic nerve stimulation

Pocket Placement

The pocket for the sacral nerve stimulation should be as close in proximity to the lead insertion site as possible. This may involve placing the pocket into the buttock or just above or below the beltline. The physician should consider the patient's body habitus, bony landmarks, and skin condition prior to creating the pocket.

For ilioinguinal and vasal nerve stimulation, the generator should be sutured to the anterior abdominal fascia in order to prevent displacement, migration, or angulation after implantation or that may occur after weight loss. Angulation of the internal pulse generator may lead to difficulty in charging (Fig. 17.8).

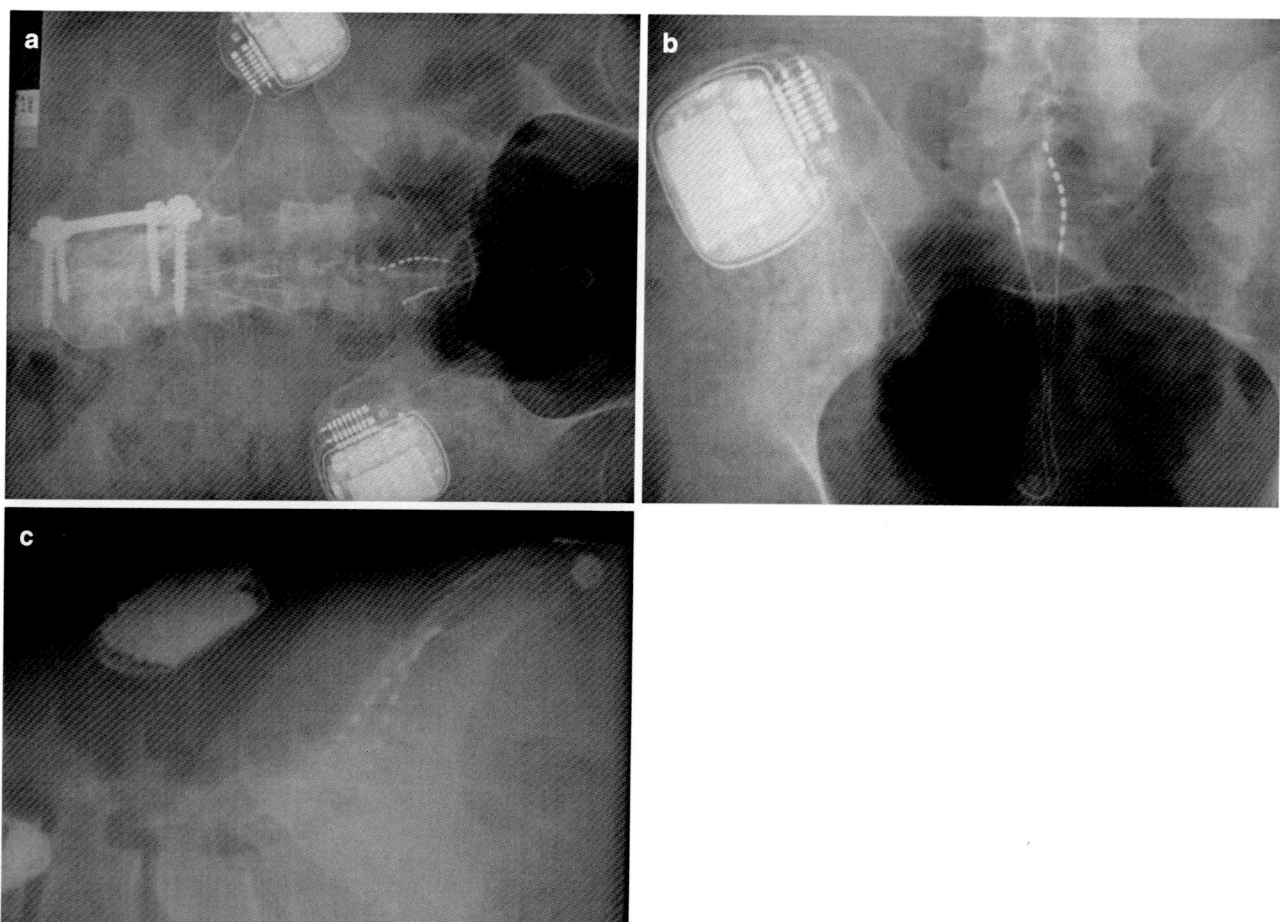

Fig. 17.8 (**a–c**) IPG location relative to lead placement and entry

17.4 Risk Assessment

1. The retrograde approach can lead to a very steep angle and may increase the risk of a wet tap or direct nerve root insult.
2. The retrograde approach can lead to difficulty passing the lead. The most common area of difficulty is at the L5–S1 level.
3. The lumbar transforaminal approach can lead to nerve root injury and an increase of the pain level. It is also difficult to anchor the lead, which may lead to migration.
4. The sacral transforaminal approach can lead to nerve root injury and increased pain. It is also difficult to anchor the lead, which may lead to migration.
5. The sacral hiatus approach may lead to infection based on the relative location to the rectum. This concern is more worrisome for the permanent device.
6. The sacral hiatus or caudal approach can cause nerve irritation that may lead to increased pain. In some cases, it is difficult to place the lead because of a stenotic or narrow canal blocking the path. An epidurogram is often helpful to identify proper needle placement and the size of the canal.
7. The neurosurgical approach can lead to bleeding and the potential for nerve damage when entering the sacrum.
8. The history of mental, physical, or sexual abuse may lead to psychological disorders that affect the long-term outcome of the device.
9. The presence of implanted mesh in the inguinal canal may preclude needle entry or stimulation.
10. Individuals of childbearing age should be counseled and advised of the risks of vasal nerve stimulation including impotence, erectile dysfunction, and damage to testis.

17.5 Risk Avoidance

1. The risk of the retrograde approach can be reduced by using a needle with a curved bevel to enter the epidural space. This risk can also be reduced by positioning the pelvis with a total elimination of the baseline lumbar lordosis.
2. Lead placement by the retrograde approach and by the lumbar transforaminal technique can beassisted by driving the lead in the midline until the lead crosses the L5–S1 junction, at which time the lead may be redirected to the desired side of capture.
3. The lumbar transforaminal approach can be difficult to achieve and should be attempted only in those who are an expert at the procedure of transforaminal injection. The risk can be reduced if the patient is kept conversant and alert during lead placement and lead movement.
4. The sacral transforaminal approach can be improved by placing several pillows below the pelvis to reduce the amount of lordosis. The procedure can be improved by keeping the patient alert and by carefully adjusting the fluoroscopic beam to improve the view of the foramen.
5. When using the sacral hiatus or caudal approach, the patient should be widely prepared and draped with a potent cleanser on at least six occasions. The preparation should involve the buttocks, anal region, and perineum.
6. The reduction of space in the sacral hiatus can lead to difficulty in passing the lead. The use of smaller leads and 17-gauge needles may help overcome this issue. If the obstruction continues, the physician should consider an alternative route of lead placement.
7. The neurosurgical approach should be performed with caution and the surgeon should carefully expose the nerve roots as they enter the foramen. If there are any structural anomalies that are known prior to moving forward, the surgeon should consider placing the leads with the patient under sedation to ensure ongoing communication and warning of any paresthesia.
8. Ilioinguinal lead placement involves risks including direct damage to inguinal, ilioiohypogastric, genitofemoral, femoral, and lateral femoral cutaneous nerves, as well as possible damage to abdominal contents and viscera. This procedure should therefore be performed with extreme caution. Ultrasound guidance may be employed to mitigate this risk (Gofeld & Christakis 2006).
9. Vasal neurostimulator lead placement carries inherent risk of vascular damage within the spermatic cord and should therefore be performed with extreme caution. Ultrasound guidance may be employed to mitigate this risk. The patient should be made aware of this risk (Parekattil et al. 2013).
10. In pelvic pain patients, it is important for the patient to be given a full psychological evaluation prior to moving forward. Psychological comorbidity is not an absolute contraindication, but the treatment and counseling may improve the longterm outcome with the device.

Conclusions

Stimulation of the sacral, ilioinguinal, and vasal nerves can lead to decreased pain, improved function, and improved quality of life. The nerves are technically difficult to access by conventional percutaneous methods. The patients should be carefully selected, the sacral and pelvic anatomy carefully reviewed, and the patient should be educated regarding expectations and risks.

Suggested Reading

Gofeld J, Christakis M. Sonographically guided ilioinguinal nerve block. J Ultrasound Med. 2006;25:1571–5.

Parekattil SJ, Gudeloglu A, Brahmbhatt JV, Priola KB, Vieweg J, Allan RW. Trifecta nerve complex: potential anatomical basis for microsurgical denervation of the spermatic cord for chronic orchialgia. J Urol. 2013;190:265–70.

18 Selective Nerve Root Stimulation: Facilitating the Cephalocaudal "Retrograde" Method of Electrode Insertion

Kenneth M. Alò, Darnell Josiah, and Erich O. Richter

18.1 Introduction

Selective nerve root stimulation (SNRS) as a method was first presented in 1998 [1–3] and was published in 1999 [4, 5]. Despite advances at that time in dual electrode technology and patient controlled programming, "anterograde" spinal cord stimulators (SCSs) were unable to consistently produce and maintain paresthesia in the neck, pelvic, and foot dermatomes [6, 7]. As well some individual lower extremity dermatomes lacked SCS paresthesia coverage. Thus, selective, cephalocaudal, "retrograde" electrode placement was developed to improve capture in these targets [4]. Safety concerns limited cervical in vivo application [3, 5]; however, lumbosacral placement gained interest in the evaluation of many difficult-to-treat conditions [8–19]. Despite initial enthusiasm and success, many encountered technical difficulty entering the lumbar intralaminar space from the superior to inferior or cephalocaudal, "retrograde" direction [17, 20, 21]. Subsequently this author began teaching a needle entry technique utilizing a lateral intralaminar approach (Figs. 18.1, 18.2, 18.3, 18.4, 18.5, 18.6, 18.7, 18.8, 18.9, and 18.10). This mimics the "single-shot epidural" needle placement applied commonly by interventional practitioners. This facilitates entry of the stimulation electrode into the epidural midline, and standardizes entry of the needle below the conus at L2–3.

K.M. Alò
The Methodist Hospital Research Institute,
5318 Weslayan #182, Houston, TX 77005, USA
e-mail: aglioolio@gmail.com

D. Josiah, MD • E.O. Richter (✉)
Department of Neurosurgery, West Virginia University Hospitals,
PO Box 9183, Morgantown, WV 26506, USA
e-mail: djosiah@hsc.wvu.edu; eorichter@hsc.wvu.edu

T.R. Deer, J.E. Pope (eds.), *Atlas of Implantable Therapies for Pain Management*, DOI 10.1007/978-1-4939-2110-2_18

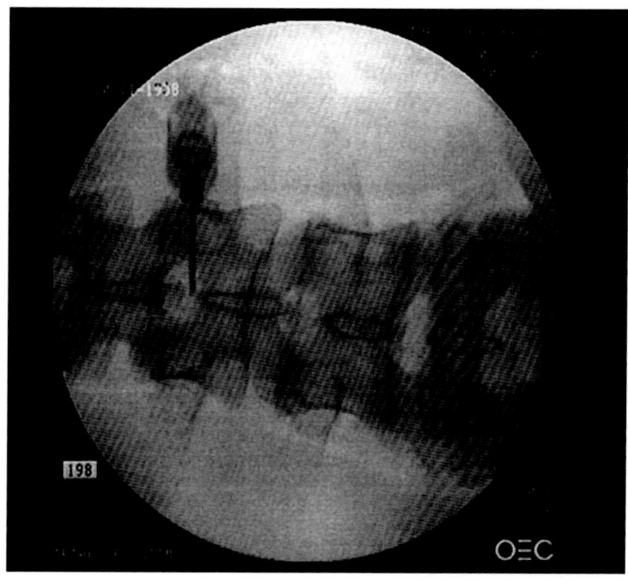

Fig. 18.1 S2–3 Retrograde: L2–3 epidural "lateral" approach (anteroposterior [AP] view)

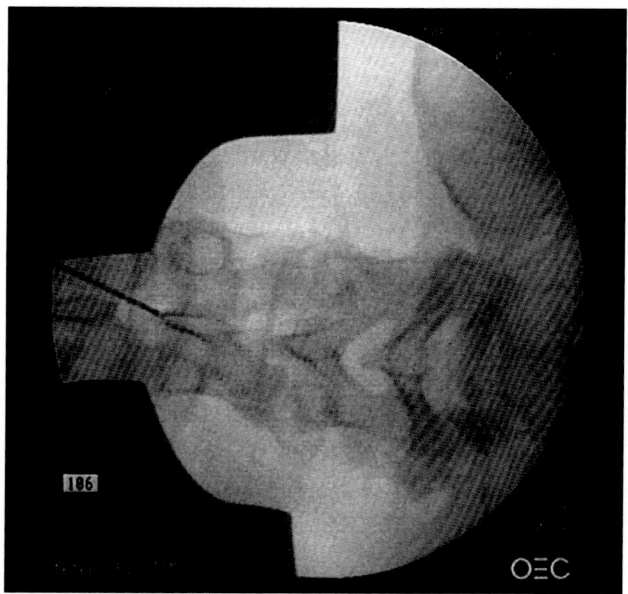

Fig. 18.2 S2–3 Retrograde: L2–3 needle tip in steep caudal view to limit hand exposure

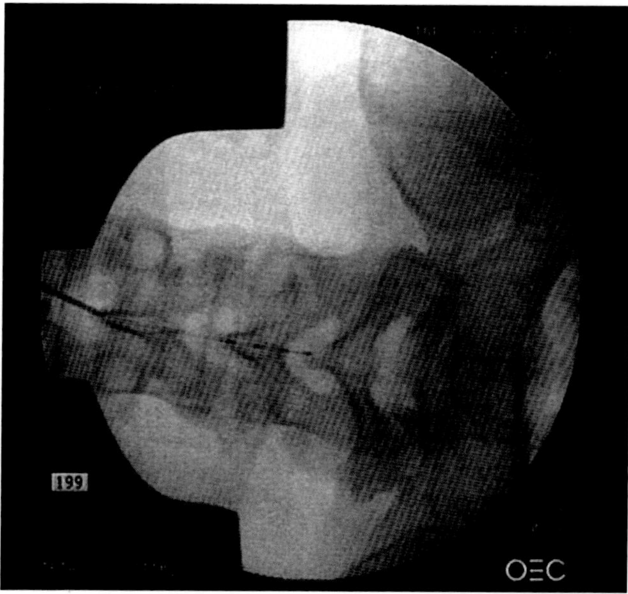

Fig. 18.3 S2–3 Retrograde: electrode directed caudally in the midline

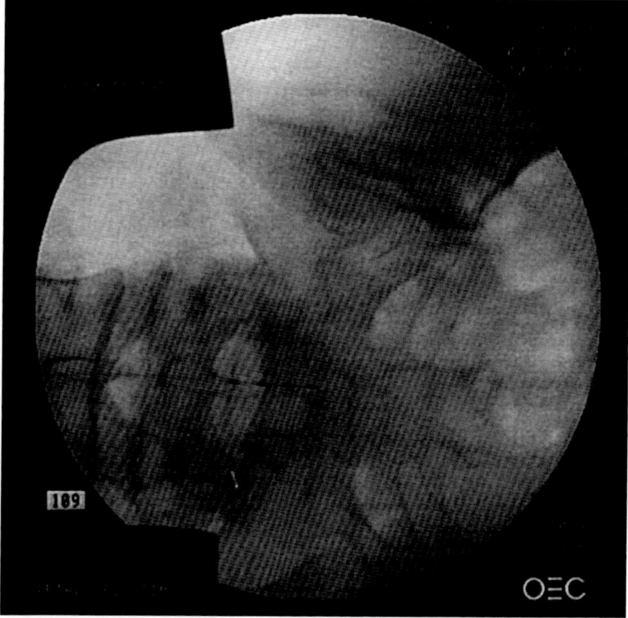

Fig. 18.4 S2–3 Retrograde: electrode crossing S1 level in midline

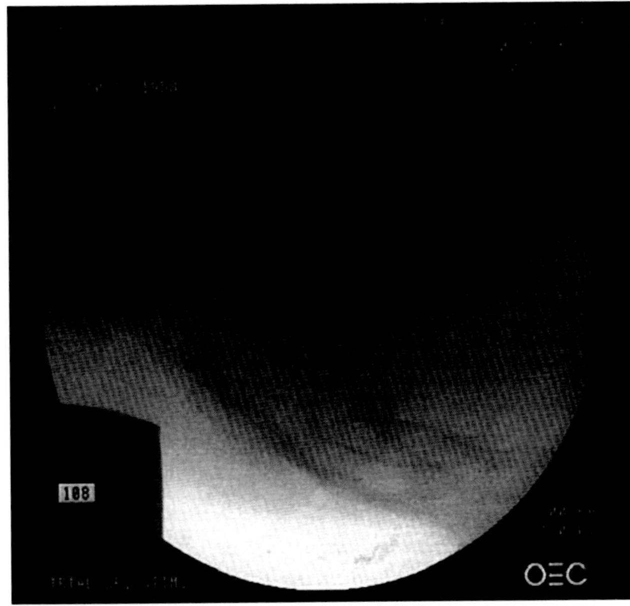

Fig. 18.5 S2–3 Retrograde: S1 level electrode posterior on lateral view

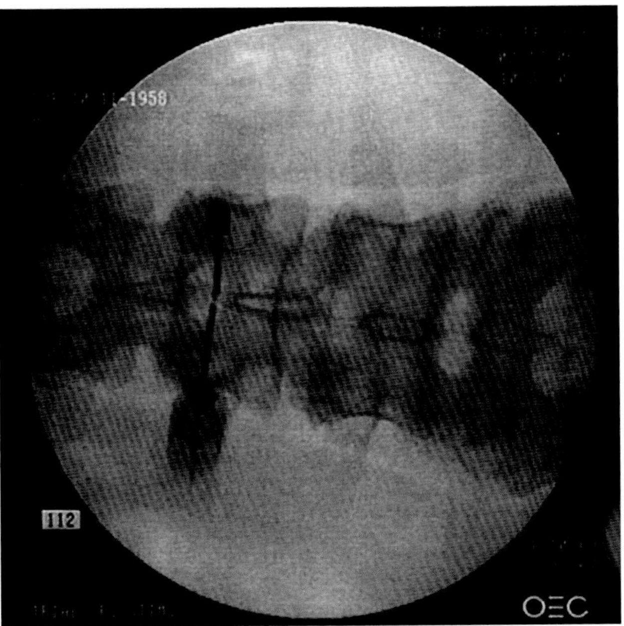

Fig. 18.7 S2–3 Retrograde: dual L2–3 epidural "lateral" approach (AP view)

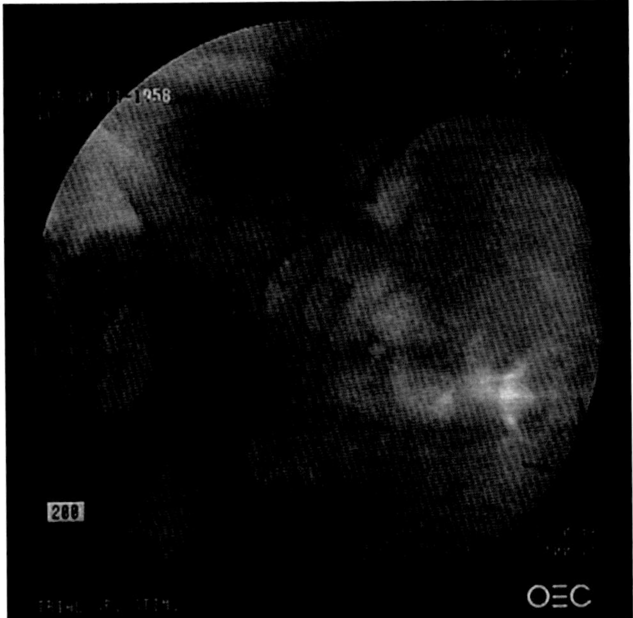

Fig. 18.6 S2–3 Retrograde: electrode rotated to right S2–3 foramen: stimulating right S2–4 roots

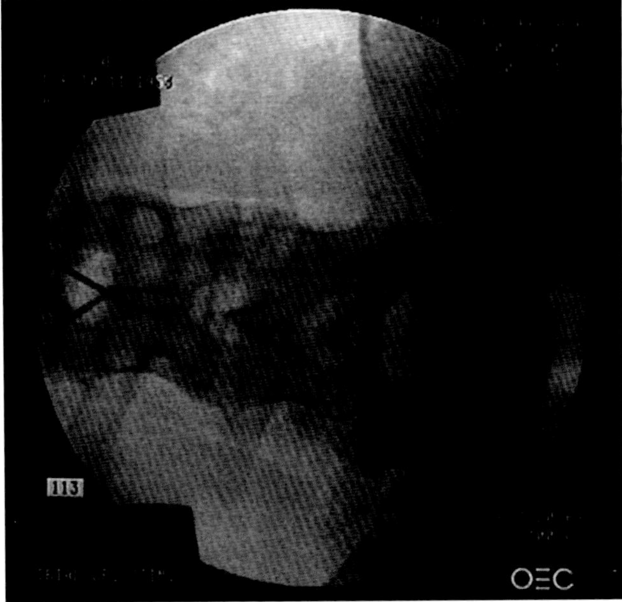

Fig. 18.8 S2–3 Retrograde: dual L2/3 needle tips in steep caudal view to limit hand exposure

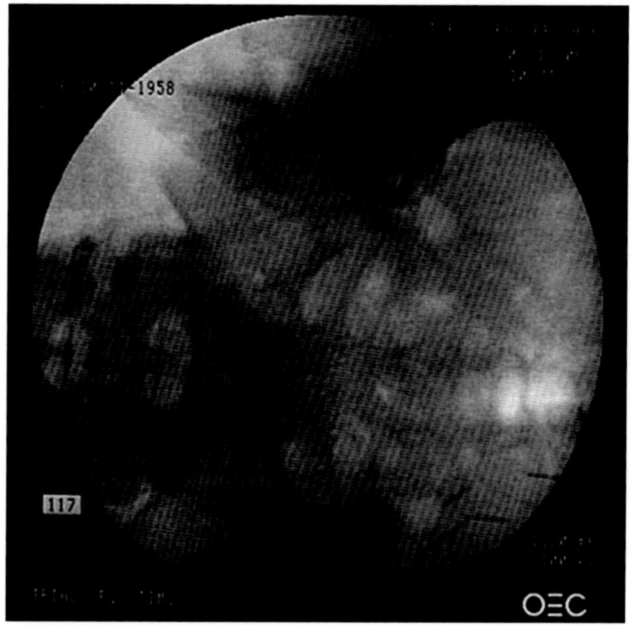

Fig. 18.9 S2–3 Retrograde: dual electrodes at final S2–3 foramen stimulating S2–4 roots

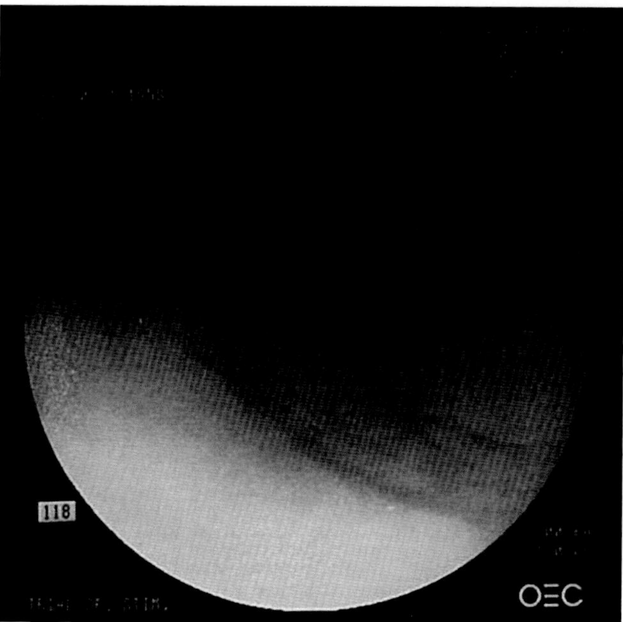

Fig. 18.10 S2–3 Retrograde: dual electrodes at S2–3 stimulating S2–4 roots (lateral view)

18.2 Technical Overview

18.2.1 Cephalocaudal Lumbosacral Electrode Placement: Foot and Pelvic Root Placement

To stimulate the foot, a quadrapolar electrode enters the midline at L2–3 crossing over the L3–4 disc space before it is then rotated to, but not through, the L4 foramen (Figs. 18.11 and 18.14). This positioning allows the electrode to remain "in line" with the ipsilateral L4, L5, and S1 roots. It is then programmed at the foramen with an anode and up to three proximal contacts as cathodes. This allows depolarization of all three roots as they course cephalad lateral to medial. A second electrode can be applied if needed depending on the stimulation pattern obtained (Fig. 18.11). Given the reduced cerebrospinal fluid and proximity to the root, most patients feel initial paresthesia at low thresholds (1.0–1.5 V), with maximal tolerable intensity approximately 1.5 times that level (1.5–2.5 V).

To stimulate the pelvic roots, a quadrapolar electrode enters the midline at L2–3 and remains there until it crosses S1 before it is rotated to, but not through, the ipsilateral S2 foramen. A second electrode is positioned in the same fashion contralaterally for bilateral pathology (Figs. 18.1, 18.2, 18.3, 18.4, 18.5, 18.6, 18.7, 18.8, 18.9, and 18.10). These electrodes are also programmed with a distal anode at the foramen, and up to three cathodes over the proximal S2–4 roots, respectively. This allows an anatomical placement for stimulating all of the following conditions: urge incontinence, neurogenic bowel dysfunction, urgency-frequency syndromes (including detrusor dysfunction), pudendal neuralgia, vulvadynia, and interstitial cystitis [15, 16]. This may be done as well with small paddle style electrodes through a small S1 laminotomy (Fig. 18.12). To ease placement of the paddle toward the S2 foramen, a Penfield 3 can be used at the laminotomy to elevate the electrode into position (Fig. 18.13). Given the relative lack of cerebrospinal fluid at the S2 level, most patients feel initial paresthesia at low thresholds (0.7–1.2 V) with maximal tolerable intensity approximately 1.5 times that level (1.2–1.7 V).

When programming both foot and pelvic electrode placements, varying pulse width is perceived as increasing or decreasing regional paresthesia coverage, and varying frequency as altering character and intensity of paresthesia. The clinical parameter effects and thresholds of these electrodes are physiologically those of intraspinal, epidural, peripheral nerve stimulators.

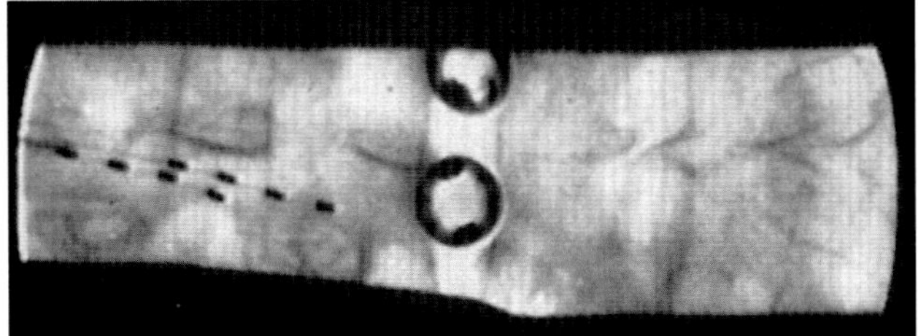

Fig. 18.11 Unilateral left leg/foot stimulation with two quadrapolar, selective, cephalocaudal electrodes. Distal electrode terminates at the L4 foramen stimulating the L4–S1 roots with an anode at the foramen, and three proximal cathodes. The proximal electrode stimulates the L3 and L4 roots programmed the same way. As pulse width is increased, geographic paresthesia coverage is increased in the left L3–S1 dermatomes

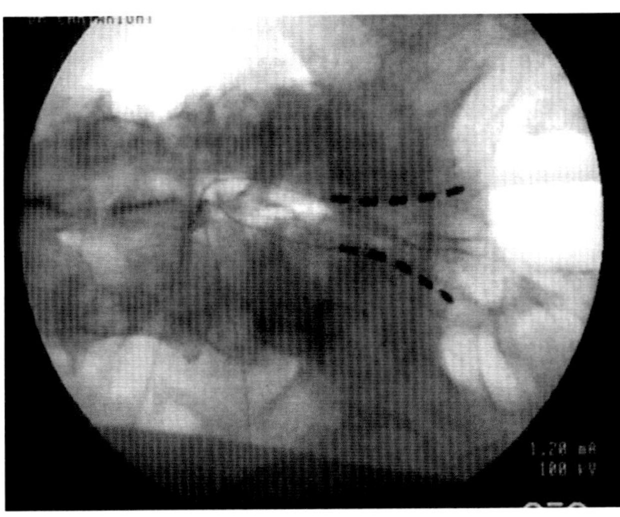

Fig. 18.12 Bilateral pelvic stimulation with 3.8-mm quadrapolar, selective, cephalocaudal paddles (S1 laminotomy). Distal contacts are anodes at each S2 foramen, and proximal three contacts are each cathodes

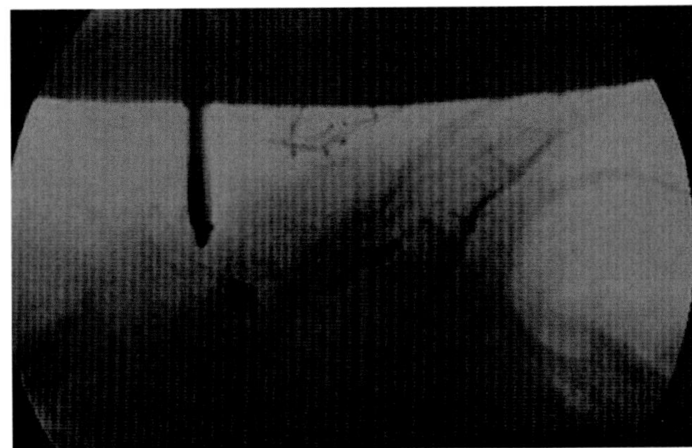

Fig. 18.13 Lateral radiograph of Fig. 18.12. Penfield 3 elevating tool assisting with placement of 3.8-mm paddles toward the S2 foramen

18.2.2 Cephalocaudal Lumbosacral Electrode Placement: Coccygeal Root Placement

To stimulate the coccyx, a quadrapolar electrode enters the midline at L2–3 and remains there until the tip rests at S3 (Fig. 18.13). If the tip of the electrode is advanced to close to the sacral hiatus, painful stimulation may be seen, in particular if scarring from a previous coccygectomy is encountered. Programming follows the same distal anode, proximal cathode configuration to achieve paresthesia into the distal S4 and S5 dermatomes. Wide pulse widths assist in recruiting both the left and the right S4 and S5 roots, which are close to the midline at this level (with single or dual quadrapolar electrodes).

18.2.3 Cephalocaudal Lumbosacral Electrode Placement: Individual Lower Extremity Root Placement

To stimulate the individual lower extremity roots, a quadapolar electrode enters the midline at L2–3 and is rotated to, but not through, the foramen at the root level(s) of interest (Figs. 18.14, 18.15 and 18.16). Programming and activation thresholds are much like those for foot placement, with the possibility of slightly increased activation and maximal intensity thresholds, owing to the relative increase of cerebrospinal fluid above L5. When programming individual lower extremity root electrodes (just as coccygeal, pelvic, and foot), varying pulse width is perceived as increasing or decreasing regional paresthesia coverage, and varying frequency as altering character and intensity of paresthesia.

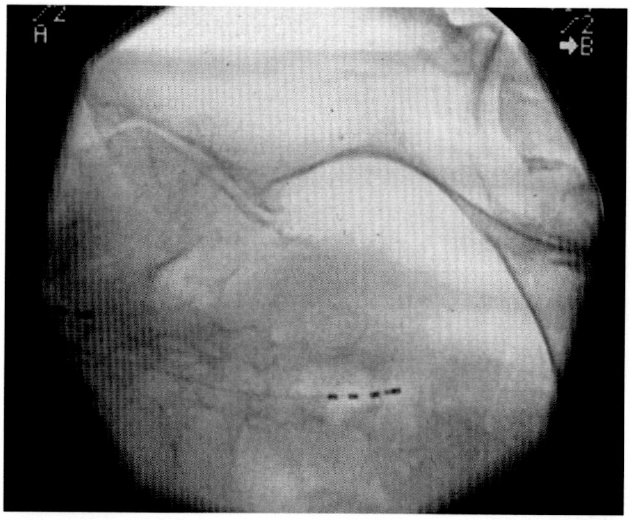

Fig. 18.14 Midline quadrupolar, selective, cephalocaudal electrode for coccygodynia. Programming a distal anode and up to three proximal cathodes with a wide pulse width (>200) provided paresthesia capture of the bilateral S4 and S5 roots

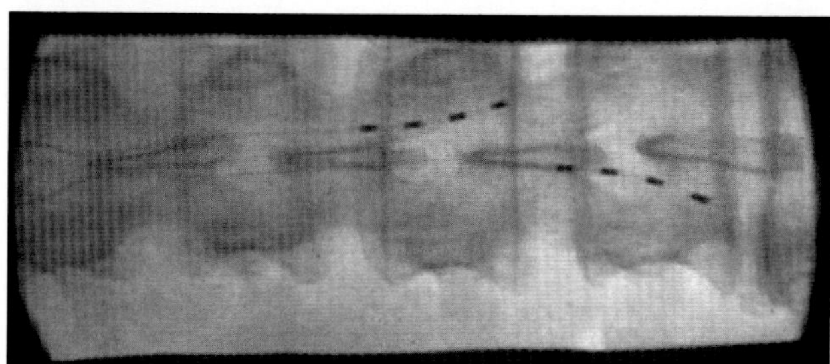

Fig. 18.15 Individual quadrupolar, selective, cephalocaudal root electrodes for lower extremity radicular pain. Right electrode at the foramen of L3 (capturing the L3–5 roots), and left at the foramen of L4 (capturing the L4–S1 roots). Both programmed with a distal anode at the foramen, and up to three cathodes proximally

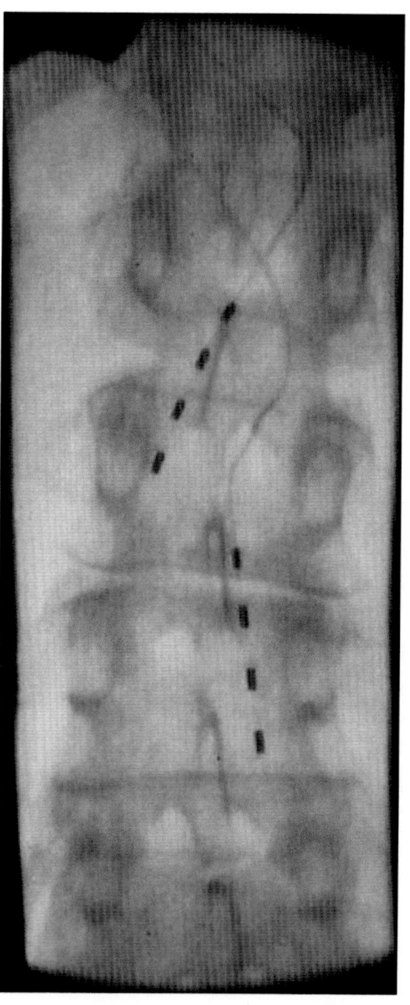

Fig. 18.16 Individual quadrapolar, selective, cephalocaudal root electrodes for lower extremity radicular pain. Right electrode just medial to the foramen of L3 (capturing L3–S1), and left at the foramen of L2 (capturing L2 and L3 roots). Both programmed with a distal anode at the foramen, and up to three proximal cathodes

18.2.4 Contraindications

Relative contraindications to perform cephalocaudal electrode insertion include previous spinal epidural operation, spondylolisthesis, spina bifida, and epidural lipomatosis. Absolute contraindications include lack of informed consent, coagulopathy, lack of adequate training, and infection. Experienced interventionalists, noting that in vivo cephalocaudal cervicothoracic placements have not been routinely performed to date, should carefully consider needle or electrode placements above L2–3.

Conclusions

The cephalocaudal, "retrograde" method of electrode insertion remains an important technique for the interventional neuromodulation specialist. With prudent application of the modified placement and programming approach described, this strategy can facilitate SNRS of many conditions involving the L2–S5 anatomy.

References

1. Alò KM, Yland MJ, Redko V. Retrograde intraspinal peripheral neurostimulation: a novel anatomic approach. In: Proceedings of the International Neuromodulation Society, Lucerne, Number 87; 1998.
2. Alò KM, Yland MJ, Redko V. Selective lumbar and sacral nerve root stimulation in the treatment of chronic pain. In: Proceedings of the International Neuromodulation Society, Lucerne, Number 89; 1998.
3. Alò KM, Feler CA, Oakley J, Yland MJ. An in vitro study of electrode placement at the cervical nerve roots using a trans-spinal approach. In: Proceedings of the International Neuromodulation Society, Lucerne, Number 90; 1998.
4. Alò KM, Yland MJ, Redko V, Feler C, Naumann C. Lumbar and sacral nerve root stimulation (NRS) in the treatment of chronic pain: a novel anatomic approach and neuro stimulation technique. Neuromodulation. 1999;2:23–31.
5. Alò KM, Oakley J, Feler C, Yland MJ. A study of electrode placement at the cervical and upper thoracic nerve roots using an anatomic trans-spinal approach. Neuromodulation. 1999;2:222–7.
6. Alò KM, Holsheimer J. New trends in neuromodulation for the management of neuropathic pain. Neurosurgery. 2002;50:690–704.
7. Alò KM. New techniques in neurostimulation analgesia. In: Casasola OD, editor. Techniques in regional anesthesia and pain management: special issue on emerging therapies in chronic pain management. 2001. p. 30–6.
8. Alò KM, Feler CA, Whitworth L. Long-term follow-up of selective nerve root stimulation for interstitial cystitis: review of results. Abstracts of the World Pain Meeting 2000, San Francisco; 2000.
9. McDonald JS, Alo KM. Pain of urogenital origin. In: Loeser J, editor. Bonica's management of pain. 3rd ed. Section E: Pain in pelvis, perineum, and genitalia. Philadelphia: Lippincott Williams & Wilkins; 2001. p. 1448–61.
10. Alò K, Yland M, Redko V, Feler C, Naumann C. Selective nerve root stimulation in the treatment of chronic pain. Fortschritte in Anaesthesie, Intensive, Notfall, Und Schmerztherapie. 1999; 1:38.
11. Alò KM, Yland MJ, Redko V, Feler C, Naumann C. Selective lumbar and sacral nerve root stimulation in the treatment of chronic pain: an anatomic approach. Abstract Book: St. Antoni Arlberg Austrian Annal anesthesiology and pain management meeting, German, 4 Feb 1999.
12. Alò KM, McKay E. Selective nerve root stimulation (SNRS) for the treatment of intractable pelvic pain and motor dysfunction: a case report. Neuromodulation. 2001;4:19–23.
13. Alò KM, Zidan AM. Selective nerve root simulation (SNRS) in the treatment of end-stage, diabetic, peripheral neuropathy: a case report. Neuromodulation. 2000;3:201–8.
14. Alò KM, Gohel R, Corey CL. Sacral nerve root stimulation for the treatment of urge incontinence and detrusor dysfunction utilizing a cephalocaudal intraspinal method of lead insertion: a case report. Neuromodulation. 2001;4:53–8.
15. Alò KM, McKay E. Sacral nerve root stimulation for the treatment of intractable pelvic pain: clinical experience. In: Jose De Andres, editor. Bound version proceedings Puesta Al Dia En Anestesia Regional Y Tratamiento Del Dolor. 2003;VI:247–51.
16. Alò KM, McKay E. Sacral nerve root stimulation for the treatment of urge incontinence and detrusor dysfunction utilizing a cephalocaudal intraspinal method of lead insertion: a case report. In: Jose De Andres, editor. Bound version proceedings Puesta Al Dia En Anestesia Regional Y Tratamiento Del Dolor. 2003;VI:251–6.
17. Feler CA, Whitworth LA, Brookoff D, Powell R. Recent advances: sacral nerve root stimulation using a retrograde method of lead insertion for the treatment of pelvic pain due to interstitial cystitis. Neuromodulation. 1999;2:211–6.
18. Kothari S. Neuromodulatory approaches to chronic pelvic pain and coccygodynia. Acta Neurochir Suppl. 2007;97:365–71.
19. Worsoe J, Rasmussen M, Christensen P, Krogh K. Neurostimulation for neurogenic bowel dysfunction. Gastroenterol Res Pract. 2013;2013:563294.
20. Alò KM, Bennett D, Oakley JC, et al. Fluoroscopy manual for pain management: chapter: radiologic considerations for neurostimulation lead placement: lumbar/sacral placement. In: Tina McKay Best, editor. Pain management innovations. Evergreen; 2000. p. 31–37, 38–44.
21. Richter EO, Abramova MV, Aló KM. Percutaneous cephalocaudal implantation of epidural stimulation electrodes over sacral nerve roots—a technical note on the importance of the lateral approach. Neuromodulation. 2011;14:62–7.

19 Neurostimulation for the Treatment of Anterior Abdominal Pain

Nameer R. Haider and Timothy R. Deer

19.1 Introduction

Abdominal pain is a common disease state that affects millions of people globally. Unlike other painful areas of the body, pain in the abdomen can be visceral or somatic, and even further, with vicerosomatic convergence, the presentation can be very complex. Many patients suffer from pain of the anterior abdominal wall after surgical procedures, such as hernia repairs, cesarean sections, cholecystectomy, appendectomy, bowel surgeries, and from chronic conditions, such as endometriosis. Furthermore, after multiple abdominal surgeries, adhesions may form within the tissues of the abdominal wall leading to localized neuropathic pain. This neuropathic pain is secondary to nerve entrapment or direct nerve trauma. Treatment of such painful conditions is often difficult and complex. Recently, transversus abdominis plane blocks with local anesthetic have been utilized to treat such painful conditions. This method, although often efficacious temporarily, is not seen as a long-term solution in most cases. More definitive pain relief of anterior abdominal pain may be achieved by implantation of a neurostimulator.

N.R. Haider, MD
Minimally Invasive Pain Institute, Washington, DC, USA
e-mail: drhaider@killpain.com

T.R. Deer, MD (✉)
The Center for Pain Relief, 400 Court Street, Suite 100, Charleston, WV 25301, USA
e-mail: DocTDeer@aol.com

T.R. Deer, J.E. Pope (eds.), *Atlas of Implantable Therapies for Pain Management*, DOI 10.1007/978-1-4939-2110-2_19

19.2 Technical Overview

The visceral nociceptive pathway is much different than its somatic counterpart. The visceral nociceptive afferents have first-order neurons located in the dorsal root ganglia and extend up to more than five vertebral body segments before terminating in the ipsilateral dorsal horn of the spinal cord. There, they ascend along the ipsilateral postsynaptic dorsal column (PSDC) pathway and spinothalamic tract (STT) bilaterally (Fig. 19.1). The visceral nociceptors are widely distributed in laminae I, II, V, X, and contralaterally in laminae III and X.

Divergently, the somatic nerves that supply the abdominal wall have primary afferents within the dorsal horn and ascend contralateral in the spinothalamic tract, before synapsing with thalamus and then unto the somatosensory cortex. The nerves that are within the transversus abdominis plane (the plane between the transversus abdominal muscle and the internal oblique) provide sensation to the anterior abdominal wall bilaterally. Branches of spinal nerves from T7–L1 are located within this plane.

The transversus abdominis plane (TAP) block procedure was first described in 2001 by Rafi [1] as a blind landmark technique targeting the lumbar triangle of Petit (Fig. 19.2).

More recently, an ultrasound-guided subcostal approach has been utilized to place the stimulating leads in the plane between the internal oblique and the transversus abdominis muscles. A third method of lead placement has been described in this area that involves a percutaneous nerve stimulator to guide placement of a small novel lead. This device, StimRouter (Bioness; Valencia, CA) is now in U. S. Food and Drug Administration (FDA) studies.

19.2.1 The Percutaneous Method of Epidural Stimulation

In some settings physicians have chosen to treat this complex problem with spinal cord stimulation (SCS). Once the epidural needle is in place, the lead is targeted to the nerves that are involved in the generation of pain. The traditional approach involves placing the lead at the level of T4–7. This is often done in parallel or a staggered array. If these lead arrays are successful in controlling abdominal pain, no further adaptations are needed. In many settings, the pain best treated by this method is visceral in nature. Kapural et al. [2] have shown the most common lead placement for this abnormality is at T5 or T6. This pattern often leads to total coverage of the entire abdomen. In selected patients the paresthesia is unpleasant or does not adequately cover the patient's pain. In these cases the epidural approach is not the ideal treatment option.

19.2.2 The Method of Transversus Abdominis Plane Stimulation

The anatomical boundaries of the lumbar triangle of Petit are external oblique muscle anteriorly, latissimus dorsi posteriorly, and iliac crest inferiorly. This may act as the landmark in order to facilitate the placement of neurostimulator leads in the neurovascular plane.

Ultrasound-guided access to the transversus abdominis neurovascular plane may be performed using an oblique subcostal approach or a horizontal approach at the midaxillary line between the postal margin and the iliac crest. Prior to attempting this method the physician should be well versed in ultrasound imaging and the anatomy of the musculature of this region.

Hydrodissection of the transverse abdominis plane with normal saline may be employed to facilitate placement of neurostimulator leads. However, utilizing this approach may limit the ability to stimulate the surrounding tissues until there has been absorption of the fluid.

Using a needle with a plastic stylet, the needle should be bent to mimic the convexity of the anterior abdominal wall in order to place the lead electrode in the transversus abdominal plane along this convexity. This may be more easily facilitated by advancing the lead from a lateral to a medial direction. Furthermore during permanent placement of leads, careful dissection to the anterior abdominal wall should be performed before needle entry and placement in order to ensure that all contacts of the lead placed within the transversus abdominis plane.

Another option for lead placement is the use of an introducer sheath to separate tissue planes and allow adequate room for lead placement and program. Novel sheaths exist for this method.

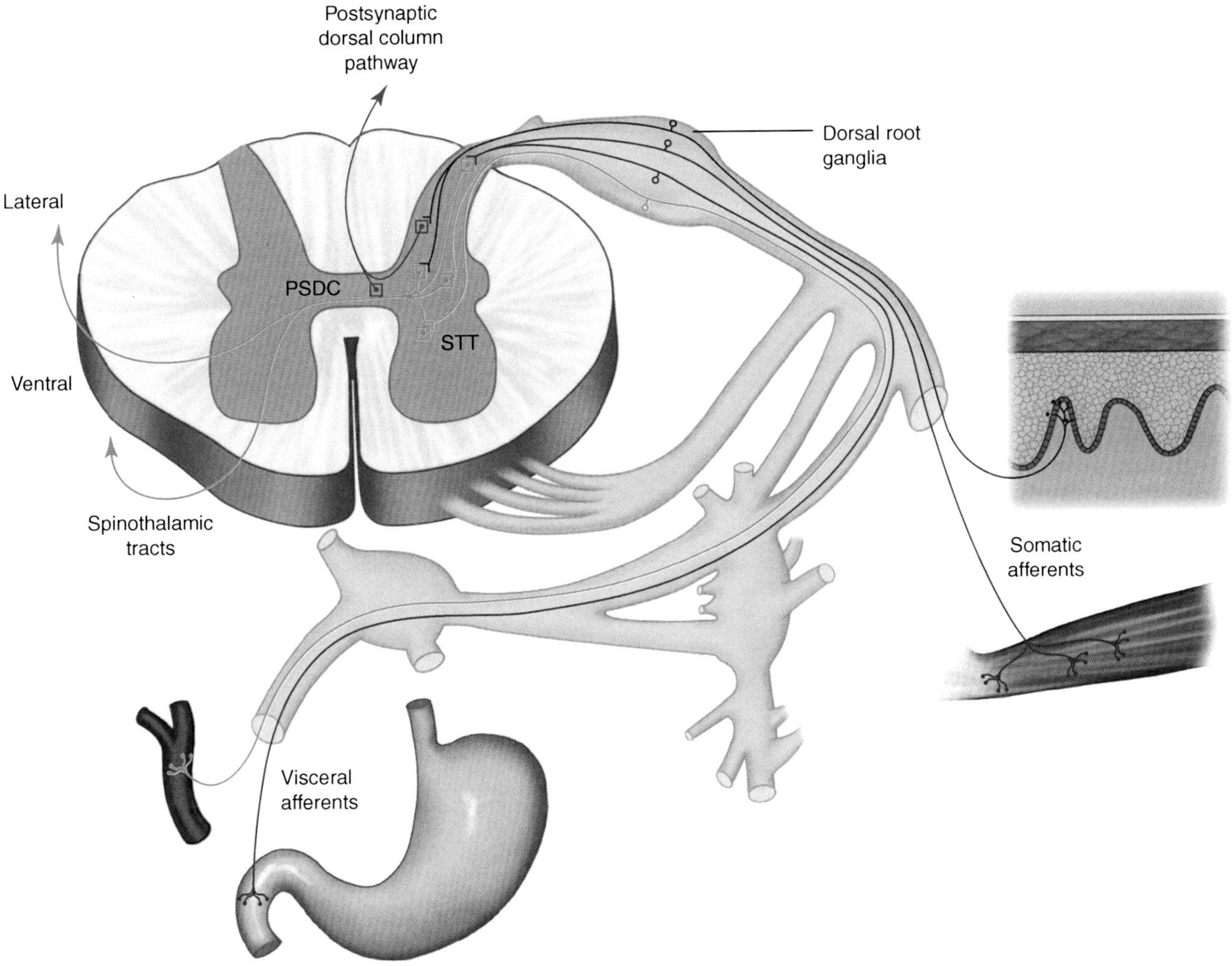

Postsynaptic
dorsal column
pathway
Dorsal root
ganglia
Lateral
PSDC
STT
Ventral
Spinothalamic
tracts
Somatic
afferents
Visceral
afferents

Fig. 19.1 The postsynaptic dorsal column pathway. Importantly, these fibers ascend ipsilaterally within the spinal cord

External oblique
muscle
Transversus
abdominis
muscle
Internal oblique

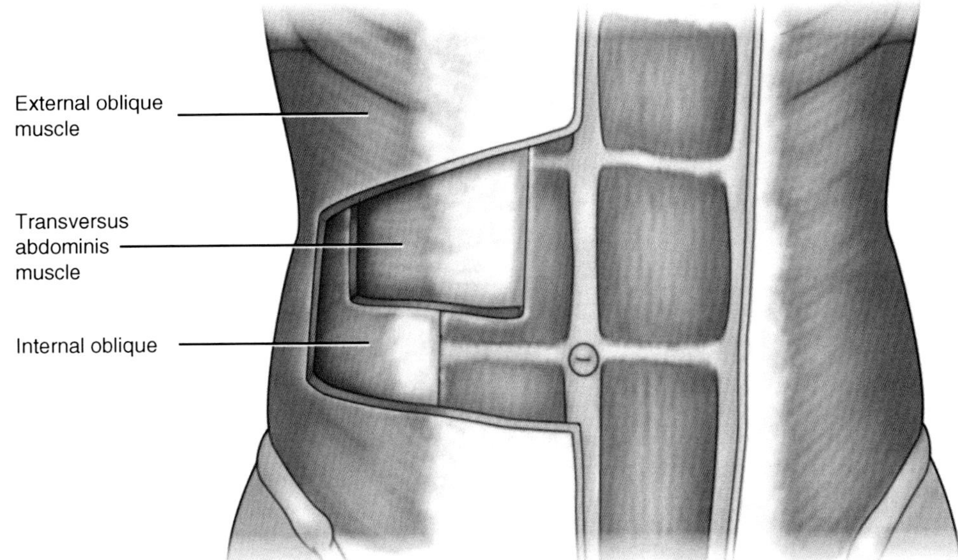

Fig. 19.2 The transversus abdominal plane is between the internal oblique and the transversus abdominis muscles

19.3 Risk Assessment

1. The patient may be at high risk with epidural lead placement or major neurosurgical interventions may be a candidate for transversus abdominis plane lead placement. The risks are limited, but careful preoperative planning, as well as extensive knowledge of the regional anatomy, is necessary.
2. Skin infection is the most common problem with peripheral nerve stimulation, but it is limited in its potential severity.
3. Nerve injury of a peripheral nerve or its fibers is possible and may lead to increased pain.
4. Injury to vascular structures is possible and may lead to ischemic injury, although the ability to directly visualize the surgical field reduces this risk.
5. Skin erosion may occur when the lead, anchor, or generator irritates the skin causing a cellulitis and potential skin breakdown.
6. Pain and a component of the device may be due to a decreased use of the device, increase function, and need to revise the system.

19.4 Risk Avoidance

1. The patient should be alert and awake during the placement and the needle or lead should be redirected if the patient complains of paresthesia. Only the entry site should be anesthetized; an area where the lead is to be implanted adjacent to the nerve should not be anesthetized in order to prevent injury.
2. The use of needle with a plastic stylet will optimize placement of the needle on the abdominal wall convexity.
3. Nonabsorbable suture may be used for the anchoring.
4. The bony structure should be carefully examined prior to device implantation. The IPG pocket should be in a location that receives the least amount of tissue pressure or movement during the patient's daily activities. Placement of the generator in close proximity to the anterior superior iliac spine and anterior rib margins should be avoided. In newly developing peripheral leads the need for a generator may be avoided. Options may be skin-based power sources or remote blue tooth technology.
5. The IPG that is usually placed above the belt line in order to avoid undue pressure that may lead to skin erosion.
6. If pain persists after implantation, options include use of topical anesthetics, topical patches, compounded pain creams, padding, and surgical revision.
7. Use of ultrasound guidance allows for direct visualization of all anatomical structures including bowel and abdominal viscera, needle, and the lead, thereby increasing the safety margin and optimizing lead placement.

19.5 Conclusions

Anterior abdominal wall pain can be a debilitating condition causing extreme suffering for this patient population. Neurostimulation in both the epidural space and the transversus abdominis plane may be employed to control these painful conditions. The possibility of hybrid targets and smaller self-contained peripheral nerve stimulation leads should be entertained in future studies.

19.6 Supplemental Images

See Figs. 19.3, 19.4, 19.5, and 19.6.

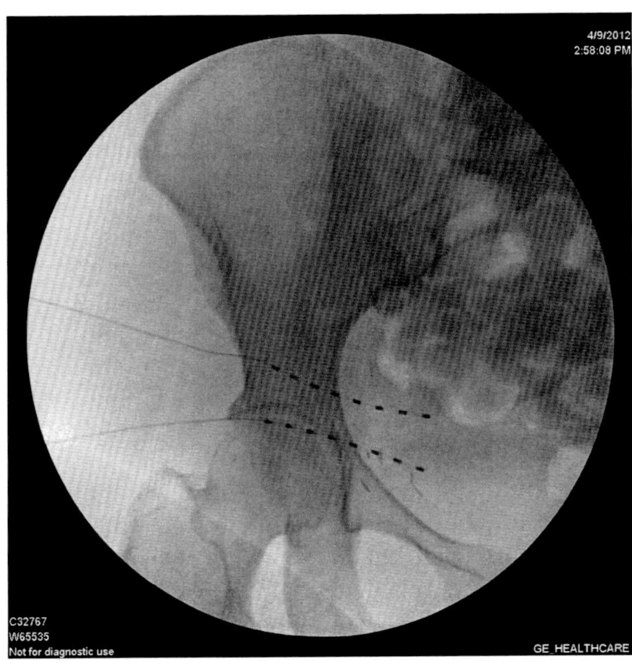

Fig. 19.3 Abdominal TAP stimulation, AP view

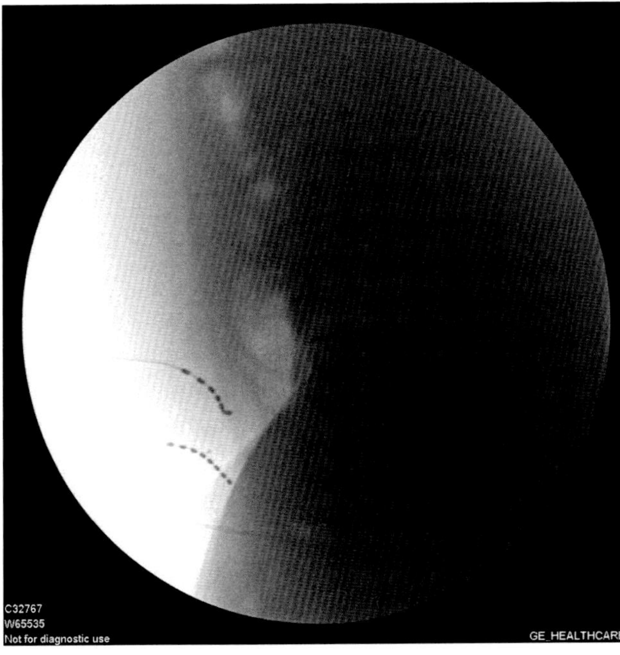

Fig. 19.4 Abdominal TAP stimulation, lateral view

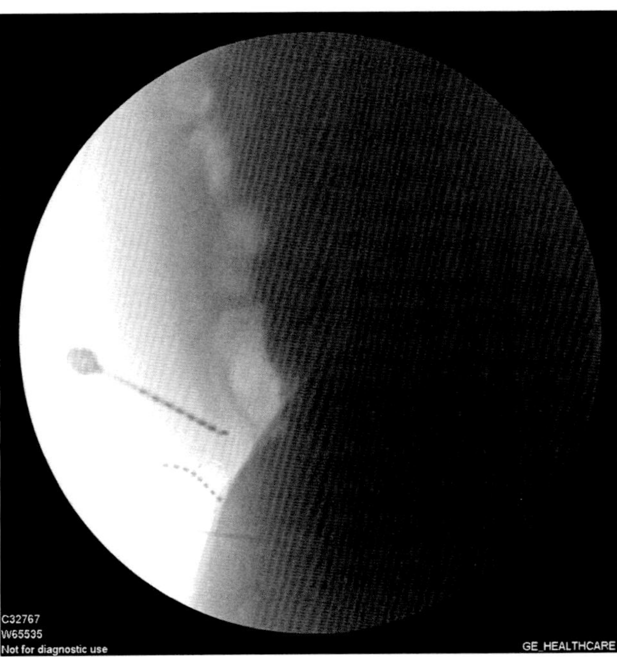

Fig. 19.5 Abdominal TAP stimulation, lateral view with needle

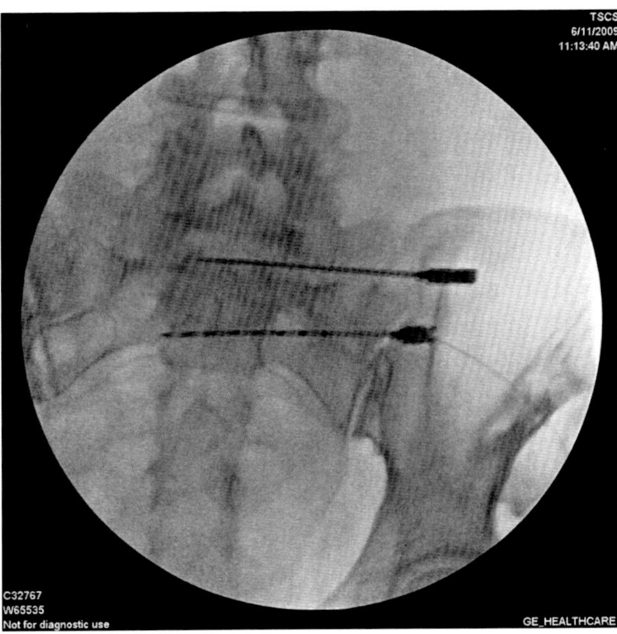

Fig. 19.6 TAP stimulation, AP view with needles

References

1. Rafi AN. Abdominal field block: a new approach via the lumbar triangle. Anaesthesia. 2001;56:1024–6.
2. Kapural L, Deer T, Yakovlev A, Bensitel T, Hayek S, et al. Technical aspects of spinal cord stimulation for managing chronic visceral abdominal pain: the results from the national survey. Pain Med. 2010;11(5):685–91.

Suggested Reading

Deer TR, Pope JE. A novel method of peripheral nerve stimulation: the tripole technique for treatment of refractory chronic intercostal nerve pain. Pain Med News. 2012;10:8–10.

Deer TR, Pope JE, Kaplan M. A novel method of neurostimulation of the peripheral nervous system: the StimRouter implantable device. Pain Manage. 2012;16:113–7.

Niraj G, Kelkar A, Powell R. Ultrasound-guided subcostal transversus abdominis plane block. Int J Ultrasound Appl Technolo Perioper Care. 2010;1:9–12.

Petersen PL, Mathiesen O, Torup H, Dahl JB. The transversus abdominis plane block: a valuable option for postoperative analgesia? A topical review. Acta Anaesthesiol Scand. 2010;54:529–35.

Wiisanen M, Hartwig JW. Transversus abdominis plane block. Medscape. http://emedicine.medscape.com/article/2000944-overview.

20 Electromyographic/Somatosensory-Evoked Potential Monitoring During Thoracolumbar Spinal Cord Stimulation

Erich O. Richter, Marina V. Abramova, Darnell Josiah, and Kenneth M. Aló

20.1 General Uses of Neurological Monitoring in Spine Surgery

Intraoperative neurophysiological monitoring has become a routine procedure in complex spine surgery. Somatosensory-evoked potential (SSEP) recording has been advocated to monitor the functional integrity of the nervous system during surgical manipulation [1–4]. When stimulated, sensory afferents give rise to signals carried via the dorsal columns (DCs) within the spinal cord to the medial lemniscus and spinocerebellar tracts, ending in the primary somatosensory cortex [5]. SSEP monitoring does not involve the motor pathways, which in some clinical situations can lead to false-negative results and postoperative neurological deficits undetected intraoperatively [6–12]. Dermatomal SSEP testing allows for assessment of individual nerve roots during surgery and has been shown to be more sensitive [11, 13]. However, the sensitivity and specificity of this method varies and is inferior to electromyographic (EMG) monitoring [13–15]. EMG has become the standard of practice in complex spine surgery, providing surgeons with accurate feedback about individual nerve root activity during surgical manipulation of neural structures and the presence of malpositioned screws [12, 16–19].

E.O. Richter (✉) • D. Josiah, MD
Department of Neurosurgery, West Virginia University Hospitals, PO Box 9183, Morgantown, WV 26506, USA
e-mail: eorichter@hsc.wvu.edu; djosiah@hsc.wvu.edu

M.V. Abramova
Department of Neurosurgery, Louisiana State University Health Sciences Center, New Orleans, LA 70112, USA
e-mail: mva774@yahoo.com

K.M. Aló
The Methodist Hospital Research Institute, 5318 Weslayan #182, Houston, TX 77005, USA
e-mail: aglioolio@gmail.com

T.R. Deer, J.E. Pope (eds.), *Atlas of Implantable Therapies for Pain Management*, DOI 10.1007/978-1-4939-2110-2_20

20.2 Neurological Testing to Implant Spinal Cord Stimulation Devices

We devote this chapter to a technique that allows the comfort and safety of general anesthetic while determining the physiological midline (PM) by objective neurophysiological testing [20, 21].

The identification of PM using evoked potentials was introduced by Claudio Feler, who obtained a patent for a device to perform the mapping [US 6,027,456]. Although the device did not gain widespread usage, a few centers adopted this methodology using standard intraoperative electrophysiological monitoring equipment. To obtain the optimal coverage over painful areas, two major criteria must be met: the applied stimulation should be positioned longitudinally along the DC and the PM must be identified. When general anesthesia is used, intraoperative neurophysiological monitoring with evoked potentials becomes the only way to determine the PM. Stimulation of various portions of the dorsal spinal cord produces paresthesia in a given distribution in the awake patient and produces a reliable pattern of SSEPs and motor unit action potentials (MUAPs) of the EMG in the patient under anesthesia. In addition, the output data may include interpolations between specific measured points for optimal assessment of applied stimulation between evaluated lateral positions [US 6,027,456].

These fundamental findings have been implemented in practice by the senior author (KA) who began using this approach in 1999, noting a marked outcome improvement over the previous fluoroscopically guided technique. In this technique MUAPs via EMG activation are used to determine the PM by examining the symmetry of the evoked potentials with presumed midline stimulation. In addition it became clear that objective MUAPs via EMG activation of specific muscles corresponded with postoperative induced paresthesia in particular regions depending on laminectomy level. For example, EMG activation of the external oblique muscle from a T9 to T10 thoracic paddle consistently correlates with low back paresthesia (Fig. 20.1). These correlations are summarized in Table 20.1. These concepts can be readily employed as a basis for cervical and sacral placement of electrodes. The application of EMG/SSEP for cervical and sacral spinal cord stimulation (SCS) is further explored in later chapters.

The general concept of using intraoperative EMG in the placement of the SCS on the PM of the spinal cord is similar with respect to the two- and three-column paddle configuration and differs in terms of whether the "expected" pattern should be symmetrical (the middle column of a three-column array) or "equally asymmetrical" (a two-column array). We have just begun PM evaluation with this technique using the newest five-column array (Penta, St. Jude Medical, Plano, TX).

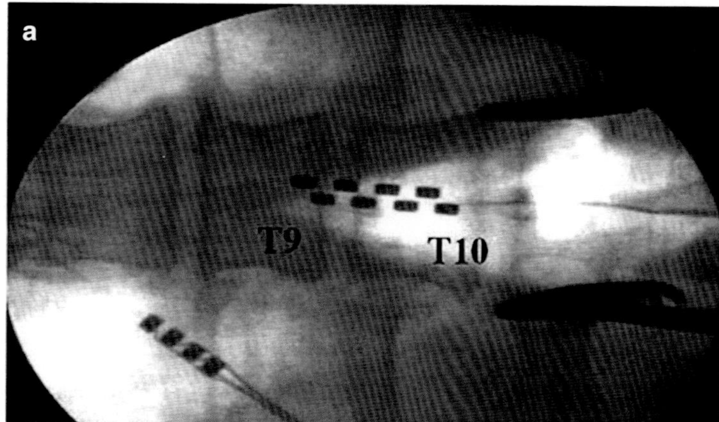

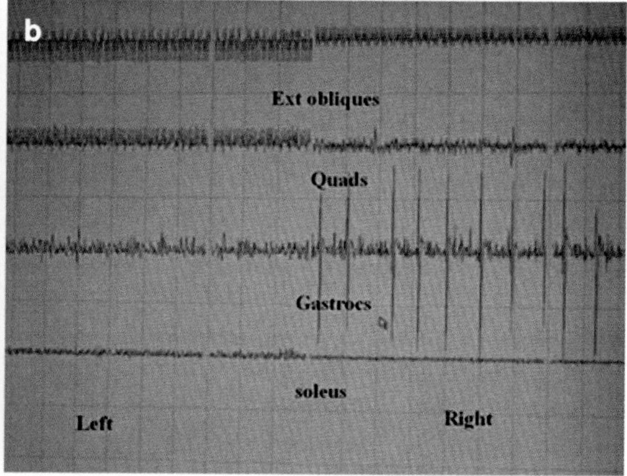

Fig. 20.1 Intraoperative view of thoracic paddle lead implantation. (**a**) The electrode is behind the body of T9 and T10. Stimulation is right sided with the cathode at the second position and the anode at the third. (**b**) With right-sided stimulation, there is right-side gastrocnemius activation, which will correlate with an S1 dermatomal paresthesia

Table 20.1 Correlations between EMG activation of specific muscles with postoperative induced paresthesia—thoracic paddle electrode at T9–10 (laminectomy T10–11)

EMG activation, muscle group	Induced paresthesia
External oblique	Low back
Tibialis anterior	L4
Vastus lateralis	L5
Gastrocnemius	S1

20.3 Technique of Midline Positioning of the Spinal Cord Stimulator: Tripolar Paddle

Once the three-column paddle (Fig. 20.2) is placed in the dorsal epidural space, the superior midline contact is stimulated at minimal settings and the EMG trace recording associated with the dermatomal level of stimulation is monitored. The stimulus intensity is gradually increased until MUAPs are seen on EMG. The lowest stimulus intensity needed to elicit a motor response is referred to as the threshold stimulus. MUAPs will be seen bilaterally at the threshold stimulus if the midline contact of the SCS is in line with the PM of the spinal cord. If MUAPs are seen unilaterally, the threshold intensity for that side is recorded and the stimulus is further increased to elicit a response on the other side. A difference in threshold stimulus intensity between the left and the right sides indicates that the SCS is lateral to the PM. Medial/lateral repositioning of the SCS is only necessary, however, if the difference in threshold intensity between the two sides is greater than 2 mA. In this case the paddle may not be perfectly flat on the lateral x-ray (Fig. 20.3a), thus dissection of the lateral recesses or proximal/superior lamina is further performed until the electrode is perfectly aligned with vertebrae on a lateral view (Fig. 20.3b). This ensures optimal electrode column symmetry and programmability relative to the PM. Of course, as a last resort, the laminotomy can be extended to a full laminectomy to allow perfect alignment of the paddle on the PM. In this case tissue must typically be identified to suture the electrode in place to prevent migration. These tenants hold true for all paddle (one-, two-, three- and five-column) array configurations.

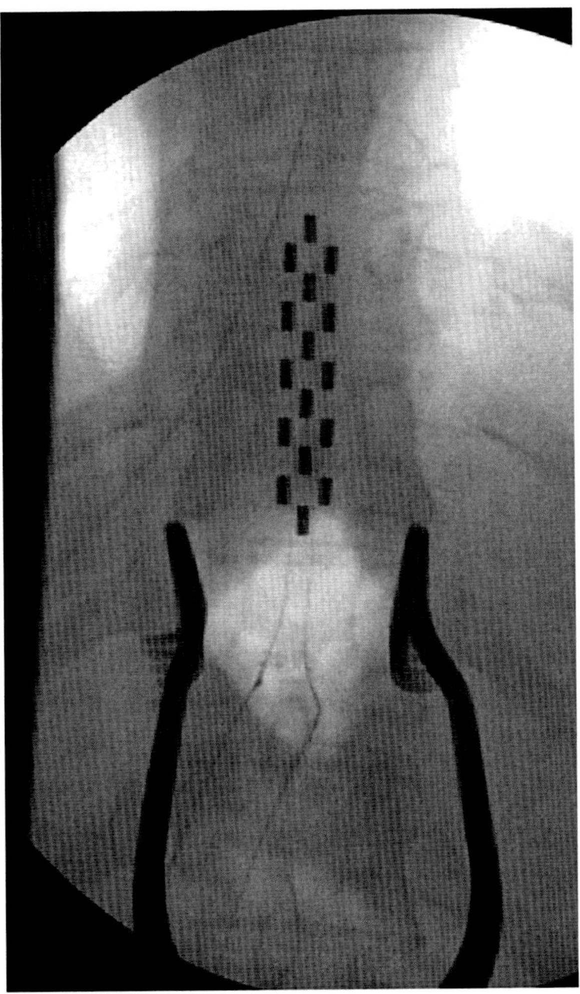

Fig. 20.2 Intraoperative image of initial placement of a three-column paddle electrode. Self-retaining retractors are seen providing exposure. The middle column of the paddle lies under the image of the spinous processes, and the array is relatively symmetrical with respect to the pedicles. This is a reasonable starting position to begin physiological mapping

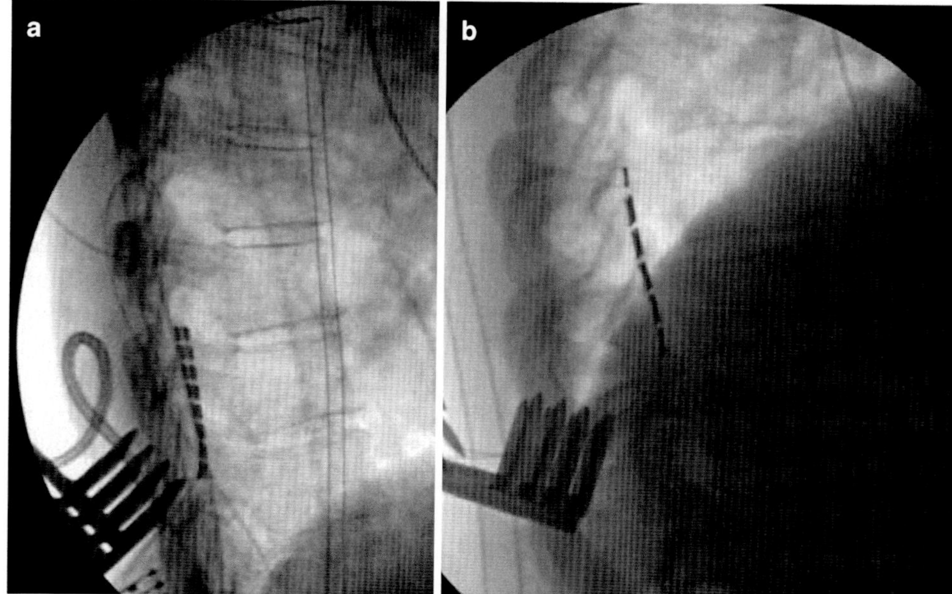

Fig. 20.3 Lateral intraoperative views. (**a**) Lead placed off the midline. (**b**) Perfect alignment on the midline

20.4 New Frontiers of Intraoperative EMG Application

There appears to be a correlation between the muscles with objective EMG activation during intraoperative monitoring and the subjective paresthesia obtained postoperatively as described in Table 13.1. Thus this may be explored to generate a precise model of paresthesia coverage and create a functional dermatomal mapping of perceived stimulation threshold after the surgery. Furthermore the EMG activation threshold may be a reliable predictor of the patient's perceived paresthesia threshold. It has been the author's experience that EMG activation correlated with pain control at amplitudes lower than the paresthesia threshold (i.e., subthreshold stimulation) and that occasionally persistent EMG activation intra- and postoperatively may be seen lasting as long as 15 min after the stimulation is discontinued. These patients typically respond extremely well to the stimulation therapy. It seems likely that these patients are the occasional patients who use their stimulation only intermittently, often having effective long-term pain relief while using their system only for a portion of each day.

Conclusions

EMG and SSEP monitoring are well-accepted modalities of neurophysiological testing in traditional spine surgery, but their application relative to implantation of neuromodulatory systems, in particular epidural paddle electrode systems, is comparatively new. Given the limitations associated with other methods of implantation, however, we expect that the techniques described in this chapter will continue to gain acceptance and improve outcomes by objectively localizing neurophysiological stimulation targets.

References

1. Mostegl A, Bauer R. The application of somatosensory-evoked potentials in orthopedic spine surgery. Arch Orthop Trauma Surg. 1984;103:179–84.
2. Spielholz NI, Benjamin MV, Engler GL, Ransohoff J. Somatosensory evoked potentials during decompression and stabilization of the spine. Methods and findings. Spine (Phila Pa 1976). 1979;4:500–5.
3. Ryan TP, Britt RH. Spinal and cortical somatosensory evoked potential monitoring during corrective spinal surgery with 108 patients. Spine (Phila Pa 1976) . 1986;11:352–61.
4. Perlik SJ, Van Egeren R, Fisher MA. Somatosensory evoked potential surgical monitoring. Observations during combined isoflurane-nitrous oxide anesthesia. Spine(Phila Pa 1976). 1992;17:273–6.
5. Ryu H, Uemura K. Origins of the short latency somatosensory evoked potentials in cat—with special reference to the sensory relay nuclei. Exp Neurol. 1988;102:177–84.
6. Ben-David B, Haller G, Taylor P. Anterior spinal fusion complicated by paraplegia. A case report of a false negative somatosensory-evoked potential. Spine (Phila Pa 1976). 1987;12:536–9.
7. Ben-David B, Taylor PD, Haller GS. Posterior spinal fusion complicated by posterior column injury. A case report of a false-negative wake-up test. Spine(Phila Pa 1976). 1987;12:540–3.
8. Wagner W, Peghini-Halbig L, Maurer JC, Perneczky A. Intraoperative SEP monitoring in neurosurgery around the brain stem and cervical spinal cord: differential recording of subcortical components. J Neurosurg. 1994;81:213–20.
9. Dunne JW, Silbert PL, Wren M. A prospective study of acute radiculopathy after scoliosis surgery. Clin Exp Neurol. 1991;28:180–90.
10. Meyer Jr PR, Cotler HB, Gireesan GT. Operative neurological complications resulting from thoracic and lumbar spine internal fixation. Clin Orthop Relat Res. 1988;237:125–31.
11. Toleikis JR, Carlvin AO, Shapiro DE, Schafer MF. The use of dermatomal evoked responses during surgical procedures that use intrapedicular fixation of the lumbosacral spine. Spine(Phila Pa 1976). 1993;18:2401–7.
12. Holland NR, Kostuik JP. Continuous electromyographic monitoring to detect nerve root injury during thoracolumbar scoliosis surgery. Spine(Phila Pa 1976). 1997;22:2547–50.
13. Owen JH, Padberg AM, Spahr-Holland L, Bridwell KH, Keppler L, Steffee AD. Clinical correlation between degenerative spine disease and dermatomal somatosensory-evoked potentials in humans. Spine(Phila Pa 1976). 1991;16(6 Suppl):S201–5.
14. Rodriquez AA, Kanis L, Rodriquez AA, Lane D. Somatosensory evoked potentials from dermatomal stimulation as an indicator of L5 and S1 radiculopathy. Arch Phys Med Rehabil. 1987;68:366–8.
15. Yazicioğlu K, Ozgul A, Kalyon TA, Gündüz S, Arpacioğlu O, Bilgic F. The diagnostic value of dermatomal somatosensory evoked potentials in lumbosacral disc herniations: a critical approach. Electromyogr Clin Neurophysiol. 1999;39:175–81.
16. Bose B, Wierzbowski LR, Sestokas AK. Neurophysiologic monitoring of spinal nerve root function during instrumented posterior lumbar spine surgery. Spine(Phila Pa 1976). 2002;27:1444–50.
17. Weiss DS. Spinal cord and nerve root monitoring during surgical treatment of lumbar stenosis [review]. Clin Orthop Relat Res. 2001;384:82–100.
18. Beatty RM, McGuire P, Moroney JM, Holladay FP. Continuous intraoperative electromyographic recording during spinal surgery. J Neurosurg. 1995;82:401–5.
19. Owen JH, Kostuik JP, Gornet M, et al. The use of mechanically elicited electromyograms to protect nerve roots during surgery for spinal degeneration. Spine (Phila Pa 1976). 1994;19:1704–10.
20. Parker SL, Amin AG, Farber SH, et al. Ability of electromyographic monitoring to determine the presence of malpositioned pedicle screws in the lumbosacral spine: analysis of 2450 consecutively placed screws. J Neurosurg Spine. 2011;15:130–5.
21. Kumar K, Lind G, Winter J, et al. Spinal cord stimulation: placement of surgical leads via laminotomy-techniques and benefits (Aló KM. EMG/SSEP during SCS implant surgery). In: Krames E, Peckham PH, Rezai AR, editors. Neuromodulation. Amsterdam: Elsevier; 2009. p. 1008–9.

Suggested Reading

Aló KM, Holsheimer J. New trends in neuromodulation for the management of neuropathic pain [review]. Neurosurgery. 2002;50:690–703; discussion 703–4.

Boswell MV, Iacono RP, Guthkelch AN. Sites of action of subarachnoid lidocaine and tetracaine: observations with evoked potential monitoring during spinal cord stimulator implantation. Reg Anesth. 1992;17:37–42.

Holsheimer J, Barolat G, Struijk JJ, He J. Significance of the spinal cord position in spinal cord stimulation. Acta Neurochir Suppl. 1995;64:119–24.

Holsheimer J, den Boer JA, Struijk JJ, Rozeboom AR. MR assessment of the normal position of the spinal cord in the spinal canal. AJNR Am J Neuroradiol. 1994;15:951–9.

Kleissen RF, Buurke JH, Harlaar J, Zilvold G. Electromyography in the biomechanical analysis of human movement and its clinical application. Gait Posture. 1998;8:143–58.

Kumar K, Hunter G, Demeria D. Spinal cord stimulation in treatment of chronic benign pain: challenges in treatment planning and present status, a 22-year experience. Neurosurgery. 2006;58:481–96; discussion 481–96.

Kumar K, Malik S, Demeria D. Treatment of chronic pain with spinal cord stimulation versus alternative therapies: cost-effectiveness analysis. Neurosurgery. 2002;51:106–15; discussion 115–6.

Kumar K, Taylor RS, Jacques L, et al. The effects of spinal cord stimulation in neuropathic pain are sustained: a 24-month follow-up of the prospective randomized controlled multicenter trial of the effectiveness of spinal cord stimulation. Neurosurgery. 2008;63:762–70; discussion 770.

Kumar K, Taylor RS, Jacques L, et al. Spinal cord stimulation versus conventional medical management for neuropathic pain: a multicentre randomized controlled trial in patients with failed back surgery syndrome. Pain. 2007;132:179–88.

Lang E, Krainick JU, Gerbershagen HU. Spinal cord transmission of impulses during high spinal anesthesia as measured by cortical evoked potentials. Anesth Analg. 1989;69:15–20.

Law J. Results of treatment for pain by percutaneous multicontact stimulation of the spinal cord. Paper presented at the annual meeting of the American Pain Society, Chicago, 11–13 Nov 1983.

Melzack R, Wall PD. Pain mechanisms: a new theory [review]. Science. 1965;150:971–9.

North RB, Fischell TA, Long DM. Chronic stimulation via percutaneously inserted epidural electrodes. Neurosurgery. 1977;1:215–8.

North RB, Kidd D, Shipley J, Taylor RS. Spinal cord stimulation versus reoperation for failed back surgery syndrome: a cost effectiveness and cost utility analysis based on a randomized, controlled trial. Neurosurgery. 2007;61:361–8; discussion 368–9. Erratum in: Neurosurgery. 2009;64:601.

Racz GB, McCarron RF, Talboys P. Percutaneous dorsal column stimulator for chronic pain control. Spine(Phila Pa 1976). 1989;14:1–4.

Richardson J. Facilitation of spinal cord stimulator implantation with epidural analgesia. Pain. 1996;65:277–8.

Shealy CN, Mortimer JT, Reswick JB. Electrical inhibition of pain by stimulation of the dorsal columns: preliminary clinical report. Anesth Analg. 1967;46:489–91.

Spiegelmann R, Friedman WA. Spinal cord stimulation: a contemporary series [review]. Neurosurgery. 1991;28:65–70; discussion 70–1.

Taylor RJ, Taylor RS. Spinal cord stimulation for failed back surgery syndrome: a decision-analytic model and cost-effectiveness analysis. Int J Technol Assess Health Care. 2005;21:351–8.

Taylor RS. Spinal cord stimulation in complex regional pain syndrome and refractory neuropathic back and leg pain/failed back surgery syndrome: results of a systematic review and meta-analysis [review]. J Pain Symptom Manage. 2006;31(4 Suppl):S13–9.

Taylor RS, Van Buyten JP, Buchser E. Spinal cord stimulation for complex regional pain syndrome: a systematic review of the clinical and cost-effectiveness literature and assessment of prognostic factors [review]. Eur J Pain. 2006;10(2):91–101.

Villavicencio AT, Leveque JC, Rubin L, Bulsara K, Gorecki JP. Laminectomy versus percutaneous electrode placement for spinal cord stimulation. Neurosurgery. 2000;46:399–405; discussion 405–6.

Washburn S, Monroe CD, Cameron T. A review of articles published on spinal cord stimulation treatment for chronic pain: 1981–2008. NANS meeting, Las Vegas, 4–7 Dec 2008.

21 Electromyographic/Somatosensory Evoked Potential Monitoring During Sacral Neuromodulation

Erich O. Richter, Marina V. Abramova, Darnell Josiah, and Kenneth M. Aló

21.1 Introduction

Sacral root neuromodulation has been employed for the treatment of idiopathic overactive bladder, fecal incontinence, urgency-frequency syndromes, interstitial cystitis, pudendal neuralgia, vulvodynia, coccygodynia, and a variety of chronic pelvic pain (CPP) syndromes [1–13]. A direct, single root stimulation device received U.S. Food and Drug Administration (FDA) approval for the treatment of urinary urgency and frequency, urinary incontinence in 1997, and urinary retention in 1999 [6], but many centers have had more success with retrograde longitudinal placement within the spinal canal. The ventral rami of S2–4 provide innervation of the pelvis. The S3 sacral level contributes to the innervation of the anterior perineal muscles [14], making it the most frequent target in treatment of pelvic dysfunction and a typical target for the single root percutaneous device. These portions of the nervous system have traditionally been very difficult to target with traditional methods over the dorsal columns in the spinal cord. The conus medullaris is a highly mobile structure, which is nearly enveloped in the nerve roots of the cauda equina. Accordingly, placement of epidural stimulating electrodes over the conus has traditionally been plagued by extreme variability in the effects of stimulation, not only from patient to patient but also in the same patient over time. At the conus level, the dorsal cerebrospinal fluid layer is relatively thick and serves as an insulator for the spinal cord; the conus is very mobile, which increases the risk of lead migration, and finally, owing to the presence of large afferent fibers, the sacral stimulation may produce undesired paresthesia in additional regions [14].

Intraoperative neurophysiological monitoring with somatosensory-evoked potential (SSEP) and electromyographic (EMG) monitoring are widely used in traditional spinal neurosurgery [14–25]. In this chapter, we focus on the use of neuromonitoring techniques for placement of sacral root stimulation electrodes. These techniques of implantation are specific to the anatomy of sacral root stimulator implantation within the epidural space of the spinal canal and are not specific to the clinical indication for the electrode placement, although the targeting of individual electrodes will have characteristic patterns for each disorder. The radiology of the sacral region is often difficult to reliably interpret, and the depth of muscle dissection to approach the lumbosacral junction makes direct surgical approaches under strict local anesthetics impractical at most centers. Accordingly, techniques to reliably identify the stimulation of individual sacral nerve roots by neurophysiological methods in a patient under general anesthetic are particularly helpful.

E.O. Richter (✉) • D. Josiah, MD
Department of Neurosurgery, West Virginia University Hospitals, PO Box 9183, Morgantown, WV 26506, USA
e-mail: eorichter@hsc.wvu.edu; djosiah@hsc.wvu.edu

M.V. Abramova
Department of Neurosurgery, Louisiana State University Health Sciences Center, New Orleans, LA 70112, USA
e-mail: mva774@yahoo.com

K.M. Aló
The Methodist Hospital Research Institute, 5318 Weslayan #182, Houston, TX 77005, USA
e-mail: aglioolio@gmail.com

T.R. Deer, J.E. Pope (eds.), *Atlas of Implantable Therapies for Pain Management*, DOI 10.1007/978-1-4939-2110-2_21

21.2 Technical Overview

21.2.1 Technique for Sacral Placement

Stimulation of multiple specific nerve roots of the cauda equine is best accomplished through an intraspinal, epidural, "retrograde" technique. The details of retrograde access have been addressed in other publications [1–13]. In this chapter, we focus on the use of intraoperative monitoring techniques to verify effective placement [26]. Most centers place temporary trial electrodes with the patient awake under local anesthetic, and accordingly, these techniques are seldom used for trial implantations. For open placement of permanent electrodes, the patient is positioned prone, on some form of soft support that allows the abdomen to remain free of compression to minimize epidural bleeding. We use gel chest rolls, but some centers use the Wilson frame or similar equipment. It is critical that whatever equipment is used not obstruct the ability to obtain high-quality fluoroscopic visualization from all angles. In the direct open approach, the lumbosacral junction is identified on lateral imaging, and a midline incision is used to create a subperiosteal dissection to expose the superior edge of the S1 lamina, and the L5–S1 interspace. The ligamentum flavum is released from the S1 lamina, and frequently a small laminotomy is created to define these planes and expose the dura. A small, blunt, angled dissector is used to free the initial portion of the epidural space, and then a single-column electrode is passed into the epidural space and turned laterally toward the foramen of interest distally, usually the S2 or S3 foramen. The marked angle of the sacral canal back toward the surgeon can make this placement difficult, and a curved instrument such as a Penfield #3 is often indispensable in helping the electrode transition into an appropriate trajectory (Fig. 21.1). The Penfield is placed into the epidural space, and the single-column paddle is passed over it and directed by it into the epidural space.

For pelvic pain, the electrode is typically rotated off the midline toward the S2 foramen. For coccygodynia it generally remains midline, but stops at the S3 level (more caudal placements frequently produce painful stimulation). Other disorders may require other targeting. When the electrodes appear appropriately positioned on anteroposterior and lateral fluoroscopy, attention is turned to the physiological assessment of electrode position. When the nerve roots are stimulated, SSEP or motor unit action potentials (MUAPs) via EMG serve as the main monitoring tool used to verify accurate position of the electrodes over the roots of interest. The dermatomal distribution of postoperative paresthesia can be predicted from the pattern of intraoperative stimulation activation and is clearly associated with the specific pattern of responses coming from the muscles of the lower extremities. For example, the placement of an S2–3 paddle may result in EMG activation in adductor hallucis muscle (Fig. 21.2), which will correlate with an S2–3 paresthesia. The typical correlation pattern between muscles in the lower extremity and induced postoperative paresthesia is represented in Table 21.1.

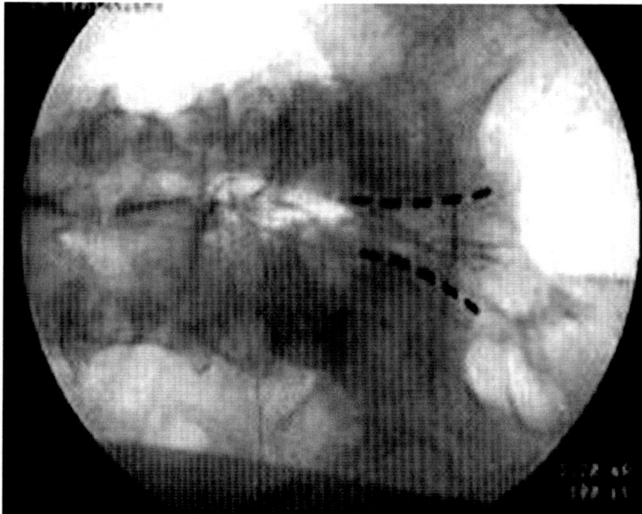

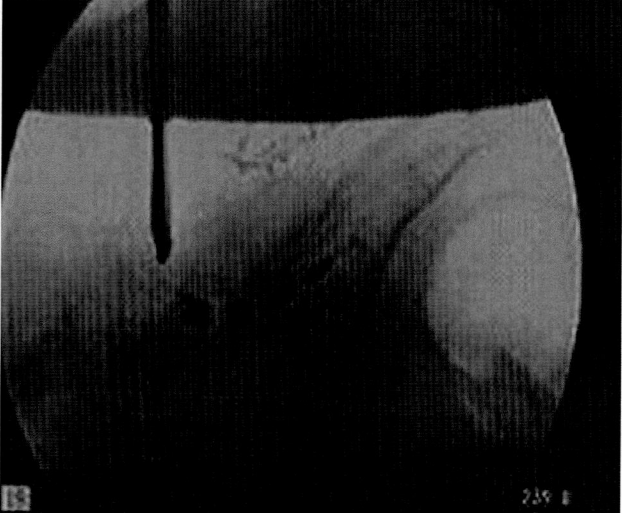

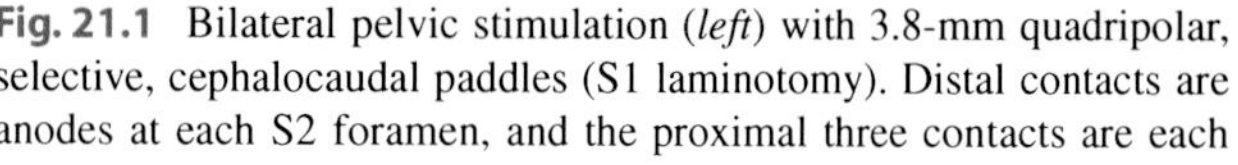

Fig. 21.1 Bilateral pelvic stimulation (*left*) with 3.8-mm quadripolar, selective, cephalocaudal paddles (S1 laminotomy). Distal contacts are anodes at each S2 foramen, and the proximal three contacts are each cathodes. Lateral radiograph (*right*). Penfield 3 elevating tool assisting with placement of 3.8-mm paddles toward the S2 foramen

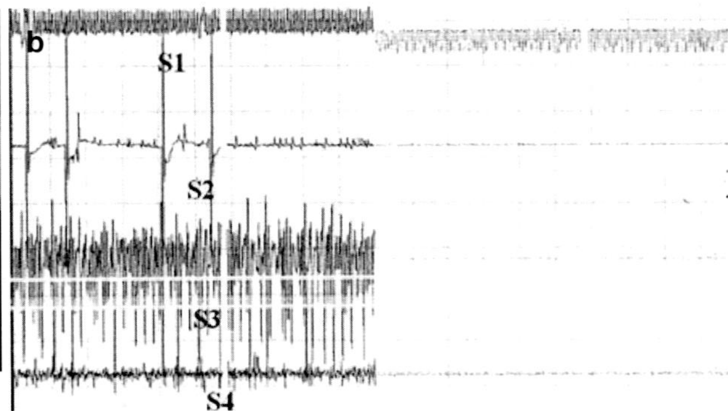

Fig. 21.2 Permanent retrograde implantation of sacral root paddle leads. Stimulation is left sided, with the cathode at the second position and the anode at the third (*left*). In this older tracing (*right*), the stimulation in the second left contact produces primarily adductor hallucis activation, solely on the left side (**a**). This correlated with the postoperative paresthesia felt in the S3 perineal region (**b**)

Table 21.1 Correlation between EMG activation of specific muscles with postoperative-induced paresthesia-sacral paddle(s) S2–3 (laminectomy S1)

EMG Activation, Muscle Group	Induced paresthesia
Gastrocnemius	S1 (undesired)
Adductor hallucis	S2–3
Perianal	S4

Conclusions

With the accumulation of knowledge and experience on intraoperative neuromonitoring with SSEP and EMG techniques, new applications such as intraoperative verification of neuromodulatory electrode placement under general anesthesia have emerged. In this chapter, we have reviewed the use of such techniques to determine effective stimulation of individual sacral roots when placing electrodes in the intraspinal, epidural space from a retrograde or open approach. As an objective method SSEP/EMG monitoring is an attractive alternative to awake methods in open cases owing to the significant muscle mass at the lumbosacral junction, which makes such awake cases quite uncomfortable and relatively impractical. With the increasing prominence of sacral root neuromodulation as an important treatment modality across a number of prevalent conditions, we expect that these techniques will become more widespread over coming years.

References

1. Aló KM, Feler CA, Whitworth L. Long-term follow-up of selective nerve root stimulation for interstitial cystitis: review of results. In: Abstracts of the World Pain Meeting 2000, San Francisco, July 2000.
2. Aló KM, McKay E. Selective nerve root stimulation (SNRS) for the treatment of intractable pelvic pain and motor dysfunction: a case report. Neuromodulation. 2001;4:19–23.
3. Aló KM, McKay E. Sacral nerve root stimulation for the treatment of intractable pelvic pain: clinical experience. In: De Andres J, editor. Bound version proceedings Puesta Al Dia En Anestesia Regional Y Tratamiento Del Dolor, vol. VI. 2003. p. 247–51.
4. Aló KM, McKay E. Sacral nerve root stimulation for the treatment of urge incontinence and detrusor dysfunction utilizing a cephalocaudal intraspinal method of lead insertion: a case report. In: De Andres J, editor. Bound version proceedings Puesta Al Dia En Anestesia Regional Y Tratamiento Del Dolor, vol. VI. 2003. p. 251–6.
5. Feler CA, Whitworth LA, Brookoff D, Powell R. Recent advances: sacral nerve root stimulation using a retrograde method of lead insertion for the treatment of pelvic pain due to interstitial cystitis. Neuromodulation. 1999;2:211–6.
6. Kohli N, Rosenblatt PL. Neuromodulation techniques for the treatment of the overactive bladder [review]. Clin Obstet Gynecol. 2002;45:218–32.
7. Sherman ND, Amundsen CL. Current and future techniques of neuromodulation for bladder dysfunction [review]. Curr Urol Rep. 2007;8:448–54.
8. Steinberg AC, Oyama IA, Whitmore KE. Bilateral S3 stimulator in patients with interstitial cystitis. Urology. 2007;69:441–3.
9. Whitmore KE, Payne CK, Diokno AC, Lukban JC. Sacral neuromodulation in patients with interstitial cystitis: a multicenter clinical trial. Int Urogynecol J Pelvic Floor Dysfunct. 2003;14:305–8; discussion 308–9.
10. Ramsay LB, Wright Jr J, Fischer JR. Sacral neuromodulation in the treatment of vulvar vestibulitis syndrome. Obstet Gynecol. 2009;114:487–9.
11. Kothari S. Neuromodulatory approaches to chronic pelvic pain and coccygodynia. Acta Neurochir Suppl. 2007;97:365–71.
12. Aló KM, Gohel R, Corey CL. Sacral nerve root stimulation for the treatment of urge incontinence and detrusor dysfunction utilizing a cephalocaudal intraspinal method of lead insertion: a case report. Neuromodulation. 2001;4:53–8.
13. Iachetta RP, Cola A, Villani RD. Sacral nerve stimulation in the treatment of fecal incontinence—the experience of a pelvic floor center: short term results. J Interv Gastroenterol. 2012;2:189–92.
14. Feler CA, Whitworth LA, Fernandez J. Sacral neuromodulation for chronic pain conditions. Anesthesiol Clin North America. 2003;21:785–95.
15. Bose B, Wierzbowski LR, Sestokas AK. Neurophysiologic monitoring of spinal nerve root function during instrumented posterior lumbar spine surgery. Spine (Phila Pa 1976). 2002;27:1444–50.
16. Weiss DS. Spinal cord and nerve root monitoring during surgical treatment of lumbar stenosis [review]. Clin Orthop Relat Res. 2001;384:82–100.
17. Holland NR, Kostuik JP. Continuous electromyographic monitoring to detect nerve root injury during thoracolumbar scoliosis surgery. Spine(Phila Pa 1976). 1997;22:2547–50.
18. Beatty RM, McGuire P, Moroney JM, Holladay FP. Continuous intraoperative electromyographic recording during spinal surgery. J Neurosurg. 1995;82:401–5.
19. Owen JH, Kostuik JP, Gornet M, et al. The use of mechanically elicited electromyograms to protect nerve roots during surgery for spinal degeneration. Spine(Phila Pa 1976). 1994;19:1704–10.
20. Mostegl A, Bauer R. The application of somatosensory-evoked potentials in orthopedic spine surgery. Arch Orthop Trauma Surg. 1984;103:179–84.
21. Spielholz NI, Benjamin MV, Engler GL, Ransohoff J. Somatosensory evoked potentials during decompression and stabilization of the spine. Methods and findings. Spine(Phila Pa 1976). 1979;4:500–5.
22. Ryan TP, Britt RH. Spinal and cortical somatosensory evoked potential monitoring during corrective spinal surgery with 108 patients. Spine(Phila Pa 1976). 1986;11:352–61.
23. Parker SL, Amin AG, Farber SH, et al. Ability of electromyographic monitoring to determine the presence of malpositioned pedicle screws in the lumbosacral spine: analysis of 2450 consecutively placed screws. J Neurosurg Spine. 2011;15:130–5.
24. Yazicioglu K, Ozgul A, Kalyon TA, Gunduz S, Arpacioglu O, Bilgic F. The diagnostic value of dermatomal somatosensory evoked potentials in lumbosacral disc herniations: a critical approach. Electromyogr Clin Neurophysiol. 1999;39:175–81.
25. Perlik SJ, VanEgeren R, Fisher MA. Somatosensory evoked potential surgical monitoring. Observations during combined isoflurane-nitrous oxide anesthesia. Spine(Phila Pa 1976). 1992;17:273–6.
26. Aló KM. EMG/SSEP during SCS implant surgery. In: Chap: Kumar K, et al. Spinal cord stimulation: placement of surgical leads via laminotomy-techniques and benefits. In: Krames E, Peckham PH, Rezai AR, editors. Neuromodulation. San Diego: Academic; 2009. p. 1008–9.

The Future of Neurostimulation

22

Timothy R. Deer and Jimmy Mali

22.1 Introduction

Neuromodulation is an exciting field that will be an integral part of treatment of pain and other diseases going forward. The future of neuromodulation continues to evolve and expand in many areas, including the understanding of the underlying mechanisms of action and the potential role of digital medicine in treating chronic disease. In the past two decades, the technological advances in this field have been impressive, but a lack of financing and collaboration has made the march forward less notable than the progress in cardiovascular electrical therapy. Currently, the application of neuromodulation is still considered to be in its infancy, but the past few years have seen some major changes to the core of the field in hardware, software, and conceptual innovations. This atlas highlights many of those changes, focusing on the near future. The long-term future will depend on innovation, investment, governmental stability and oversight, and high-level evidence. Table 22.1 describes current technology innovations.

The humble beginnings of ancient civilizations utilizing the electrophysiology of fish in order to adjust afferent sensory input to the cortex of patients has now transformed into a field of science that is boundless. Applications are breaking away from theory and becoming the forefront of options for patients with complex pain diagnoses and other disease processes. This chapter focuses on the future of neuromodulation with respect to hardware and programming, neuroanatomical targets, and novel neuromodulation strategies.

T.R. Deer, MD (✉)
The Center for Pain Relief, 400 Court Street, Suite 100, Charleston, WV 25301, USA
e-mail: DocTDeer@aol.com

J. Mali
Department of Physical Medicine and Rehabilitation, University of North Carolina School of Medicine, Chapel Hill, NC, USA
e-mail: jmali.md@gmail.com

T.R. Deer, J.E. Pope (eds.), *Atlas of Implantable Therapies for Pain Management*, DOI 10.1007/978-1-4939-2110-2_22

22.2 Current and Short-Term Advances: Miniaturization

The size of the implantable programmable generator (IPG) has been a quandary for the device companies. Larger, bulky IPGs have a greater potential for longevity and enhanced battery capacity, but a large object in the subcutaneous tissues can produce pain and cosmetic problems.

Table 22.1 Innovations in spinal cord stimulation technology

Advancement	Current use	Future impact
Rechargeable IPG	Yes	Large
Enhanced battery life	No	Important for smaller IPG
Different targets	Yes	Important for DRG-SCS
Increased frequency	Yes	Makes miniaturization difficult
Bluetooth and microwave technology	Yes	Uncertain
Improved energy conduction in leads & materials	No	Uncertain
Remote energy delivery	No	In concept, very important
Enhanced spinal cord lead arrays and Artificial Intelligence programming	No	May be the next critical step

DRG dorsal root ganglia, *IPG* implantable programmable generator, *SCS* spinal cord stimulation

22.3 Modern Advances and Future Enhancements

22.3.1 Stimulation Frequency

For more than four decades, the current has been delivered to implants either as a constant current or a constant voltage mode with frequencies that are considered "low" or normal, unusually ranging from 30 to 100 Hz. In recent years, this situation has been an area of investigation. In the United States, investigators in an early pilot study found that stimulation at high frequencies of 10 kHz could improve pain without eliciting a paresthesia. This finding led to an interest in investigating a new mode of spinal cord stimulation (SCS), termed HF10, which has now advanced to approval in the European Union (EU) and Australia. Interesting evidence from multiple centers in those two regions have shown improvement in patients with axial back pain and failed back surgery. There has also been efficacy in patients who had earlier failed conventional frequency stimulation.

The lead placement for HF10 has been shown to be similar to that for conventional SCS. Because no paresthesia has been elicited, the trialing has the advantage of being efficient, but not being able to get immediate feedback from the patient is a disadvantage. Interestingly, the use of 5000 Hz in Switzerland was found not to create pain relief, as compared to sham stimulation. This finding suggests that a particular neurotransmission change may occur at 10 kHz that is unique to that frequency.

In the future, investigations may include ultra-high frequency (Ultra HF) or more research into the basic science of the effect of frequency on neural plasticity and neurotransmitters.

22.3.2 Waveform Delivery

Waveform Shape: In addition to innovations with frequency, new devices will have changes in the way waveforms are delivered. For decades, the traditional waveforms have been rectangular. These conventional waveforms have been used in all devices in the field, including those targeting deep brain, the vagal nerve, peripheral nerves, and the spinal cord.

Some new, non-rectangular waveforms have been investigated in recent years, including triangular waveforms and other novel attempts. Each of these has suggested an improvement in energy efficiency.

Waveform Programming: In recent years, work by De Ridder and others has led to an interest in the programming of the waveform. This work is seated in the neurophysiology of the brain and the "language of the brain" in regards to conventional tonic waveform delivery verses a focus on the "burst" delivery. This landmark work has been based on preliminary work by prominent neurophysiologists that suggested three types of neuronal communication in the brain: regular spiking, fast spiking, and bursting. The theory of burst stimulation involves changing current delivery to accommodate to these different brain nerve systems. In this mode, there is a 40 Hz burst mode with five spikes at 500 Hz per burst. The pulse width is fixed at 1 ms, with 1-ms interspike interval delivery. The delivery is in a constant current mode. This burst-type stimulation is free of paresthesia in over 85 % of patients and has shown statistically significant improvement in axial back pain when compared with conventional tonic stimulation. The ability to go back and forth from tonic SCS to burst SCS may lead to lower failure rates and improved long-term cost efficiency.

22.3.3 Closed-Loop Feedback Systems

The use of closed-loop neurostimulation has been studied in the treatment of seizure disorders, and now is being applied to SCS and the treatment of pain. These results have been promising and have shown improved efficacy and outcomes. In the treatment of pain, researchers in Australia have used closed-loop systems to provide internal stimulation feedback that may enable the system to change its programming and response automatically, thus improving outcomes, reducing system variability, and improving patient pain relief and satisfaction.

22.3.4 Material Engineering

An engineering focus going forward will be on the materials used for leads, contacts, and wiring. New design concepts have included micro-texturing and new metal use. Goals of this engineering include MRI compatibility, improved efficiency, and the ability to deliver more complex programming. Part of this materials engineering is also important for the ability to make more complex arrays while simultaneously limiting battery size and improving energy efficiency.

Table 22.2 Traditional and selected evolving targets for neurostimulation

Site	Clinical evidence	Used in clinical treatment
Dorsal columns	Strong	Yes
Peripheral nerve field	Evolving	Yes
Deep brain	Strong in Parkinson's	Yes
Motor cortex	Evolving	Investigational
Vagus nerve	Evolving	Yes
Dorsal root ganglion	Strong	Yes
Occipital nerve	Moderate and evolving	Yes
Supraorbital nerve	Evolving	Yes
Sphenopalatine ganglion	Evolving	Yes (investigational)
Tibial nerve	Evolving in incontinence	Investigational
Sacral nerves	Strong in incontinence	Yes
Hybrid: Epidural with PNfS	Evolving	Yes (investigational)

PNfS peripheral nerve field stimulation

22.3.5 Current and Future Neuroanatomical Targets

In the current field of neurostimulation, common targets are the dorsal columns of the spinal cord, the peripheral nerves, and the brain, with targets in the cortex, the thalamus, and other deep brain structures. Table 22.2 examines current targets and newly approved and clinically evolving targets.

22.3.5.1 Dorsal Root Ganglia

The dorsal root ganglia (DRG) is the primary anatomical structure for communicating primary afferent peripheral stimulus and transferring this stimulus to the higher pain centers. Many have called this spinal structure "the Grand Central Station" of the body in regard to pain transmission. Considering previous attempts at injecting the DRG, using pulsed radiofrequency, and stimulating the DRG with conventional leads, it is not surprising that SCS of this structure would lead to pain relief, but the ability to stimulate the DRG has been challenging. When previous attempts at stimulation failed, the reason was poorly understood. The DRG could not be stimulated with conventional SCS leads without capturing the nerve root, dorsal entry root zones, and motor fibers. The invention of a novel lead and delivery system tailored to deliver current specifically to the DRG led to success and the eventual approval of this therapy in the EU and Australia. Current studies are under way in the United States. The European and Australian experience suggests success with DRG-SCS in relieving pain in areas of the body where conventional SCS has failed in the past, including the groin, foot, chest wall, and axial back.

22.3.5.2 Vagus Nerve

Vagal nerve stimulation has been clinically utilized for the treatment of epilepsy and depression, and recently it has been studied for new indications. Interestingly, the possibility of treating headache has shown clinical promise. The common method of providing this therapy has been implantation of a device, but recent work on transcutaneous stimulation is evolving.

22.3.5.3 Occipital Nerve

Weiner first described stimulation of the occipital nerve for the treatment of pain in the head. This description led to work in the area of peripheral nerve stimulation (PNS) to treat headache and face pain and ushered in advancements in lead placement and programming. Experimental studies have been very promising in the areas of migraine, cluster headache, and C2 radiculitis. These studies have shown promise and have led to EU approval for migraine. In the United States, approval is pending, and it is hoped that approval soon will allow improved patient access.

22.3.5.4 Supraorbital Nerve

The supraorbital nerve is a target for stimulation in patients with severe pain of the face. This nerve, a branch of the ophthalmic division of the trigeminal nerve, is often a factor in cluster headaches, post–herpetic neuralgia neuritis, and frontal headaches. The use of combined PNS of the occipital nerve and the supraorbital nerve has been reported in severe headache treatment. The combination of these targets could be key in improving outcomes.

22.3.5.5 Sphenopalatine Ganglion

The sphenopalatine ganglion (SPG) is an extracranial structure in the pterygopalatine fossa. The role of this ganglion in pain causation and treatment has been debated; it may involve the parasympathetic nervous system.

Novel devices to treat headache disorders in which the SPG is involved may show promise. Much like the DRG-SCS system, treatment involving this complex target may require a specific device.

22.4 Thoughts About the Future

22.4.1 The Field of Neuromodulation

The use of neuromodulation will continue to grow and change the lives of many patients around the world. The goal of the International Neuromodulation Society is to enhance outcomes, improve patients' lives, and advance treatment for both pain and other disease states. A major 10-year goal identified in 2014 is the globalization of neuromodulation, to allow education and access in Third World nations, which have been underserved in this arena. This mission will be critical in enhancing the lives of millions and the well-being of humankind.

22.4.2 The Device of the Future for Pain

Table 22.3 lists some the features likely to be found on future devices for the management of pain.

Table 22.3 Features of future devices for management of pain

Feature	Availability
Positionality control	Current: DRG, HF, motion sensors
DRG targeting	Current: DRG-SCS
High frequency	Current: HF10
Bluetooth programming	Current
Microwave programming	Current
Burst stimulation	Current
MRI compatibility	Current
Percutaneous paddles	Current
Artificial Intelligence programming	5 years
Remote programming	Near future
Miniature generators	Continuing process
Genetic programming	Futuristic

DRG dorsal root ganglia, *HF* high frequency, *SCS* spinal cord stimulation

Suggested Reading

Cecchini AP, Mea E, Tullo V, Curone M, Franzini A, Broggi G, et al. Vagus nerve stimulation in drug-resistant daily chronic migraine with depression: preliminary data. Neurol Sci. 2009;30 Suppl 1:S101–4.

De Ridder D, Vanneste S, Plazier M, van der Loo E, Menovsky T. Burst spinal cord stimulation: toward paresthesia-free pain suppression. Neurosurgery. 2010;66:986–90.

Deer TR, Grigsby E, Weiner RL, Wilcosky B, Kramer JM. A prospective study of dorsal root ganglion stimulation for the relief of chronic pain. Neuromodulation. 2013;16:67–72.

Foutz TJ, McIntyre CC. Evaluation of novel stimulus waveforms for deep brain stimulation. J Neural Eng. 2010;7(6):066008.

Mauskop A. Vagus nerve stimulation relieves chronic refractory migraine and cluster headaches. Cephalalgia. 2005;25:82–6.

McJunkin T, Lynch P, Deer TR, Anderson J, Desai R. Regenerative medicine in pain management. Pain Med News. 2012;10:35–8.

Narouze S, Kapural L. Supraorbital nerve electric stimulation for the treatment of intractable chronic cluster headache: a case report. Headache. 2007;47:1100–2.

Rasche D, Tronnier V. Implementation of a new lead and stimulation device for spinal cord stimulation with MRI-safety-first implantation worldwide and initial clinical experience [Abstract]. Berlin: International Neuromodulation Society; 2013.

Tepper SJ, Rezai A, Narouze S, Steiner C, Mohajer P, Ansarinia M. Acute treatment of intractable migraine with sphenopalatine ganglion electrical stimulation. Headache. 2009;49:983–9.

Tiede J, Brown L, Gekht G, Vallejo R, Yearwood T, Morgan D. Novel spinal cord stimulation parameters in patients with predominant back pain. Neuromodulation. 2013;16:370–5.

Vaisman J, Markley H, Ordia J, Deer T. The treatment of medically intractable trigeminal autonomic cephalalgia with supraorbital/supratrochlear stimulation: a retrospective case series. Neuromodulation. 2012;15:374–80.

Vallejo R. High-frequency spinal cord stimulation: an emerging treatment option for patients with chronic pain. Tech Reg Anesth Pain Manag. 2012;16:106–12.

Van Buyten JP, Al-Kaisy A, Smet I, Palmisani S, Smith T. High-frequency spinal cord stimulation for the treatment of chronic back pain patients: results of a prospective multicenter European clinical study. Neuromodulation. 2013;16:59–66.

Weiner RL, Reed KL. Peripheral neurostimulation for control of intractable occipital neuralgia. Neuromodulation. 1999;2:217–21.

Spinal Cord Stimulation of the Dorsal Root Ganglion for the Treatment of Pain

23

Greg A. Bara and Timothy R. Deer

23.1 Introduction

The treatment of chronic pain conditions has gone beyond traditional options such as pharmacotherapy and behavioral and physical therapy to include injections and other minimally invasive interventions. This algorithm in many cases also includes open surgical resection to free the nerve or stabilize the spine. Still, no panacea for the treatment of chronic pain has yet been found. The pain treatment algorithm is often unsuccessful, and the desperate patient is left in pain, leading to an increasingly huge burden on society and the health care economy.

Recent advances in biomedical engineering have transformed the field of neuromodulation and have given rise to many new technologies. This technology update includes advanced electrode geometry, as in percutaneously implantable paddle leads; built-in accelerometers for adaptive stimulation during changes in body position; and new methods of current delivery, such as progressive stimulation patterns with high-frequency and burst stimulation.

Spinal cord stimulation (SCS) has become an important part of the pain algorithm, but unfortunately it often is found at the end. Strong evidence has shown its value for chronic, intractable pain, including complex regional pain syndrome (CRPS) and failed back surgery syndrome (FBSS). Other conditions such as pain of the axial lower back, groin, foot, and chest wall, as well as monoradicular pain syndromes, remain more complicated and cannot be addressed by conventional neuromodulation techniques in many clinical settings. This need to expand the field of SCS to improve outcomes has given rise to novel and exciting advanced technology targeting a new structure that plays a crucial role in the pathophysiology of chronic neuropathic pain: the dorsal root ganglion (DRG).

G.A. Bara
Department of Neurosurgery, University Hospital Dusseldorf, Moorenstr 5, Düsseldorf 40225, Germany
e-mail: gregbara@me.com

T.R. Deer, MD (✉)
The Center for Pain Relief, 400 Court Street, Suite 100, Charleston, WV 25301, USA
e-mail: DocTDeer@aol.com

T.R. Deer, J.E. Pope (eds.), *Atlas of Implantable Therapies for Pain Management*, DOI 10.1007/978-1-4939-2110-2_23

23.2 History and Background

The DRG's ability to modulate pain perception and its crucial role in the development and maintenance of chronic pain has been closely studied. The DRG is located in the lateral epidural space within the spinal foramen. It contains the cell bodies of the primary sensory neurons transducing sensory information from peripheral nerve endings to the central nervous system via unmyelinated Aδ and large C fibers. Pathophysiologically, a peripheral nerve injury is associated with hypersensitization and cross-excitation by impulse traffic in nearby neurons in this structure, which is thought to be a major contributing factor for the development of neuropathies. The result is an exacerbated neural firing rate, the electrophysiological correlate of a chronic pain state, which often includes hyperalgesia and allodynia.

Treatment that targets the DRG has a long tradition in interventional pain therapy: Dorsal root rhizotomies showed a high failure rate owing to traversing incoming pain fibers via the ventral rootlets, so they were superseded by dorsal root ganglionectomies. This open surgical procedure requires an invasive far lateral laminectomy, a foraminotomy, or both, to expose the ganglion. However, even in purely monoradicular pain syndromes, a multilevel approach with ganglionectomy of the somatotopically matched DRG and its neighboring rostral and caudal ganglia is required because of the divergence of incoming sensory input and the concept of neurointegrative pathways within the spinal cord. This procedure thus has potential morbidity. Radiofrequency (RF) and pulsed RF techniques have been used more widely, but unfortunately the durability of any positive outcomes are limited to 3–6 months. Various electrophysiological animal studies have shown that RF therapy induces short-lasting cellular activity changes. The fact that RF techniques have caused minimal complications despite their high-energy tissue delivery suggests that the DRG can be an attractive and robust target for neuromodulatory techniques, however.

Anatomically, the DRG is situated bilaterally with 7 cervical, 12 thoracic, 5 lumbar, and 4 sacral structures. In the vast majority of healthy individuals, the DRG is located interior to the foramen and under the medial and lateral borders of the vertebral pedicle. Radiculopathies are associated with more proximal locations of the DRG, and in this population, the position of the DRG may be seen to vary depending on the spinal level: DRGs on level L5 are usually intraforaminal, with more than 75 % on both sides, whereas on level S1, it is mostly intraspinal, with more than 80 % on both sides, and is intraforaminal in only a few cases.

Three key features must be noted:

- Given the strict dermatomal organization of the DRG, the area of paresthesia and the efficacy of stimulation can be estimated by previous interventions such as periradicular injections and pulsed RF stimulation. The convergent and divergent nature of the structures allows stimulation to be accurate at more than one potential level.
- Quadripolar DRG neurostimulation leads are generally free of positional changes around the ganglion, given the relative lack of isolating cerebrospinal fluid (CSF) around the ganglion and the relative lack of tissue conformation due to gravity. This anatomical structure allows for positional stability regardless of whether the patient is standing, sitting, or lying.
- Despite the dermatomal organization of the DRG, afferent information is cross-connected to adjacent levels owing to divergence of incoming sensory input and the concept of neurointegrative pathways within the spinal cord. Placing leads on nonadjacent ipsilateral levels may achieve overlapping coverage.

23.3 Technical Overview

Suitable candidates for DRG stimulation consist of patients with neuropathic pain syndromes of the limbs or trunk. Once identified as proper candidates, the patients undergo the usual psychological evaluation and preoperative anesthesia workup. Potential infection risks, bleeding factors, and other comorbidities must be addressed and successfully managed before surgery can be performed.

Once stable, the patient can be taken to the operating room. The anesthetic of choice is initiated and the patient is placed in prone position on the operating table. The patient's skin is properly prepped with solutions that are appropriate based on local pathogens, and drapes are widely placed. Kyphosation of the lumbar spine allows an easier puncture of the spinal canal and can be supported via a roll or inflatable balloon placed under the lumbar spine. A fluoroscope is placed over the site of puncture in an anteroposterior (AP) position. The clinician should ensure that the spinous processes are aligned correctly in the AP line to reveal an ideal puncture site according to the targeted DRG.

As for conventional SCS, the needle is placed epidurally under fluoroscopy. The lead placement is based on preoperative planning. If the implanter is trained and experienced, lead placement is relatively straightforward. The physician must learn to place the sheath near the DRG of interest and then to inject the lead. Preplanning the approach and angle of puncture according to fluoroscopic landmarks is crucial in delivering the lead. We recommend a contralateral one-level or two-level approach for the targeted DRG: For the two-level contralateral approach, the skin puncture site should be the contralateral pedicle two levels below the targeted DRG, and the tip of the needle should enter the epidural space in midline at the site of the spinal process one level below, the needle pointing to the targeted DRG (Fig. 23.1). In case of the one-level contralateral approach, the implanter may choose a steeper angle (Fig. 23.2).

Using fluoroscopic guidance and loss-of-resistance technique, the epidural space of the spinal canal is punctured with the bevel of the needle (a modified 14G Tuohy) facing towards the targeted DRG at an angle of approximately 30°. Once loss of resistance is achieved, complete insertion into the epidural space can be verified by inserting a guide wire through the needle.

The quadripolar DRG stimulation lead and its delivery system should be prepared at this point. The curved stylet must be inserted into the flexible lead from the back, and the lead must be loaded into a curved sheath from the front. Make sure the stylet is completely inserted into the lead (Fig. 23.3) and that the lead is completely inserted into the sheath. The ball tip end of the lead should be flush against the sheath and tightened down with the lead stabilizer until the lead does not slide within the sheath.

Prior to placing the sheath, the implanter should determine the length of the lead required to extend from the targeted foraminal level to the site for the internal pulse generator (IPG). Using a 90-cm lead in the lumbar region may cause difficulty in coiling the excess lead, whereas a 50-cm lead used in the upper thoracic region may not be long enough to reach the IPG implantation site, with a potential risk of dislocation. In this situation, a lead extension should be considered to bridge the additional length.

Depending on the puncturing angle, the implanter can choose between a smaller and a larger curved sheath. The steering wing on the sheath lines up with the bend of the sheath and allows later steering. The lead and its delivery system are inserted through the needle into the epidural space and advanced towards the targeted foraminal opening.

As noted above, planning the trajectory of the needle is crucial for delivering the lead. If the approach to the foraminal opening is not adequate, it may be useful to choose a more accurate trajectory, with a new puncture site and angle. When retracting the sheath, the steering wing should be aligned with the bevel of the needle to prevent damaging the sheath.

With the distal end of the sheath in or at the targeted foramen, loosen the lead stabilizer and advance the lead so that it moves into the foramen. Ideally, contacts No. 2 and 3 should be just below the pedicle where the DRG is expected to be (Fig. 23.4).

Correct lead position can be confirmed with a lateral fluoroscope image to show lead placement at the dorsal but not ventral ganglion (Fig. 23.5). Intraoperative testing is helpful to verify the area of paresthesia, as well as the lack of motor artifacts. When the lead is correctly placed, programming is often very straightforward.

Once the lead is successfully in place, the implanter can retract the sheath to anchor the lead within the spinal canal. Advancing the lead further into the epidural space allows the implanter to place a lasso-shaped strain relief (Fig. 23.4). At this point, the implanter can remove the delivery sheath by gently pulling back the sheath near the needle. A fluoroscopic marker is placed at the tip of the sheath, helping to verify the sheath's position in respect to the lead and needle. The implanter should hold forward pressure on the lead while retracting the sheath to prevent lead migration, by retracting the stylet beyond the tip of the sheath into the needle. The implanter then should turn away the sheath from the opening of the foramen and advance the lead to create a loop in the epidural space. The trial leads can be placed through a needle and secured to the skin with occlusive dressing, or a staged approach can used. In the staged method, once the leads are in place, a skin incision is made at the insertion site of the electrodes. (The Tuohy needle can be left in place to protect the electrode from the scalpel at this point.) The fascia is prepared towards the insertion site of the leads. The

Tuohy needle is removed, and an anchor is placed. The anchor is sutured to the fascia and the lead to minimize the risk of dislocation. See Fig. 23.6

At this point, the lead is connected to an extension lead, externalized, and connected to an external pulse generator. A trial is performed, which may last between 3 and 30 days, depending on the clinical protocol.

To verify the integrity of the electrical circuit, lead impedances should be checked after lead placement and connection to the external pulse generator. Standard postinterventional impedances range between 600 and 1,500 mOhm. Impedances higher than usual indicate lead breakage and may require an exchange. Impedances lower than expected indicate an intraspinal lead placement, which usually does not occur because of the relative lack of CSF surrounding the DRG.

Standard programming usually starts with a bipolar stimulation of contacts No. 2 and 3, which should ideally be placed just below the pedicle where the DRG is expected. In case of an electrode placement on level L5, contact No. 4 can be activated to steer the electric field towards a potentially intraspinal S1 ganglion. The frequency is set to 2 Hz with a 200 μs pulse width. The amplitude is gradually increased, starting from 300 μA up to 800 μA until paresthesia is induced. Subthreshold or paresthesia-inducing stimulation are reported to offer successful pain reduction and may be chosen, depending on the patient's compliance and preference.

When the patient achieves acceptable pain relief and wishes to move forward with a permanent implant, the patient is brought back to the operating room. In the staged approach, the extension leads are removed. In the traditional approach, after the successful trial, the leads are removed prior to the permanent therapy and freshly placed. The IPG is placed in an epifascial gluteal or abdominal pocket and connected to the leads. Once the connection is secured and tested, all wounds are closed carefully. See Fig. 23.7.

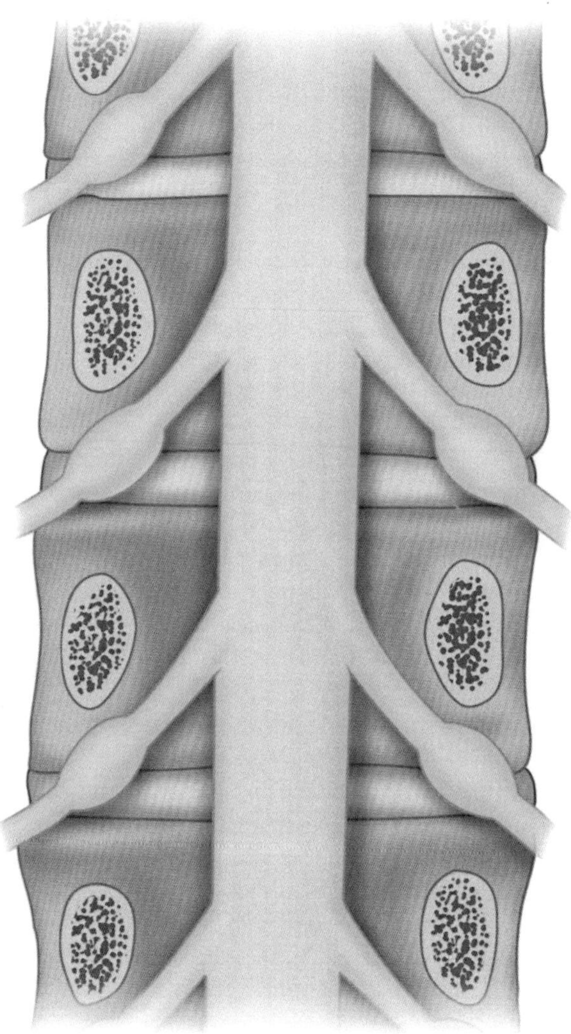

Fig. 23.1 Location of the dorsal root ganglion (DRG) as compared to the pedicle

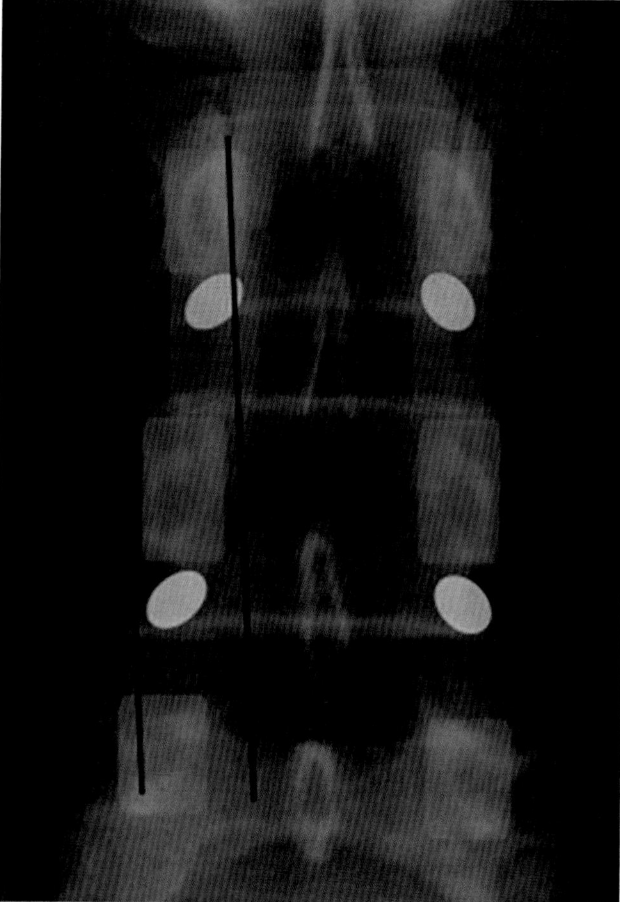

Fig. 23.2 Radiographic of DRG location. *Blue* indicates pedicle; *red* indicates neuroforamen; *yellow* indicates DRG

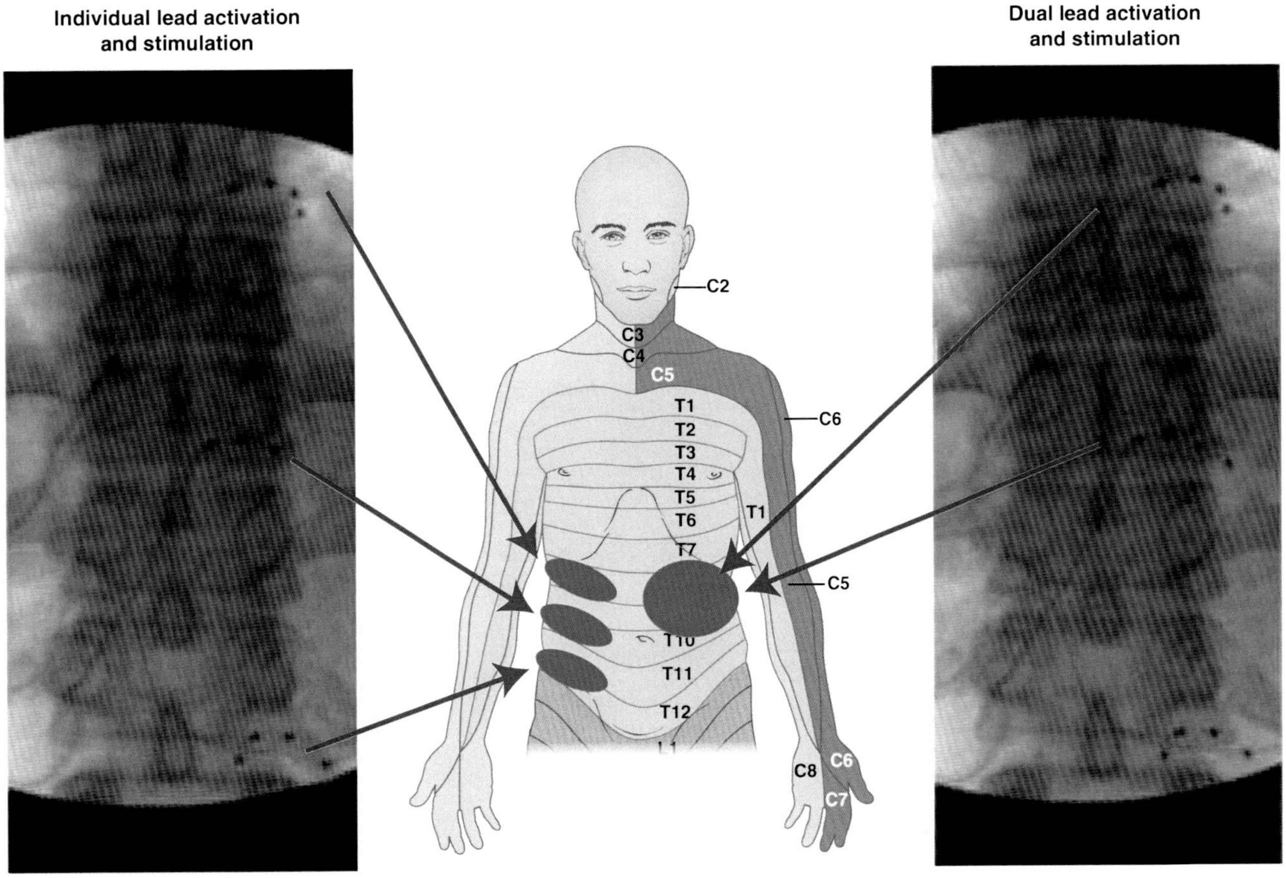

Individual lead activation and stimulation

Dual lead activation and stimulation

C2
C3
C4
C5
T1
T2
T3
T4
T5
T6
T7
T10
T11
T12
C6
T1
C5
C8
C6
C7

Fig. 23.3 Convergence and divergence of the afferent nociceptive input to the spinal cord can be exploited to provide therapeutic coverage over larger or smaller regions

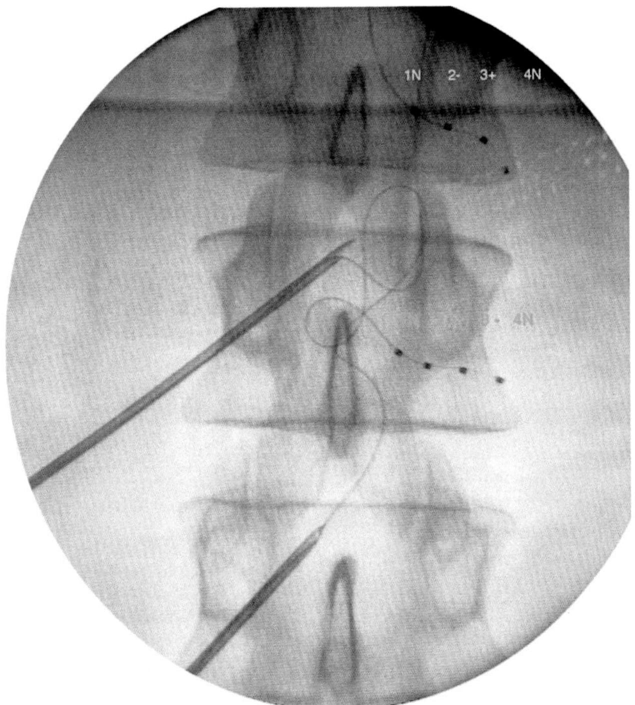

Fig. 23.4 AP radiograph demonstrating needle trajectory and lead placement in the superior/posterior portion of the foramen, with created stress relief loop

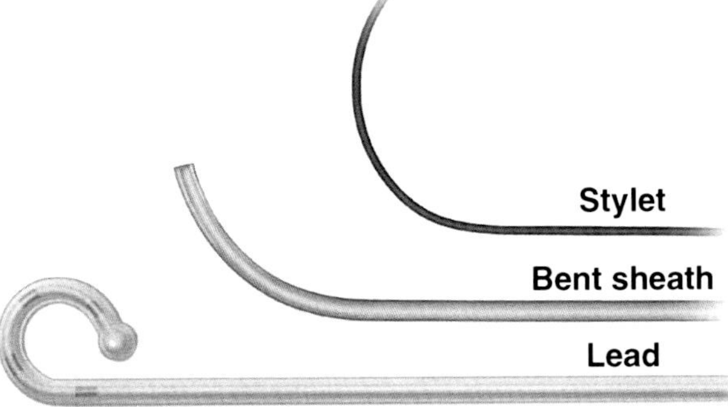

Fig. 23.5 The lead/stylet/sheath system to deploy the lead into the foramen overlying the DRG

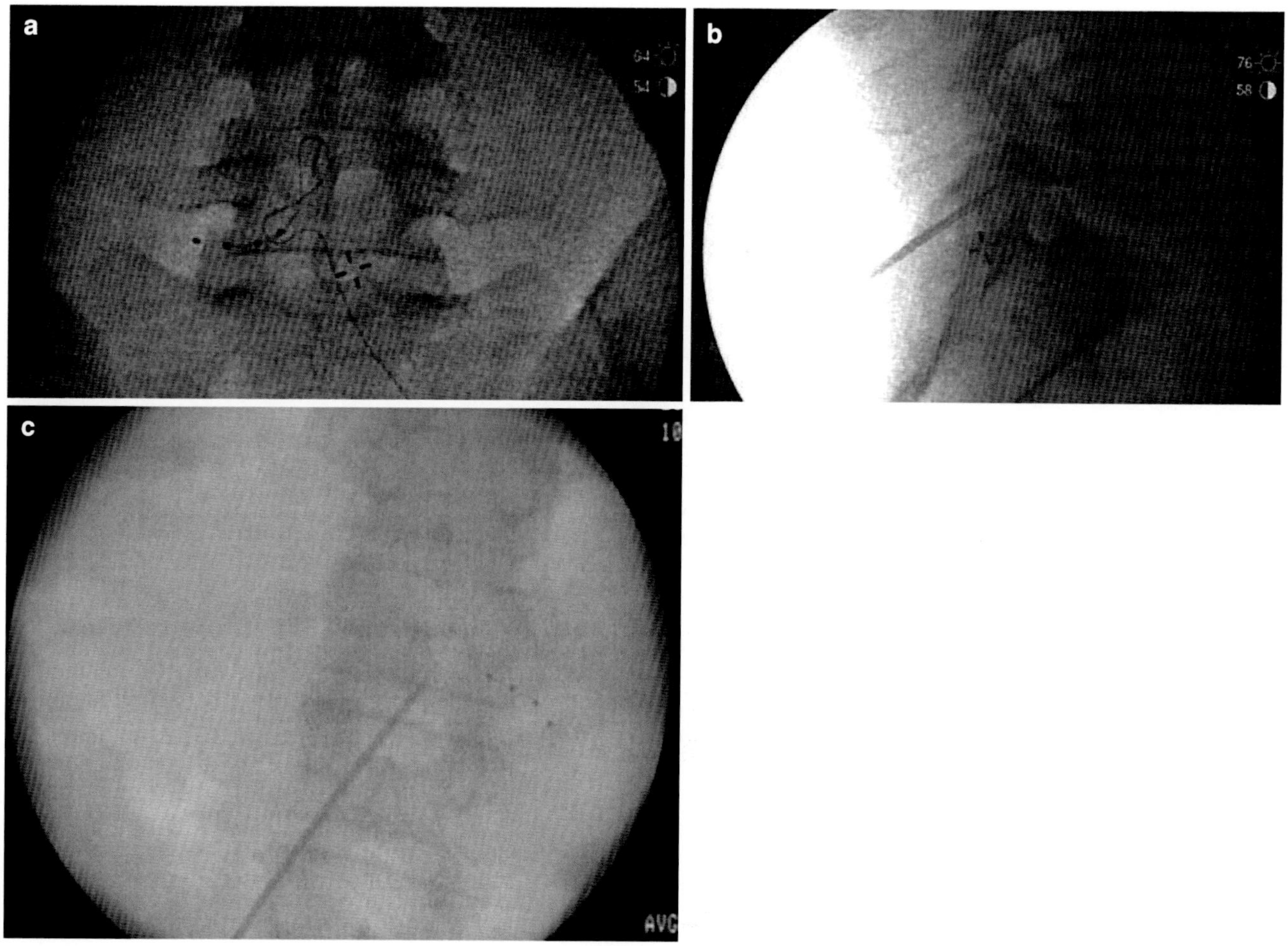

Fig. 23.6 Radiographs of the AP (**a**) and lateral (**b**) lead placement at the left L5 DRG (**c**) needle and lead placement at the right L3 DRG

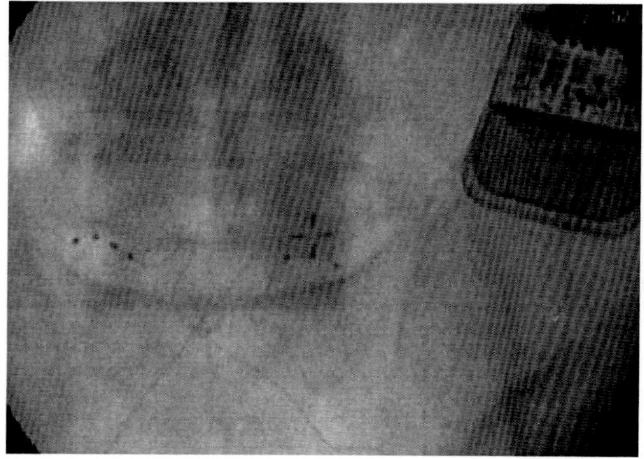

Fig. 23.7 AP radiograph of bilateral L5 DRG placement and IPG

23.4 Risk Assessment

The risk profile of DRG-SCS is very similar to the profile for traditional SCS. Preliminary studies have not reported serious or life-threatening complications or adverse outcomes:

- Lead placement at the correct ganglion and anchoring are crucial for the efficacy of therapy. Suboptimal intraoperative lead placement or postoperative lead migration may preclude sufficient pain relief.
- Very rare but serious complications (as with any spinal epidural approach) include spinal hematoma leading to severe neurological dysfunction including weakness, paresthesia, paralysis, or cauda equina compression syndrome.
- The most commonly reported complication is wound infection. Infections may result in sepsis and require immediate device explantation. The staged method of trialing appears to be associated with more infections.
- Pocket pain is a possible complication, but it is very rare with DRG-SCS because the device is smaller than other generators, owing to its markedly lower energy requirements.
- Skin erosion seldom occurs but may lead to secondary device infection.
- Very rarely, CSF leakage may occur if the needle punctures the dura. It should be treated as for any other post–dural puncture headache.
- Conscious sedation can be associated with complications. The presence of a board certified anesthesiologist is recommended.

23.5 Risk Avoidance

The likelihood of complications can be minimized by following appropriate procedures:

- Prior to surgery, the physician should review the patient's tissue for infection or lesions in the surgical area. The surgery should be delayed if there is any doubt about the safety of moving forward.
- The physician also should review the patient's medications and ensure that all medical conditions are adequately controlled before moving forward. Drugs that affect bleeding (*eg*, warfarin) should be discussed with the proper medical specialist and discontinued if safe and advisable.
- Preoperative and intraoperative antibiotics are recommended. It is advisable to vigorously irrigate the wound prior to closure.
- Lead placement should be performed under fluoroscopic guidance in AP and lateral view. Anchoring should be performed with vigilance.
- The generator pocket should be carefully planned to allow patient comfort and to avoid tissue irritation and skin erosion.
- The patient should be awake and conversant during portions of the procedure to minimize the likelihood of nerve damage.

Conclusions

Given its importance within the nervous system in the development and maintenance of chronic pain, the DRG offers a new and fascinating intraspinal target for electrical stimulation to control pain conditions that could not be treated by conventional neurostimulation systems owing to the location and dimension of the structure.

Suggested Reading

Deer TR, Grigsby E, Weiner RL, Wicosky B, Kramer JM. A prospective study of dorsal root ganglion stimulation for the relief of chronic pain. Neuromodulation. 2013a;16:67–72.

Deer TR, Levy RM, Kramer JM. Interventional perspectives on the dorsal root ganglion as a target for treatment of chronic pain: a review. Minim Invasive Surg Pain. 2013b;1:23–33.

Hasegawa T, Mikawa Y, Watanabe R, An HS. Morphometric analysis of the lumbosacral nerve roots and dorsal root ganglia by magnetic resonance imaging. Spine. 1996;21:1005–9.

Pope JE, Deer TR, Kramer J. A systematic review: current and future directions of dorsal root ganglion therapeutics to treat chronic pain. Pain Med. 2013;14:1477–96.

24 High-Frequency Stimulation of the Spinal Cord

Greg A. Bara and Timothy R. Deer

24.1 Introduction

Spinal cord stimulation (SCS) has been an evolving electronic technology since it was first introduced into clinical practice in 1967. Unfortunately, the evolution of the technology has lagged behind other areas of medicine such as cardiac rhythm management. In the past few years, the advancements in the arena of pain treatment have accelerated. One of the biggest changes has been the advent of the use of high-frequency stimulation to treat complex axial back pain: our current understanding suggests the critical frequency for achieving pain relief appears to be 10,000 kHz. This chapter examines this exciting field of medicine.

SCS has grown in acceptance since its introduction into the chronic pain algorithm. The most common use for SCS is the management of persistent back and leg pain, mainly secondary to failed back surgery. Studies have proven the superiority of SCS in combination with conventional medical treatment over medical treatment alone in failed back surgery syndrome. Patients with a combination of lower back pain and radicular pain of the lower extremities are therefore accepted to be the best candidates for traditional SCS, but predominant chronic axial pain of the lower back still remains a problem and a huge burden for patients and for the health care economy.

High-frequency stimulation offers a novel approach for this condition by providing a much higher pulse rate than traditional SCS systems. The high-frequency waveform consists of a biphasic, charge-balanced pulse train with pulse widths usually set to 30 μs and a pulse rate of 10 kHz.

G.A. Bara
Department of Neurosurgery, University Hospital Dusseldorf, Moorenstr 5, Düsseldorf 40225, Germany
e-mail: gregbara@me.com

T.R. Deer, MD (✉)
The Center for Pain Relief, 400 Court Street, Suite 100, Charleston, WV 25301, USA
e-mail: DocTDeer@aol.com

Traditional low-frequency SCS, with frequencies up to 100 Hz, is thought to activate and drive neurons and large fibers and consecutively stop the transmission of pain according to the gate control theory. A different mechanism has been postulated for high-frequency stimulation: Preclinical studies have shown that alternating current of up to 10 kHz delivered to the sensory fibers in the spinal dorsal root and the dorsal root entry zone reduces the activity of wide dynamic range (WDR) dorsal horn neurons of the spinal cord. The output of the WDR neurons crosses and ascends to the thalamus via the spinothalamic and paleospinothalamic tracts and is critical for pain perception. WDR neurons have been shown to be hyperactive in chronic pain conditions. High-frequency SCS modulates overall excitability and leads to conduction blockade and preinjury states. The high dosage of energy transmitted into the spinal cord has been shown to be safe and effective in preclinical animal studies and in clinical patient studies. Histological animal studies have show no pathological consequences of high-frequency stimulation.

Two key features must be noted:

- High frequency delivers electrical stimulation to the spinal cord without the sensation of paresthesia while minimizing the common side effects of SCS—mainly recruitment and stimulation of nonpain areas, resulting in patient discomfort. Low-frequency stimulation is thought to provide the best pain relief when the intraoperatively tested paresthesia covers the pain area. This goal is difficult to achieve when it comes to chronic axial lower back pain, a condition mostly represented in dermatomes L1 and L2. Typically this level corresponds to intraspinal segmental levels T8–T9. As the distance between the epidural space and the dorsal columns is increased at the needed levels, a stimulation to provide concordant paresthesia would lead to uncomfortable stimulation paresthesia of the legs and mainly the chest wall. High-frequency SCS systems offer not only reduced pain and increased disability performance scores but also high patient satisfaction and an improvement of sleep disturbances

T.R. Deer, J.E. Pope (eds.), *Atlas of Implantable Therapies for Pain Management*, DOI 10.1007/978-1-4939-2110-2_24

because the stimulation is paresthesia-free. Further, as uncomfortable stimulation is not a concern, it may allow patients to drive automobiles.

- The leads for high-frequency SCS are placed anatomically and equally for back and leg pain. All current studies have shown the electrode placement to differ from conventional SCS. Optimal placement is considered to be the "sweet spot" between T8 and T11. Usually two electrodes are placed approximately at the anatomical midline, staggered to have an maximum number of contacts over the T9-10 area. Owing to anatomical placement, no intraoperative paresthesia testing is required. Creating paresthesia coverage is usually very time-consuming and requires a cooperative patient during implantation to adjust the lead locations according to the patient's feedback. Because this feedback is not needed, the whole implantation can be performed under deep sedation or general anesthesia, leading to shorter and more predictable surgical times, reduced patient anxiety, and improved physician satisfaction.

24.2 Technical Overview

The technique for implantation of a high-frequency SCS system is very similar to the technique for conventional SCS. The patient is evaluated preoperatively, and proper control of infection risks, bleeding factors, and other comorbidities are addressed. The patient is placed in prone position on the operating table, and the anesthesia of choice is initiated. The patient is properly prepped with solutions that are appropriate based on local pathogens, and drapes are widely placed. Kyphosation of the lumbar spine allows easier puncture of the spinal canal and can be supported via a roll or inflatable balloon placed under the lumbar spine. A fluoroscope is placed over the site of puncture in an anteroposterior (AP) position. The spinous processes need to align correctly in an AP line to reveal an ideal puncture site, which is usually the L1-2 window. With fluoroscopic guidance and loss-of-resistance technique, the epidural space of the spinal canal is punctured with a modified Tuohy needle. The first lead is pushed forward through the lumen of the Tuohy needle and can be maneuvered with the guide wire to the right anatomical position. The lead should be placed in midline position with its first contact being placed at the upper rim of the vertebral body T8. Puncture of the epidural space is performed a second time, and again the lead is pushed forward through the Tuohy needle and steered with the guide wire to the correct position in anatomical midline position between vertebral bodies T8 and T11. Both leads should be staggered to have a maximum number of contacts over the T9-10 area (Fig. 24.1). Because paresthesia testing is not required, the correct lead position is confirmed with a lateral fluoroscope to verify a dorsal lead placement. The impedances are checked to ensure the integrity of the stimulation system, and the leads are verified to be in the epidural space before completing the procedure. Usually impedances are around 1000 Ω. Impedances that are higher than usual may indicate lead fracture, whereas impedances lower than usual may indicate intraspinal lead placement.

The trial leads can be placed through a needle and then secured to the skin with occlusive dressing, or a staged approach can be used. In the staged method, once the leads are in place, a skin incision is made at the insertion site of the electrodes. The Tuohy needle can be left in place to protect the electrode from the scalpel at this point. The fascia is prepared towards the insertion site of the leads. The Tuohy needle is removed and an anchor is placed. The anchor is sutured to the fascia and the lead to minimize the risk of dislocation. The lead is connected to an extension lead, externalized, and connected to an external pulse generator. A trial is performed, usually lasting 7 days (depending on the clinical protocol). Frequencies for stimulation can vary from 2 to 10 kHz, with amplitudes 2–4 mA, and pulse widths 30–40 μs. Usually, the contacts above and below the T9-10 intervertebral disc are activated. The standardized stimulation protocol starts with a frequency of 10 kHz, an amplitude of 2 mA, and a pulse width of 30 μs. The amplitude is gradually increased during the trial phase. Pain reduction usually is initiated within the first 24–48 h after the start of stimulation.

When the patient achieves acceptable amounts of pain relief and wishes to move forward with a permanent implant, the patient is brought back to the operating room and the extension leads are removed. The internal pulse generator is placed in an epifascial gluteal or abdominal pocket and connected to the leads. Once the connection is secured and tested, all wounds are closed carefully.

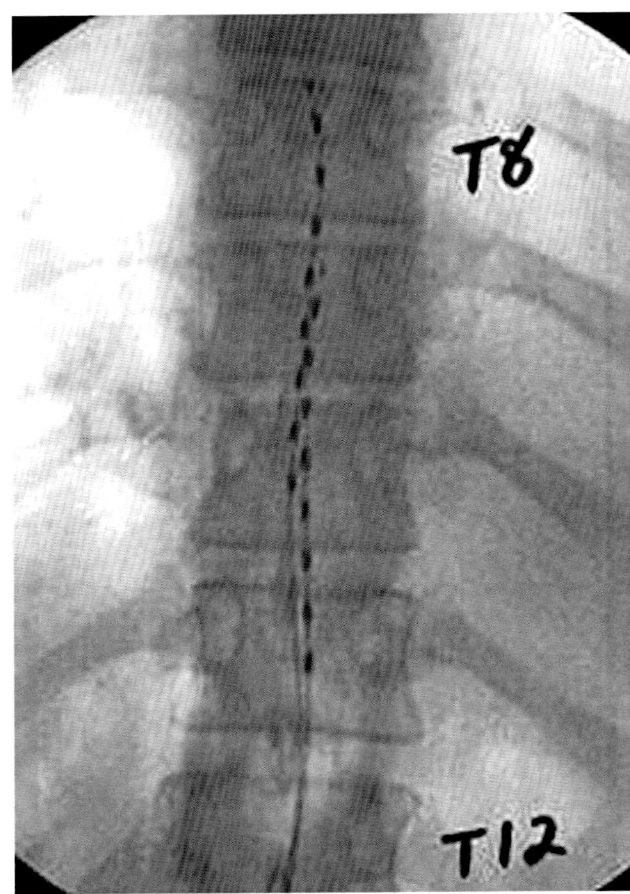

Fig. 24.1 Radiograph of correct lead placement at vertebral levels T8 to T11, the "sweet spot."

24.3 Risk Assessment

The risk profile of high-frequency SCS is very similar to the profile of traditional low-frequency SCS. Preliminary studies have not reported serious or life-threatening complications or adverse outcomes, but physicians should be aware of possible complications:

- Optimal lead placement and anchoring are crucial for the efficacy of therapy. Suboptimal intraoperative lead placements or postoperative lead migrations prevent sufficient pain relief. Migration rates of up to 30 % have been reported in the literature, but they may be reduced to less than 5 %.
- Very rare but serious complications include spinal hematoma leading to severe neurological dysfunction including weakness, paresthesia, paralysis, or cauda equina compression syndrome.
- The most commonly reported complication is wound infection. Infections may result in sepsis and requires immediate device explantation.
- Pocket pain is commonly reported. Its occurrence may be explained by the larger size of the internal pulse generator, due to increased energy consumption of the high-frequency system.
- Skin erosion seldom occurs but may lead to secondary device infection.
- Leakage of cerebrospinal fluid (CSF) may occur, followed by CSF leakage syndrome with headache.

24.4 Risk Avoidance

The physician can reduce the rate of complications by following appropriate procedures:

- Prior to surgery, the physician should review the patient's tissue for infection or lesions in the surgical area. The surgery should be delayed if there is any doubt about the safety of moving forward.
- The physician also should review the patient's medications and ensure that all medical conditions are adequately controlled prior to moving forward. Drugs that affect bleeding (*eg*, warfarin) should be discussed with the proper medical specialist and discontinued if safe and advisable.
- Preoperative and intraoperative antibiotics are recommended. It is advisable to vigorously irrigate the wound prior to closure.
- Lead placement should be performed under fluoroscopic guidance in AP and lateral view. If anchoring is performed very accurately, pulling firmly at the lead should not change its position.
- The generator pocket should be carefully planned to allow patient comfort and to avoid tissue irritation and skin erosion.

Suggested Reading

Cuellar JM, Alataris K, Walker A, Yeomans DC, Antognini JF. Effect of high-frequency alternating current on spinal afferent nociceptive transmission. Neuromodulation. 2013;16:318–27.

Tiede J, Brown L, Gekht G, Vallejo R, Yearwood T, Morgan D. Novel spinal cord stimulation parameters in patients with predominant back pain. Neuromodulation. 2013;16:370–5.

Van Buyten JP, Al-Kaisy A, Smet I, Palmisani S, Smith T. High-frequency spinal cord stimulation for the treatment of chronic back pain patients: results of a prospective multicenter European clinical study. Neuromodulation. 2013;16:59–65.

25 Burst Stimulation: An Innovative Waveform Strategy for Spinal Cord Stimulation

Jason E. Pope and Timothy R. Deer

25.1 Introduction

Since the advent of spinal cord stimulation (SCS) or tonic spinal cord stimulation (t-SCS), developed by Norman Shealy in 1967, dorsal column stimulation has continued to evolve, primarily focused on lead innovations. Disadvantages to current SCS strategies are inherent to how it works: it requires perceived congruent therapeutic paresthesia overlying the typical painful area. Challenges include the ability to place the paresthesia in congruent areas, the positionality associated with the required perception, and the need for the patient to consider the paresthesia therapeutic. New innovations in waveform strategies are moving from the need to create a perceived paresthesia to achieve analgesia. This chapter explores one such innovation, Burst stimulation (Burst-SCS). It is important to appreciate that Burst-SCS is currently under investigation in the United States and is not approved by the U.S. Food and Drug Administration or available for use.

J.E. Pope
Summit Pain Alliance,
392 Tesconi Court, Santa Rosa, CA 95401, USA
e-mail: popeje@me.com

T.R. Deer, MD (✉)
The Center for Pain Relief, 400 Court Street, Suite 100,
Charleston, WV 25301, USA
e-mail: DocTDeer@aol.com

T.R. Deer, J.E. Pope (eds.), *Atlas of Implantable Therapies for Pain Management*, DOI 10.1007/978-1-4939-2110-2_25

25.2 Technical Overview

Current tSCS strategies rely on the delivery of energy to the spinal cord through activation of a cathode, either by alternating the current (constant voltage system) or voltage (constant current system). These systems typically deliver a frequency from 40 to 150 Hz. Burst-SCS delivers a cluster of five pulses at 500 Hz in 40 Hz intervals, where the pulse width is typically 1 μs. The amplitude is adjusted to the individual patient, as it is for tSCS. Importantly, the energy required to deliver the Burst-SCS versus tSCS is the same, in terms of battery life and recharging interval (Fig. 25.1).

It is important to briefly comment on the mechanism of action, as Burst-SCS appears to work differently than tSCS. It is hypothesized that burst-SCS works by stimulating not only the lateral pathway typically activated in tSCS but also the medial pathway, responsible for the affective component of pain. This may have implications in reducing the overall pain perception, which has been reported both anecdotally and in literature (Fig. 25.2).

It is important to note that although the Burst-SCS creates analgesia without the need for the perceived paresthesia, it requires placement within the epidural space in the same anatomic location as tSCS, namely relying on placement based on the Barolo mapping.

There is robust literature supporting Burst-SCS (Table 25.1).

The double-blind, placebo-controlled trial performed by DeRidder et al. described that Burst-SCS improved back, limb, and general pain compared to tonic or placebo. de Vos et al. described patients with typically poorly treated patient populations, including diabetic peripheral neuropathy (DPN), failed back surgery syndrome, and failed back surgery syndrome, that were poor responders to tSCS (FBSS-PR). Although Burst-SCS improved pain care in all populations studied compared to tSCS, the effect was greatest for PDN and lesser for FBSS-PR.

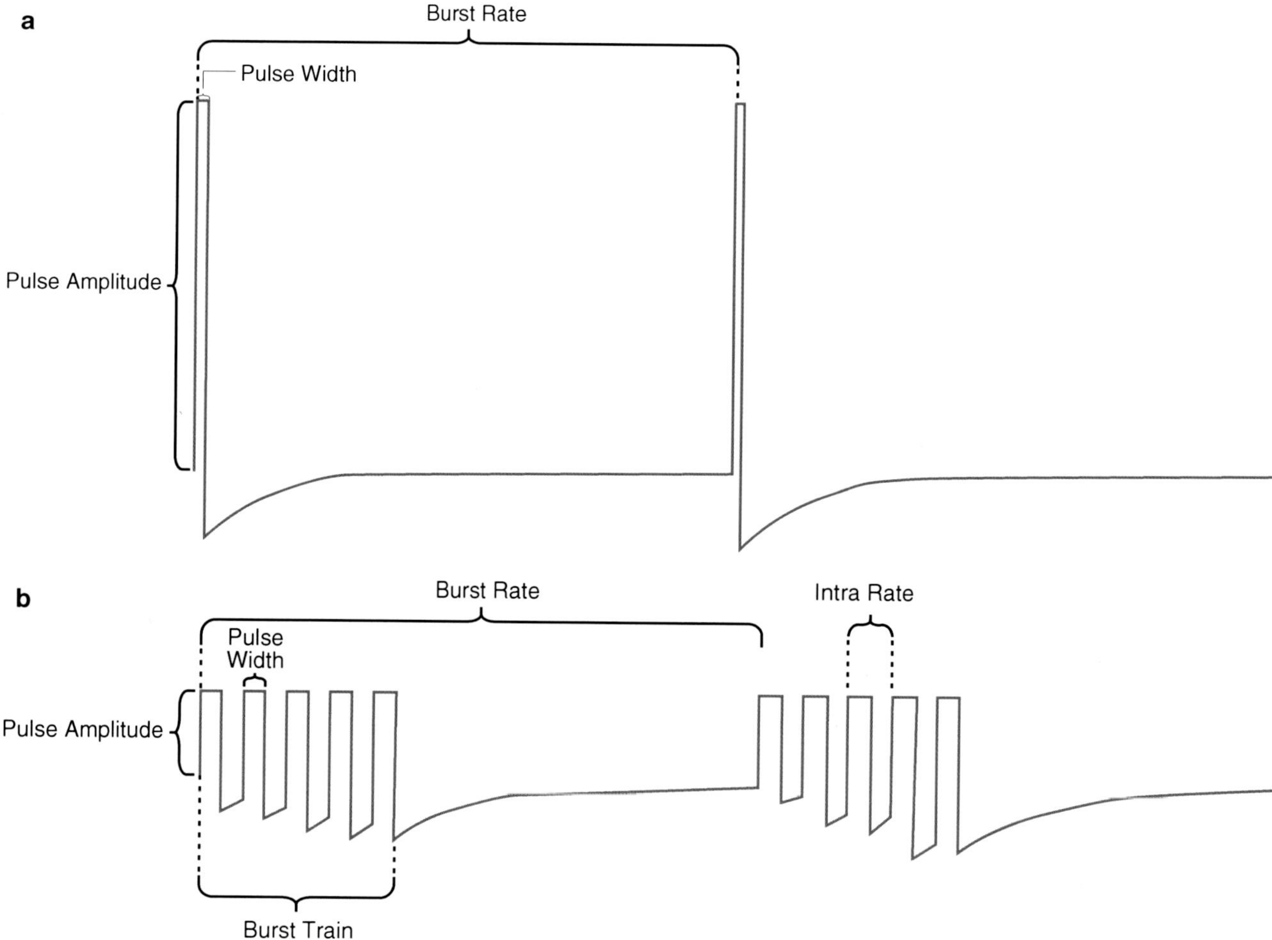

Fig. 25.1 Stimulation strategies: tonic stimulation 40 Hz (**a**); burst stimulation (**b**)

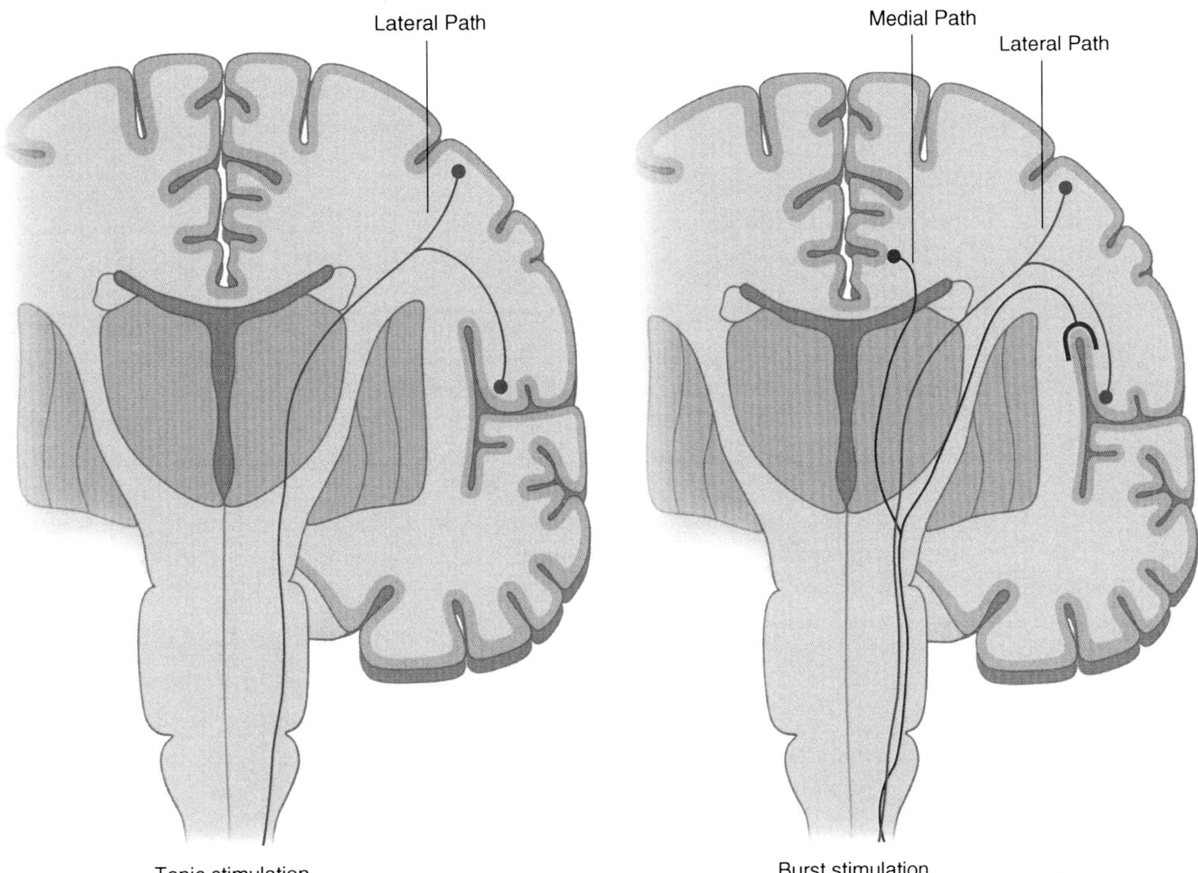

Fig. 25.2 The activation of the lateral pathway in tSCS and activation of the lateral (**a**) and the medial (**b**) pathway in Burst-SCS (*courtesy of* St. Jude Medical, Plano TX)

Table 25.1 Burst stimulation studies to date

Study	Participants	Conclusion(s)	Complications
de Vos et al. (2013)	48 patients with existing tSCS for 6 months, with PDN, FBSS, and FBSS-PR; underwent B-SCS for 2 weeks	60 % had better relief with Burst-SCS vs tSCS	None reported
De Ridder et al. (2013)	15 consecutive patients with limb and axial back pain; given Burst-SCS, tSCS, and placebo	Burst-SCS was better than tSCS or placebo in the treatment of back and leg pain	None reported
De Ridder et al. (2010)	12 patients with tSCS with paddle to treat neuropathic pain; given Burst-SCS	Burst-SCS may be better than tSCS in the treatment of neuropathic pain	None reported

FBSS failed back surgery syndrome, *PDN* peripheral diabetic neuropathy, *PR* FBSS with poor response, *SCS* spinal cord stimulation, *VAS* visual analog scale

25.3 Risk Assessment

Physicians considering the use of burst stimulation should be aware of the potential for risk:

- The procedure for employing burst stimulation relies on hardware similar to the hardware for traditional tonic stimulation, and consequently similar risks are expected. (*See* Chap. 7 on SCS lead placement.)
- Burst stimulation may decrease battery life of the equipment and increase the recharging frequency.
- Prospective published research on burst stimulation has reported no complications, though it may have been accompanied by effects that included the sense of dizziness, headache, and the sensation of "heavy legs."
- Further prospective data are required to discern the unique challenges, if any, that may accompany burst stimulation.

25.4 Risk Avoidance

- The clinician should use the same risk-mitigation techniques as for traditional spinal cord stimulation. (*See* Chaps. 5 and 11.)
- Vigilance is paramount, as burst stimulation may stimulate the perceptive and affective components of the pain experience.
- Further prospective study is needed to determine the role of burst stimulation in the neuromodulation armamentarium.

25.5 Conclusions and Future Directions

Spinal cord stimulation is in its infancy. As new software and hardware developments become reality, so too does an expansion in spinal cord stimulation disease indications. Burst stimulation may improve on the challenges inherent to tSCS, relying on the need for perceived, congruent therapeutic paresthesia. The placement of Burst-SCS in the pain care algorithm will evolve with the evidence, as it may be used as salvage therapy or potentially for first-line therapy. Perceived deficits of tSCS and the potential advantages to Burst-SCS are highlighted in Tables 25.2 and 25.3.

Burst stimulation is currently being investigated in the United States and is only available internationally. It has the potential to dramatically change the landscape of spinal cord stimulation as we know it today. Its placement in the pain care algorithm has yet to be determined.

Table 25.2 Current challenges with tonic spinal cord stimulation

Positionality of stimulation
Presence of nonresponders
Need for perceived therapeutic parasthesia and areas of coverage
Development of therapeutic tolerance

Table 25.3 Perceived advantages to burst-SCS

Reduce or eliminate the need for paresthesia stimulation
May function as salvage therapy to tonic stimulation
May eliminate the need for discrete stimulation
Reduce or eliminate positionality challenges
May offer an advantage to stimulate affective and perceptive pathways

Suggested Reading

De Ridder D, Plaizer M, Kamerling N, Menovsky T, Vanneste S. Burst spinal cord stimulation for limb and back pain. World Neurosurg. 2013;80:642–9.

De Ridder D, Vanneste S, Plaizer M, van der Loo E, Menovsky T. Burst spinal cord stimulation: toward paresthesia-free pain suppression. Neurosurgery. 2010;66:986–90.

de Vos CC, Bom MJ, Vanneste S, Lenders MW, de Ridder D. Burst spinal cord stimulation evaluated in patients with failed back surgery syndrome and painful diabetic neuropathy. Neuromodulation. 2014;17:152–9.

Pope JE, Deer TR, Amirdelfan K, Kapural L, Verrills P. New concepts for waveform and current delivery for spinal cord stimulation: burst and high frequency. Minim Invasive Surg Pain. 2015 (Epub ahead of print).

Pope JE, Falowski S, Deer TR. Advanced waveforms and frequency with spinal cord stimulation: burst and high frequency energy delivery. Expert Rev Med Devices. 2015 (Epub ahead of print).

Schade CM, Sasaki J, Schultz DM, Tamayo N, King G, Johanek LM. Assessment of patient preference for constant voltage and constant current spinal cord stimulation. Neuromodulation. 2010;13:210–7.

Washburn S, Catlin R, Bethel K, Canlas B. Patient-perceived differences between constant current and constant voltage spinal cord stimulation systems. Neuromodulation. 2014;17:28–35.

Part II

Neurostimulation: Peripheral Nerve and Peripheral Nerve Field

Stimulation of the Extraspinal Peripheral Nervous System

26

W. Porter McRoberts, Timothy R. Deer, David Abejón, and Giancarlo Barolat

Much like the carpenter's hammer, the pain interventionalist's needle begs its own substrate, and none serves like the peripheral nerve. Peripheral nerve stimulation (PNS), peripheral nerve field stimulation (PNfS), and hybrid stimulation (creating a paresthetic field of stimulation by sending current between spinal and peripheral leads at a distance from each other) are all areas of neuromodulation growing in interest from both clinical and research standpoints. The increasing use of these modalities reflects not only the efficacy, safety, and increasing technical ease with which the treatment can be delivered, but also the reports of successful relief from often obstinate and disabling pain. This surgical technique has shown growing potential in patients suffering from many severe pain conditions, including low back pain, intercostal neuralgia, ilioinguinal neuralgia, carpal tunnel syndrome, neuropathic facial pain, nerve entrapment syndromes, postsurgical nerve pain, and specific neuropathic pain isolated to confined areas of the body. This chapter seeks to tutor the neuromodulation community about the utility of the peripheral technique and its points of finesse, so that the sensitive recipient of peripheral neuromodulation is never treated bluntly, unlike the nail.

PNS and PNfS are hardly new options for patients suffering from pain involving the peripheral nervous system. Work by Wiener, Hassenbusch, Stanton-Hicks, and others showed that physicians could successfully implant devices around the peripheral nerve and create anodynic paresthesia in the innervation of the nerve. Over a decade ago, the placement of these devices required careful surgical dissection, fascial graft débridement, and placement of the lead. This complicated procedure had relatively low reimbursement and required exceptional surgical skills and significant operating room time. Newer, percutaneous methods reduced both need for surgical skill and time, and led to an improved level of access to patients, making stimulation of the peripheral nervous system a viable tool in the arsenal of the well-rounded interventionalist.

This chapter focuses further on the best selection of candidates, the technical tasks associated with implantation of devices in the peripheral nervous system, the potential pitfalls, and their solutions. For brevity, we assume that the implanter is well seasoned, with a good working knowledge of general neuromodulation.

W.P. McRoberts
Division of Interventional Spine,
Pain, and Neurosurgery,
Holy Cross Hospital,
Fort Lauderdale, FL, USA

T.R. Deer, MD (✉)
The Center for Pain Relief, 400 Court Street, Suite 100,
Charleston, WV 25301, USA
e-mail: DocTDeer@aol.com

D. Abejón
Hospital Universitario Quirón Madrid,
Calle Travesia de Suecia, 17, Madrid,
Pozuelo de Alarcón 28224, Spain
e-mail: dabejon@telefonica.net

G. Barolat, MD
Barolat Neuroscience, Presbyterian St. Lukes Medical Center,
1721 East 19th Avenue, Denver, CO 80218, USA
e-mail: gbarolat@verizon.net

T.R. Deer, J.E. Pope (eds.), *Atlas of Implantable Therapies for Pain Management*, DOI 10.1007/978-1-4939-2110-2_26

26.1 Selection of Candidates

Success in neurostimulation requires the identification of suitable candidates and then the safely targeted application of current, resulting in a change in the neural environment specific to the area of pain. In selecting candidates for PNS, PNfS, and hybrid stimulation, the physician must consider the innervation of the specific area of pain—be it cutaneous, fascial, articular, or other—and determine whether there is an opportunity to influence the area by applying current to the nerve or specific fibers that subserve the painful area. If the area is too large, or if the innervating nerve is difficult to access, then target consideration must move proximally. At a certain point, stimulation within the spinal canal may present an easier, safer, or more stable option and eclipse the peripheral nerve option, though placing electrodes within the spine presents some risk. The cord is comprised of second-order and other multiorder neurons. The peripheral nerve is the only first-order neural option, which may have implications as different frequencies and electrodes become available. Table 26.1 outlines the selection criteria for implanting a percutaneous peripheral lead. In peripheral neuromodulation, the decision to proceed from a trial to a permanent implant is no different than in spinal cord stimulation (SCS): Does the trial array confer significant pain reduction? Does the stimulation feel pleasant and acceptable? Is objective function improved during the temporary period? Contraindications include lack of significant relief from the trial phase, infection, uncorrected bleeding disorders, untreated depression or anxiety, untreated drug abuse, and the constraints of surgical access and system stability. Table 26.2 reviews the currently supported nerve targets for implanting a system for peripheral nervous system stimulation.

Table 26.1 Selection criteria for implanting the peripheral nerve stimulation system

Characteristic	Establishing the characteristic
Pain is localized to a specific nerve distribution	History and physical examination
Pain is burning or shooting in nature	History
Pain is relieved by injection of local anesthetic around the nerve(s)	Resolution of 50 % or more of the patient's pain intensity with injection of local anesthetic on two occasions
Pain has not responded to or is not appropriate for other, more conservative neuropathic treatments	Review of the records
No concomitant infection that would likely compromise the implant	History, inspection of the skin
No allergies to the materials to be implanted	History of metal allergy
No major untreated psychological factors	History and appropriate psychological evaluation
Pain is not better treated with SCS	History and physical examination

SCS spinal cord stimulation

Table 26.2 Established targets for PNS and PNfS placement

Disease	Nerve targets
Occipital neuralgia	C2 fibers at the posterior occiput
Neuritis of the face	Supraorbital, infraorbital temporo-auricular, trigeminal divisions
Upper extremity pain	Median, ulnar, radial, axillary, suprascapular
Pain of torso	Intercostal, cluneal
Pain of pelvis	Ilioinguinal, iliohypogastric, genitofemoral
Pain of lower extremity	Common peroneal, superficial peroneal, deep peroneal, lateral femoral cutaneous, tibial, saphenous, sciatic, femoral

PNfS peripheral nerve field stimulation, *PNS* peripheral nerve stimulation

26.2 Technical Overview

The use of PNS and PNfS is based on the concept that the delivery of electrical current in a controlled fashion to a specific nerve or across nerve fibers will affect the transmission of pain by influencing the firing of the A delta and C fibers, as well as potentially changing the neurotransmitters in the tissue. To make these important modifications of the nervous system, the physician must place a system in the appropriate tissue plane(s).

26.2.1 Methods of Percutaneous Trialing and Paresthetic Montage Creation

The trialing physician must first identify the areas of pain and correlating intensities, perhaps even marking them (or asking the patient to mark them) on the skin. Marking has great utility. Marking not only makes it easy to identify the nerve or nerves responsible for sensation to the area, but also clearly communicates to the physician the areas that are important to the patient—a process so seemingly simple that many gloss over the step. Missing essential areas likely contributes to significant failure of the modality.

Once the areas are clear to the physician, a decision-making process occurs, with consideration given to dense or overlapping paresthesia and its potential benefits, ease of deployment, stability of the permanent system, safety to the patient, and the ability to create a montage of paresthesia using a single implantable pulse generator (IPG). If the painful area is small (the size of a business card or less), and especially if it is superficial, a single PNfS lead may serve the area well. If the area is larger, then cross-talking (transmitting current from one lead to a different lead at a distance) one or more leads may be appropriate, as cross-talking may increase the area of paresthesia. The practice of cross-talk additionally introduces the concept that the depolarized nerve may not actually be within the direct vicinity of the electrode array. If a single nerve wholly serves the area, then consideration must be given to direct stimulation of that nerve, if possible. Often, as the nerve courses proximally it becomes mixed and deeper, and thus is more difficult to access percutaneously, being guarded by sensitive structures, muscle, or bone. The more distal the electrode array from the anchoring point, the more likely lead migration becomes. Appendicular placement may further confound the system, as nerves may be deep and encircled by dynamic muscles, and leads may have to cross joint lines. System stability is important not only in the long term but also moment to moment, because with movement of a limb and thus of stimulation relative to a nerve's braided fascicles, its often-mixed nature results in momentarily variable (and thus tenuous) results.

If the area of pain includes axial pain, or if it may be advantageous to stimulate at multiple locations along the path of pain transmission, inclusion of a spinal lead may be constructive. The spinal lead may function independently, thus generating overlapping paresthesia, or in hybrid fashion, cross-talking to the peripheral lead, be it a PNfS or direct peripheral nerve lead. Table 26.3 identifies several hybrid montages for specific pain patterns. Although this nascent technique does not yet have significant support in the literature, many seasoned implanters will testify that hybrid stimulation presents yet a different feeling and pattern of paresthesia than parallel but overlapping stimulation—a flow of paresthesia that often crosses areas of the body not stimulated by either lead alone.

Table 26.3 Combination targets for hybrid stimulation

Pain location	Spinal lead location	Peripheral lead location
Axial back/neck	Corresponding cord level	Cluneal or PNfS near cutaneous dorsal rami serving pain location
Thoracic radicular	Corresponding thoracic level	Intercostal or PNfS near pain location
Facial	Cervical (nucleus caudalis)	Corresponding nerve of the face
Shoulder	Cervical or high thoracic	Axillary or suprascapular nerve
Abdominal	Thoracic	Ilioinguinal, hypogastric, or PNfS near pain
Flank	Corresponding thoracic level	PNfS near pain location

PNfS peripheral nerve field stimulation

26.2.2 Peripheral Nerve Field Stimulation

The placement of a lead for PNfS use appears easy, and often it is, but several important pitfalls exist. Obviously, pain outside the field of paresthesia will never be reduced. Aim to create lines of current that connect through the area of pain, using the length of the array to advantage. More electrodes do not necessarily equate with better relief; at present, quadripolar arrays are usually the best compromise between redundancy and the judicious use of multiple leads. Though not studied, it is our opinion that an octapolar array rarely confers added benefit, except when possibly needed to stimulate fine or extremely important nearby nerves, as in stimulation of occipital or facial nerves. As previously mentioned, small areas may be well treated with one lead, but larger areas may need multiple leads in cross-talk fashion. Particularly hypersensitive areas or areas of anesthesia dolorosa do not respond well to leads in the immediate vicinity, but instead respond better to leads placed to bracket the area with energy cross-talked through the particularly sensitive areas.

Depth, too, must be well thought out; in PNfS, the target is the terminal sensory nerve fibers that exist deep to the basal layers of the skin within the deep dermis. Passing the needle (and thus the lead and electrode array) within the dermis is painful and may subject the lead to bacteria that live within the papillae and sweat glands. Placement of the lead too deep within the adipose of the subcutis drives up the electrical resistance of the system, and placing it deeper yet to adipose results in painful recruitment of muscle fiber. The best position is just deep to the dermis at the dermal junction with the fat. After attention to sterile preparation, a constrained wheal of local anesthetic prepares the skin for a small stab wound to permit needle entry. The needle is then directed parallel, with palpation, deep to the dermis, resulting in easy advancement with minimal resistance; though not pleasant, the patient's pain is generally manageable. Knowing the correct layer is important, and so lifting the needle will cause the skin to tent over it; horizontal depression of the needle, when it is within the correct layer, produces minimal inflection. Once deployed, the lead body is barely detectable. In some newer devices, the use of a nerve stimulator can help identify the exact target prior to deposition of the lead. Stimulation testing ensues if only limited and short-acting anesthesia is used, and comfortable programs are saved into the external pulse generator. Sometimes painful paresthesia is generated, even in the appropriate layer. In this instance, increasing the amplitude often changes the quality to pleasant. High amplitude, small paresthetic distribution, or pain may all possibly be ameliorated with slight withdrawal of the lead to stimulate appropriate fibers. Lead ligation to the skin, radiographic documentation, and wound dressing conclude the procedure. The patient is then taken to recovery for a short observation period and possible electrode programming, prior to discharge for an outpatient trial.

26.2.3 Percutaneous Permanent Implant

Once the trial has been completed with acceptable pain relief, the patient is offered a permanent implant. The physician should carefully evaluate any cosmetic or structural issues that may affect lead choice, device choice, pocket placement, and incision location. The patient is returned to the operating theater and the percutaneous lead is replaced based on pain mapping, fluoroscopy, and review of the previous films with landmarks and/or ultrasound. Often, a curve is added to the deployment needle to allow approximation of many of the curved planes of the body. As lead erosion is a concern not only at the anchor but also at the most distal tip of the lead, it is recommended to turn the bevel of the needle deep and advance the terminal few millimeters of the array deeper within the adipose. No studies have evaluated this technique, but it seems to lessen the incidence of distal tip erosion. Once the lead is in good position, an incision is made sufficiently deep to allow multilayer closure, possibly to the fascia at the area of the lead proximal to the electrodes, so that the lead can be secured without affecting the electrical fields.

Anchoring methods vary, but the aim is universal: a well-secured lead with minimal risk of erosion, migration, or lead fracture. Conventional SCS anchors used for PNfS are frequently too bulky and increase erosive risk. Using nonabsorbable sutures in a drain stitch fashion without a formal anchor is more compact, but it introduces variation, and the implanter needs to be sensitive to lead security without increasing the likelihood of lead fracture. If an anchor is chosen, it is imperative for the implanter to close the tissue in two or three planes to protect the anchor from erosion. Once the lead is secured, a pocket is made in the appropriate location. Pocket proximity to the lead array is encouraged. As with SCS, the greater the distance between the pocket and the lead array, the greater the likelihood of lead torsion, strain, fracture, and migration. If proximity is difficult, especially when the construct crosses joint lines, the use of multiple buried lead loops is recommended to permit freedom of movement without lead compromise. The smaller size of the IPGs now being produced has increased options for the pocket location. External pulse generators in development may even further reduce this concern. As with any pocket, the implanting doctor should consider the bony margins, skin condition, and body habitus before selecting an appropriate location. Programming of the device will stabilize over 6 weeks, with many patients receiving improved stimulation as fibrosis develops around the lead.

26.2.4 Direct Stimulation of and Implantations to the Peripheral Nerve

The limits of terminal nerve or field stimulation—smaller paresthetic area, difficult or multiple areas to stimulate, or simply ineffectual paresthesia—may lead to consideration of direct nerve stimulation. The recent adoption of ultrasound, especially when coupled with the following stimulating technique, has allowed the surgeon to place coaxial leads near or next to peripheral nerves with ease and increased safety. When placing more than one lead, a second and reference electrode can be placed under the skin, away from the intended neural target. With the needle stylet removed, the lead can be placed within the needle lumen with the distal (and active) electrode just outside the beveled tip. With either sensory (i.e., 50 Hz) or motor (i.e., 2 Hz) stimulation parameters, the needle and lead are directed to the target.

The history of peripheral nerve stimulation started with paddle lead placement directly on the peripheral nerve. Large and irregularly shaped or raised arrays (the only available option at the time) lead to erosion into the nerve and difficulty with lead migration and movement, especially with appendicular function. Because of lead migration or failure to capture appropriate coverage, it is still advisable to place a directional, paddle-type lead in or around the peripheral nerve in some cases, most commonly in the occipital region or in the limb targeting larger nerves such as the sciatic, femoral, common peroneal, or median nerve. This open technique is more difficult and should not be attempted without proper training. In the occiput, the tissue is expanded to allow for placement of the paddle lead after removal of the previously implanted percutaneous system. The main issues are the control of bleeding and appropriate tissue depth. The placement of a paddle lead is much more difficult in an extremity, but this problem may be mitigated by newer deployment sheaths such as the Epiducer™ (St. Jude Medical, St. Paul, MN). In typical paddle cases, the surgeon must carefully dissect to the nerve target and expose the nerve. Once the nerve is exposed, a careful graft of fascia must be performed. The fascia is secured between the nerve paddle array, and the entire complex is held with a small, nonabsorbable suture.

26.2.5 Common Nerve Targets for PNS and PNfS

Any peripheral nerve fiber, when stimulated, could produce meaningful paresthesia. The use of PNS and PNfS is more common in certain regions of the body. The most common nerve targets are noted below.

Occipital Occipital targets are well defined and have been addressed in several reports and articles over the past decade. The use of PNS for the occipital nerve was originally described in 1990s by Wiener, and has evolved. The initial description involved placing the lead horizontal to the C1 vertebra in the midline, but over time the technique has evolved and the lead is now placed through a midline incision just near the nuchal line. By placing leads bilaterally in the more superior location, it is possible to maintain better long-term contact with the nerve fibers and to reduce the risks of significant migration. Occipital leads are placed for neuritis of the greater occipital nerve and lesser occipital nerve, C2 radiculitis, transformed migraine, and cervicogenic headache.

Supraorbital Stimulation of the supraorbital nerve, a nerve derived from the trigeminal nerve, is important in the treatment of frontal pain superior to the eyebrow. Several recent, unpublished series promote the successful combined use of supraorbital and occipital stimulation for cases of headache refractory to posterior occipital stimulation alone and argue that several prospective trials of occipital stimulation would have met endpoints had 360° stimulation been employed. The most common causes of disease in the supraorbital nerve include trauma and infection. The most common infectious cause is viral, in the form of herpes zoster. The lead is placed 0.5 cm above the brow in most cases. The approach is most commonly lateral, with mapping of the nerve occurring prior to implantation. Some patients cannot tolerate the lead because of allodynia; in these cases, an approach with either a very small lead or programming current through the area, as opposed to direct lead placement on the nerve, may be indicated. The advantage of small leads is their atraumatic nature, but their disadvantage is that they do not cover as much area, and the leads may be more prone to fracture.

Infraorbital Stimulation of the infraorbital nerve, a nerve also derived from the trigeminal nerve, is important in the treatment of pain just below the eye that is of a burning and stabbing nature. Common causes of disease in this nerve are trauma and disease. The lead is placed 0.5–1.0 cm below the eye, with the exact placement based on preoperative skin mapping with a semipermanent marker from a lateral approach.

Divisions of the Trigeminal Nerve Trigeminal neuralgia is a painful condition of the face that involves one to three divisions of the nerve: ophthalmic, mandibular, and maxillary. Often, this problem is treated with oral anticonvulsants, by neurosurgical or stereotactic brainstem vascular decompression, or by nerve destruction. When these options do not give appropriate relief or are unacceptable, the interventional pain specialist may place a peripheral lead over the involved division(s). This technique involves mapping by history and examination, careful placement with mapping by landmarks and fluoroscopic guidance, and attention to proper tissue depth and anchoring techniques. High cervical SCS lead placement also may confer evoked paresthesia, especially to the lower divisions of the nerve through nucleus caudalis stimulation, but cross-talking the peripheral, facial lead to the cervical SCS lead itself also may be considered. The facial leads are often anchored behind the ear and the submandibular neck crease, with the pocket in the chest wall, trapezius area, or upper flank.

Auriculotemporal A branch of the mandibular nerve, the auriculotemporal nerve runs with the superficial temporal artery and vein, providing sensory innervation to the face and jaw. It is commonly injured by local trauma or surgery of the temporomandibular joint or parotid gland. Placement of the lead is often simple, with an understanding of the pain pattern in the face, anterior jaw, and temporal region. The lead anchoring and tunneling is performed in similar fashion to other facial leads.

Superficial Cervical Plexus The superficial cervical plexus has been described as a source of pain after trauma, radiation, or surgery. The approach of placing a lead in this region is based on pain topography, and PNfS may work best, as it can be difficult to isolate the nerves without direct tissue dissection.

Intercostal The intercostal nerves are the anterior divisions (rami anteriores; ventral divisions) of the thoracic spinal nerves from T1 to T11. The intercostal nerves are common causes of pain and disease involving neuropathic pain of the chest wall. The most common causes of pain in this region include postherpetic neuralgia, local neural trauma, and postsurgical nerve entrapment, such as that seen with postmastectomy syndrome and postthoracotomy syndrome. Treatment of this problem with oral medications can be successful. Sometimes it is treated with epidural lead placement, but higher thoracic lead placement may present stimulation difficulty secondary to the cord's anatomy, deep within cerebrospinal fluid (CSF). Additionally confounding is that these levels possess a low ratio of postsynaptic white fiber to radicular dorsal root fibers, yielding lateral root stimulation at the expense of cord stimulation. SCS success rates for this indication thus are dwarfed by those associated with failed back surgery or neuropathic limb pain. The patient should be carefully examined, and the pain topography should be well mapped. Two options exist: PNfS and direct, subcostal nerve stimulation with ultrasound placement. Again, as in the facial construct introduced above, co-stimulation or cross-talk stimulation with an SCS lead may give densely useful and comfortable paresthesia. Subcutaneous tunneling to common pocket locations is generally easy.

Ilioinguinal Burning groin pain certainly can be very disabling, resulting in decreased quality of life, inability to work, and reduced overall function. Neural trauma in any form can cause pain in this region, but the most common culprit—the knife—is guilty in most cases, either from direct insult or scar and resultant nerve entrapment. A peripheral lead can be placed by first confirming the diagnosis with examination, history, and a temporary response to nerve injection. The lead is placed in the tissue parallel to the longest axis of pain on mapping of the tissue; both PNfS and direct PNS aided with ultrasound appear to be of benefit. The generator should be near the area of the leads to reduce the risk of migration.

Genitofemoral and Iliohypogastric As with the ilioinguinal nerve, the genitofemoral and iliohypogastric nerves are often involved in chronic pain from similar causes. The use of PNS has been described for these nerves, but success has been historically difficult to achieve, though it may be improved by the use of the live, soft tissue imaging produced by ultrasound guidance. The anatomical location and course of the nerves have made it difficult to achieve good, sustained relief in these pain syndromes.

Cluneal and Nerves of the Paravertebral Region The low back is a common location of intractable pain in patients across populations. The innervation can be complicated but involves the cluneal nerve, branches of the sinuvertebral nerve, and branches of the medial and lateral branches of the dorsal primary rami. The branches of the cluneal nerves, particularly the superior cluneal nerves, are often involved in severe, burning pain of the low back. This problem commonly occurs after lumbar surgery, especially when trauma to or bone harvest from the iliac crest occurs. In many cases, the patient has successful stimulation with epidural leads, but the stimulation misses a very specific area of the lower back and buttocks. A recently published multicenter, randomized and prospective evaluation suggests that PNfS has definite benefit for low back pain from lumbar surgery. Several successful approaches exist. The most commonly performed placement of a PNfS lead in this area is based on pain mapping. The lead is placed in the subcutaneous tissue in the subdermal adipose tissue, being careful not to place it too deep (causing muscle recruitment) or too superficial (causing skin erosion or burning pain on stimulation). Additionally found to be useful is deeper or directed lead placement superficial to the bone comprising the rim of the iliac crest (being careful not to disturb the periosteum or fascial attachments of the muscular aponeurosis), and deeper placement to influence the lateral branches of the sacral nerves or of the lumbar dorsal primary rami.

Lateral Femoral Cutaneous The lateral femoral cutaneous nerve of the thigh arises from the dorsal divisions of the second and third lumbar nerves. It emerges deeply from the lateral border of the psoas major muscle, crosses the iliacus muscle obliquely, and courses superficially toward the anterior superior iliac spine. It then passes under or through the inguinal ligament and subcutaneously over the quadriceps to serve the skin of the upper thigh. This nerve, frequently damaged by trauma, injured by pressure and resulting ischemia, or injured by diabetes mellitus or other metabolic syndromes, can present the syndrome known as meralgia paresthetica. The nerve is commonly injured by compression from constrictive clothing or following weight gain. The pain is often successfully managed by oral medications, steroid injections, or topical patches or gels, but it sporadically remains severe. Recalcitrant cases may be candidates for SCS, which (for a variety of anatomic reasons) does not always succeed in providing successful stimulation. The use of PNS has been successful in some cases, including those with pain in specific areas. The lead is placed based on tissue mapping, or deeper along the visualized nerve. When placed permanently, the lead is anchored to the fascia, with the generator placed in the closest approximation to the lead(s).

Axillary, Suprascapular, Brachial Plexus, and Other Mixed Nerves The possibility of achieving pain relief and improved muscle function in nerves that contain both motor and sensory fibers has been discussed, and current studies are examining viability. The mixed nature of nerves like the axillary and suprascapular nerves may confer benefit in syndromes such as those seen with poststroke shoulder pain. Stimulation simultaneously increases the tone of formerly flaccid muscle supportive to the joint and also provides pleasant, sensory paresthesia covering a portion of the joint. These techniques remain experimental; the benefits of their use, although exciting for a large and undertreated population, remain inconclusive.

Median, Ulnar, and Radial Nerves At and distal to the elbow, the peripheral nerves of the upper extremity are superficial at many points in their courses and thus could be easily accessed with a needle. At present there are few formal reports, but growing anecdotal data support the use of PNS to treat the sensory components of the nerves of the forearm and hand. Patients who suffer from radial nerve injury or failed ulnar transposition or carpal tunnel surgery may respond very well. Ongoing studies are evaluating treatment possibilities.

Saphenous, Sural, Peroneal, and Tibial The underappreciated and often injured appendage of the lower leg appears particularly susceptible to neural injury. Metabolic syndromes, chemotherapeutic drugs, trauma, and the surgeon's knife all conspire to injure the nerves of the leg. The sciatic nerves, particularly proximal to the bifurcation, as well as the proximal femoral nerves, can be anatomically deep and guarded by mobile muscle. Their access usually requires surgical dissection and careful placement of the device with robust anchoring within the highly mobile milieu. Distal to their deep origins, these nerves course into sonographic depth and become accessible to the needle. The medial knee hosts the patellar branch of the saphenous nerve, useful for those suffering from anteromedial knee pain from either surgical or direct trauma. The anterolateral knee and inner joint is served by the quite stimulatable articular branch of the peroneal nerve. Also amenable to the technique is the superficial peroneal branch at the lateral fibular head, the deep peroneal nerve at the extensor retinaculum (the anterior tarsal tunnel), and the tibial nerve (and thus plantar nerves) proximal to the (posterior) tarsal tunnel. The common peroneal and tibial nerves can be stimulated just below the popliteal fossa, but require extensive tissue dissection. Smaller generators have made it possible to place distal generators more comfortably and nearer to the electrode array, with less need to tunnel across the hip or knee.

26.3 Risk Assessment

- The patient who may be high-risk for epidural lead placement or major neurosurgical interventions may be a better candidate for PNS. The risks are more limited, but careful preoperative planning is still necessary.
- Lead placement may injure the peripheral nerve or its fibers, leading to continued or worsened pain.
- Skin infection is the most common problem with PNS and PNfS.
- Skin erosion may occur when the lead, anchor, or generator irritates the skin, causing a cellulitis and potential skin breakdown.
- Pain at a component of the device may lead to a decreased use of the device, decreased function, and a need to revise the system.

26.4 Risk Avoidance

The risk of PNS and PNfS is limited, but it is still important to evaluate comorbidities before moving ahead with implantation of the device. Diseases such as diabetes and those involving the skin should be optimized prior to moving forward.

The skin should be examined and inspected for infection or other high-risk conditions prior to implantation. If those conditions exist, the primary care specialist or a dermatologist should be consulted prior to moving forward.

Nerve injury is very rare with the newer percutaneous techniques of lead placement. The lead usually is placed in the proximity of the nerve rather than in direct contact. The patient should be kept alert during lead placement and the needle or lead should be redirected if the patient complains of paresthesia.

The lead should be placed into the subcutaneous tissue at a level below the dermis. The physician should palpate the skin while placing the needle, and it is helpful to direct the bevel downward prior to engaging the lead. The use of leads with plastic stylets may allow for easier tissue plane identification and placement. Many implanters have begun using a technique that eliminates the use of the anchor; instead, a loop of nonabsorbable suture is used to secure the lead placement near the target nerve.

Pain at the device can be minimized by carefully examining the bony structure of the patient prior to implantation. The pocket should be in the location that receives the least amount of tissue pressure during the patient's daily activities. If pain persists, options include the use of topical anesthetics, padding, and, if other methods fail, surgical revision.

Attention to the planned course of lead tunneling is mandatory, with consideration especially of strain relief around mobile structures such as the neck and peripheral joints.

Conclusions

The interest in stimulating the peripheral nervous system to treat chronic pain has seen resurgence in recent years. New areas of research include stimulation of the motor nerves to improve function, as well as new devices that aim to stimulate only peripheral targets. The number of patients who are candidates for neuromodulation will increase exponentially if these methods are proven successful. New, prospective research is needed going forward, and careful attention to patient selection and construct planning is needed in current clinical practice.

26.5 Supplemental Images

See Figs. 26.1, 26.2, 26.3, 26.4, 26.5, 26.6, 26.7, 26.8, 26.9, 26.10, 26.11, 26.12, 26.13, 26.14, 26.15, 26.16, 26.17, 26.18, 26.19, and 26.20.

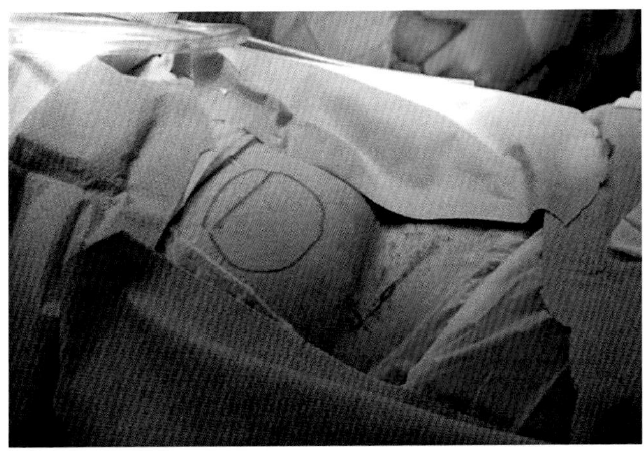

Fig. 26.1 Patient marking for the peripheral nerve stimulation (PNS) device pocket and lead target

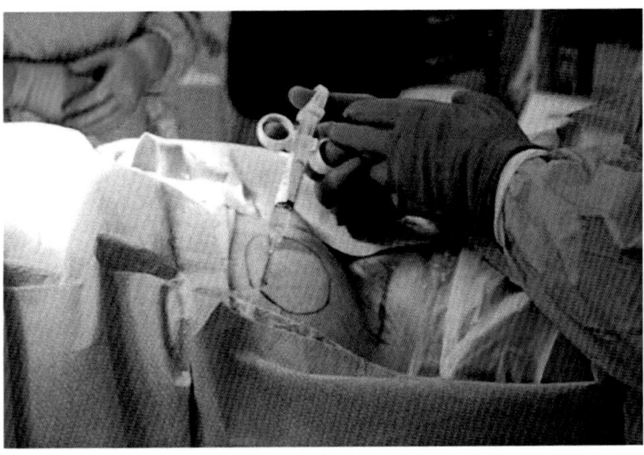

Fig. 26.2 Local anesthetic placement

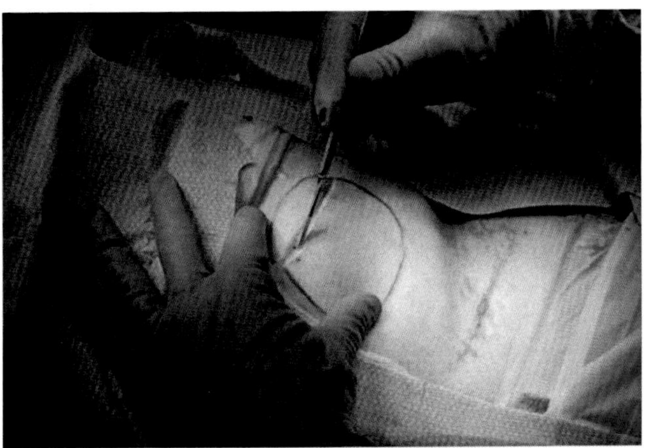

Fig. 26.3 Creation of a pocket for a PNS device

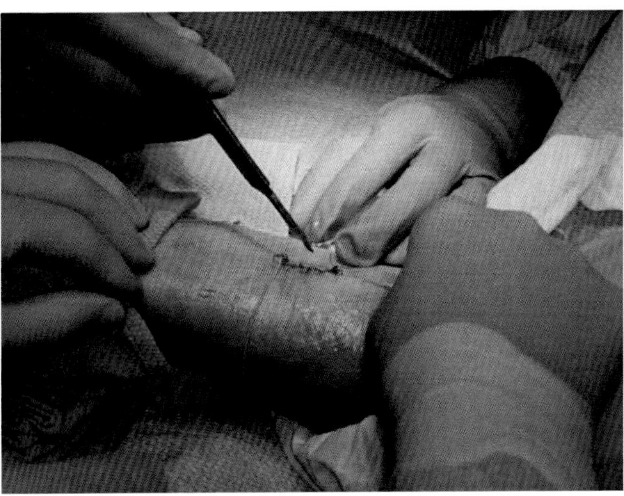

Fig. 26.4 Insertion of percutaneous leads in the area of the median nerve

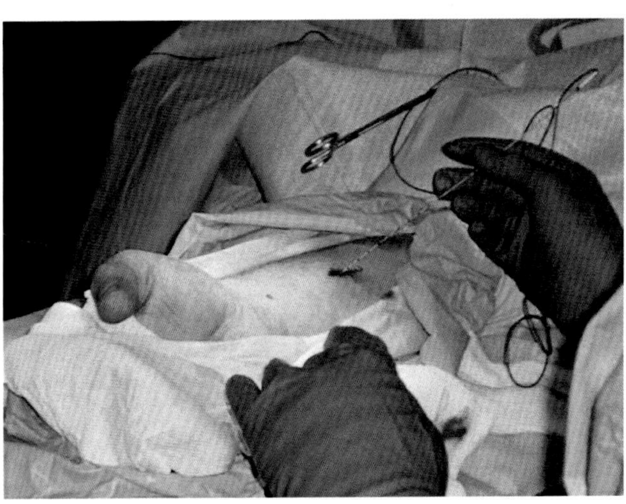

Fig. 26.5 PNS can be facilitated by identifying the nerve with a nerve stimulator, which can be used to guide the final lead placement

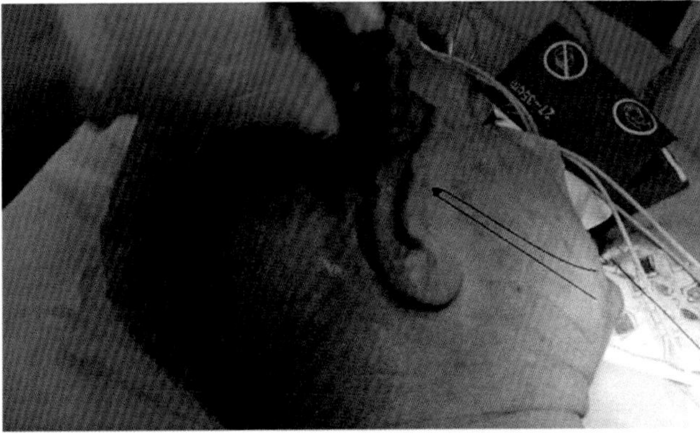

Fig. 26.6 Mapping of the neuropathic pain is helpful prior to implantation of the PNS device

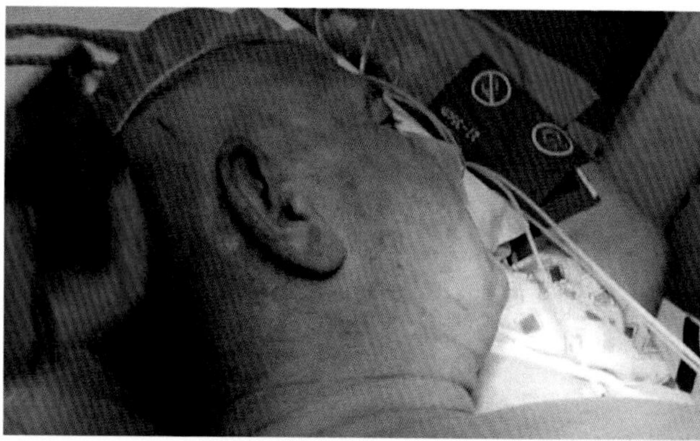

Fig. 26.7 Prepping should be well outside of the target area for implantation of the PNS device

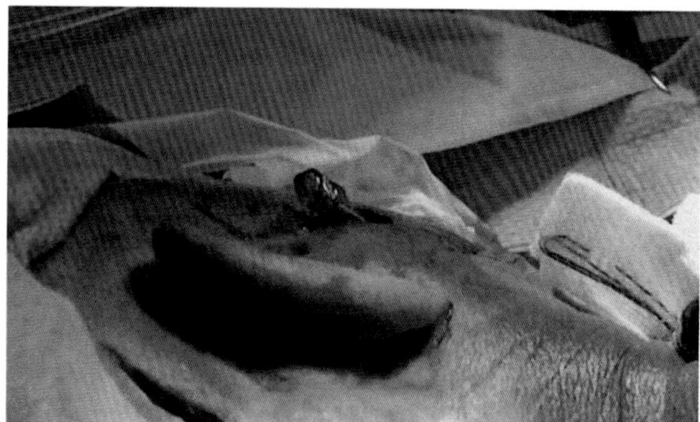

Fig. 26.8 Lateral orientation of the needle placement prior to lead delivery

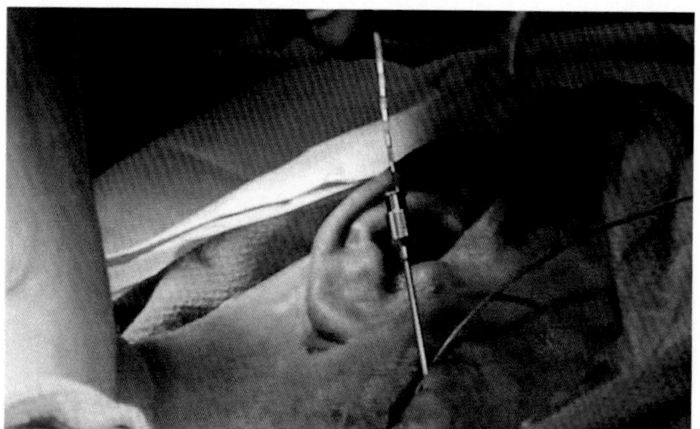

Fig. 26.9 Needle orientation and targeting is an essential part of head and neck implantation

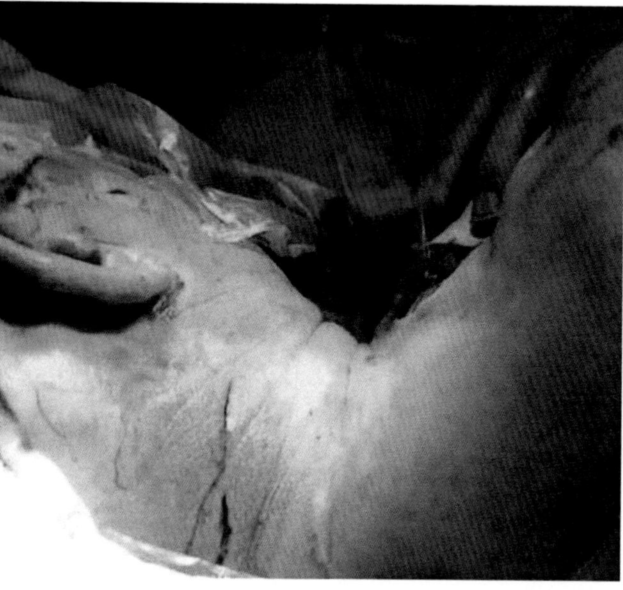

Fig. 26.10 Pectoral pocketing for head and neck implants is often desirable to reduce the risks of lead migration

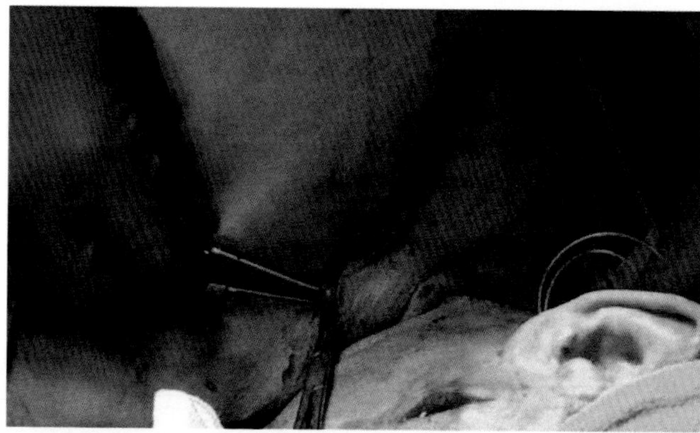

Fig. 26.11 Tunneling of the peripheral lead in the head and neck must be performed with caution to avoid the vessels in the area of the implant

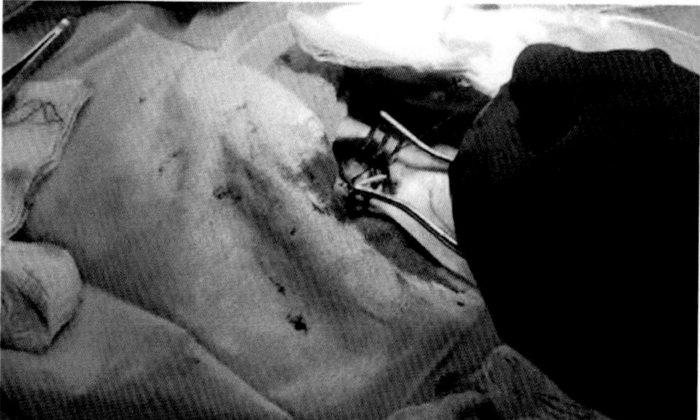

Fig. 26.12 Anchoring of the leads to the fascia behind the ear can lend extra stability to the system and can be cosmetically desirable

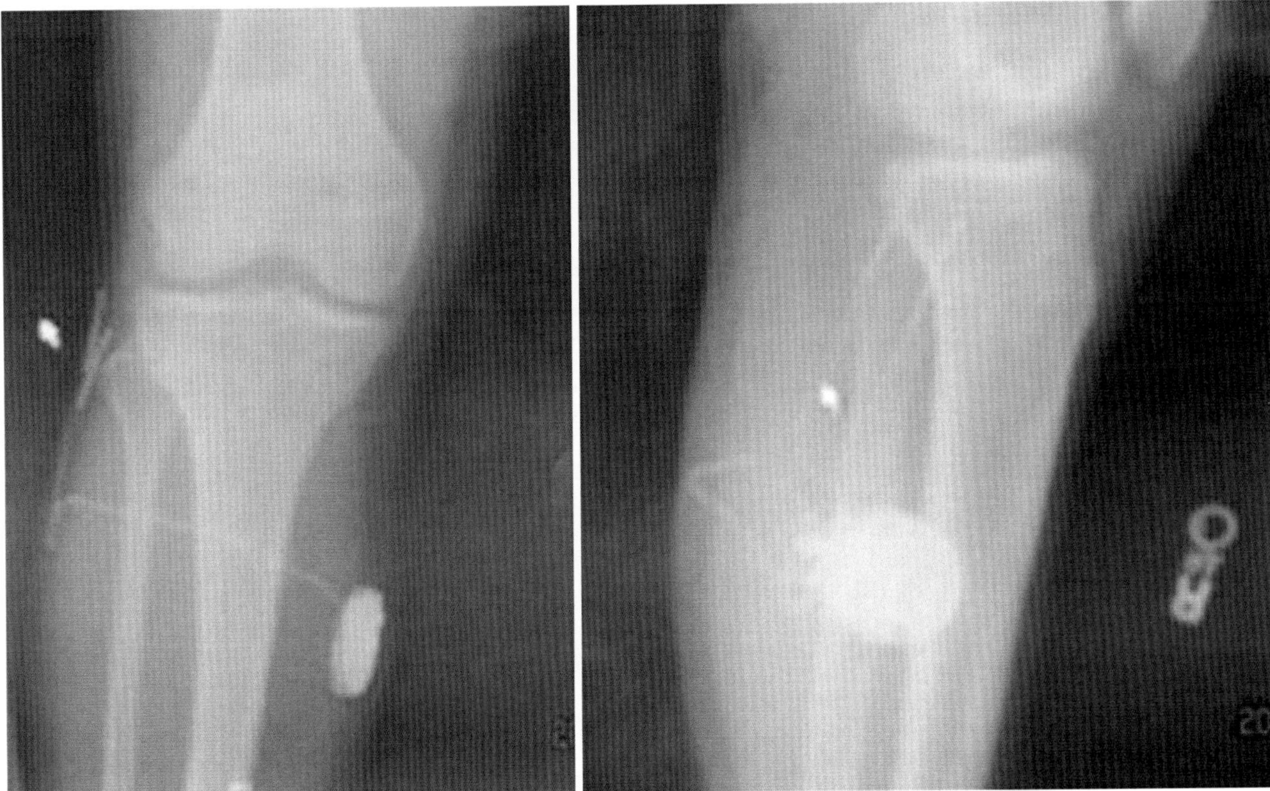

Fig. 26.13 Pocketing in an extremity

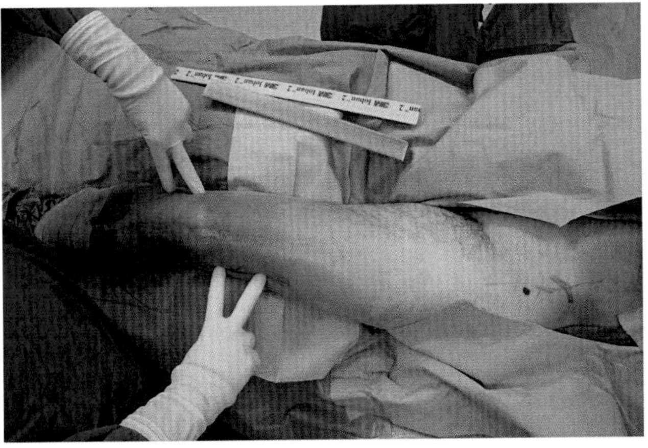

Fig. 26.14 Lead location for chronic postoperative knee pain

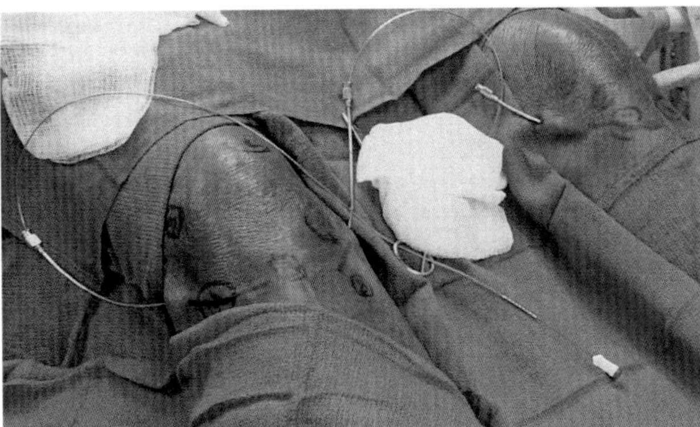

Fig. 26.15 Trialing lead location (with associated dermatographic marking) for bilateral knee pain

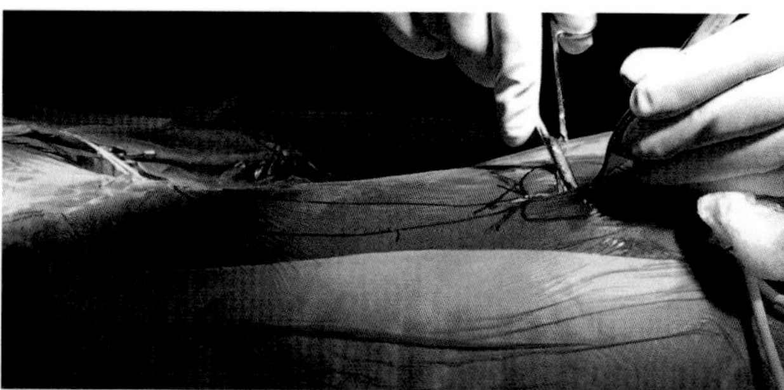

Fig. 26.16 Lead placement at the lateral fibular head for superficial peroneal nerve stimulation, with pocket creation at the anterolateral thigh

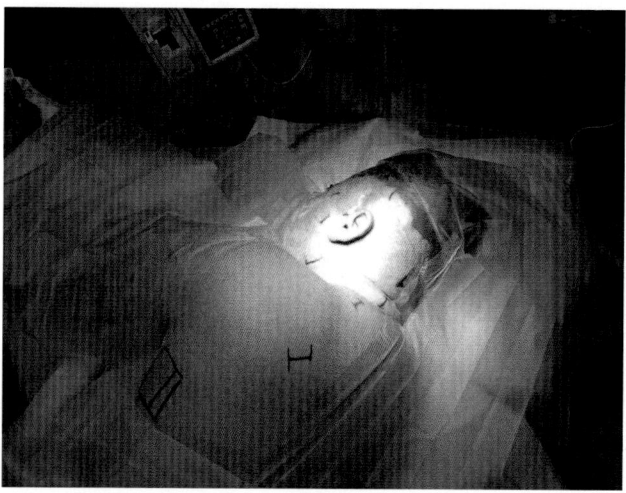

Fig. 26.17 Lead deployment, tunneling, and pocket plan for supraorbital, auricular, and occipital nerve montage

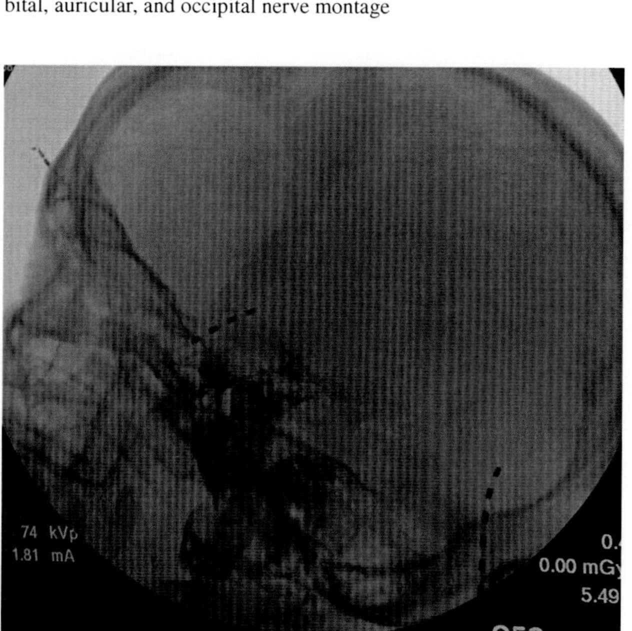

Fig. 26.18 Lateral x-ray of supraorbital, auricular, and occipital nerve construct

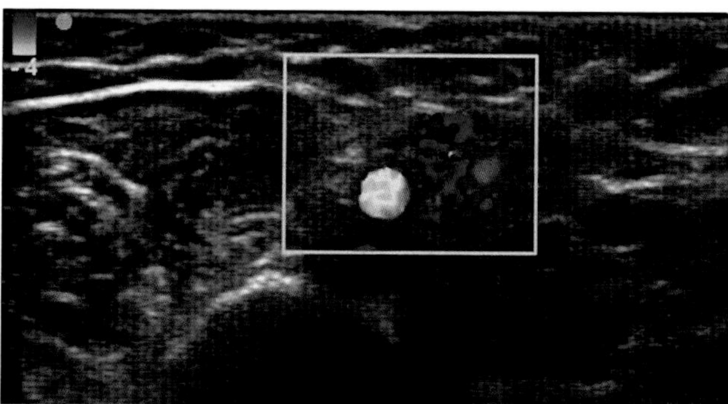

Fig. 26.19 Peripheral lead in proximity to axillary nerve and artery posterior to the shoulder under ultrasound visualization

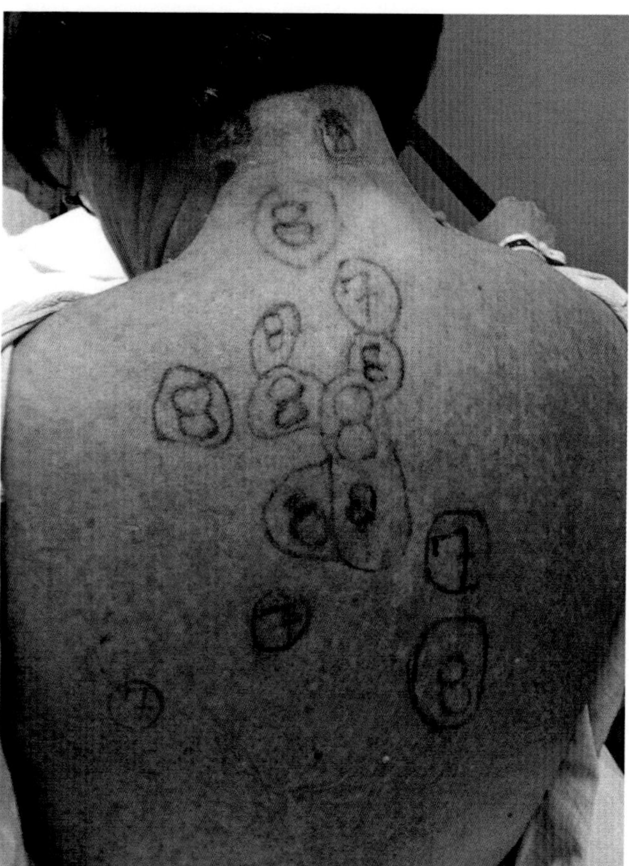

Fig. 26.20 An example of dermatographic pain mapping. It is essential to understand exactly where the patient's pain lies

Suggested Reading

Davis G. Peripheral nerve stimulation for the treatment of chronic pain. J Clin Neurosci. 2007;14:222–3.

Falco FJE, Berger J, Vrable A, Onyewu O, Zhu J. Cross talk: a new method for peripheral nerve stimulation: an observational report with cadaveric verification. Pain Physician. 2009;12:965–83.

Henderson J. Peripheral nerve stimulation for chronic pain. Curr Pain Headache Rep. 2008;12:28–31.

Huntoon MA, Burgher AH. Ultrasound-guided permanent implantation of peripheral nerve stimulation (PNS) system for neuropathic pain of the extremities: original cases and outcomes. Pain Med. 2009;10: 1369–77.

Kouroukli I, Neofytos D, Panaretou V, Zompolas V, Papasterglou D, Sanidas G, et al. Peripheral subcutaneous stimulation for the treatment of intractable postherpetic neuralgia: two case reports and literature review. Pain Pract. 2009;9:225–9.

Slavin KV, editor. Peripheral nerve stimulation. Progress in neurological surgery, vol. 24. Basel: Karger; 2011.

Sweet WH. Control of pain by direct electrical stimulation of peripheral nerves. Clin Neurosurg. 1976;23:103–11.

27 Peripheral Nerve Stimulation for the Treatment of Knee Pain

Timothy R. Deer, Jason E. Pope, W. Porter McRoberts, Paul Verrills, and Richard Bowman

27.1 Introduction

Knee pain from neuropathic pathology is a common problem after total knee replacement, arthroscopic surgery, and trauma. Treatment for this painful, lifestyle-limiting, neuropathic syndrome has included injections, pulsed radiofrequency, oral medications such as chronic opioids, physical medicine, and additional surgery. Advanced techniques, which have been successful in many patients with severe pain, have included spinal cord stimulation, intrathecal drug delivery, and most recently, dorsal root ganglion spinal cord stimulation (DRG-SCS). This focused chapter describes the techniques involved in placing a peripheral nerve stimulation (PNS) system for the treatment of neuropathic knee pain.

27.2 Anatomy

The knee and its surrounding tissue are heavily innervated. This complex network of nerves can lead to complex problems of neuropathic pain (Fig. 27.1). In some settings, the nerve pain is limited to one or two nerve distributions. The most commonly involved nerves appear to be the saphenous and sural nerves and their peripheral branches. These patients are ideal to consider for PNS of the knee. In clinical scenarios where the nerve injury leads to a more complicated, complex regional pain syndrome Type II, the use of PNS is less likely to give relief, although it could be considered as part of a combined technique with DRG-SCS where available, or with spinal cord stimulation in the United States.

T.R. Deer, MD (✉) • R. Bowman, MD
The Center for Pain Relief, 400 Court Street, Suite 100, Charleston, WV 25301, USA
e-mail: DocTDeer@aol.com

J.E. Pope
Summit Pain Alliance,
392 Tesconi Court, Santa Rosa, CA 95401, USA

W.P. McRoberts
Division of Interventional Spine, Pain, and Neurosurgery, Holy Cross Hospital, Fort Lauderdale, FL, USA

P. Verrills
MetroPain Group, Caulfield, South VIC, Australia

T.R. Deer, J.E. Pope (eds.), *Atlas of Implantable Therapies for Pain Management*, DOI 10.1007/978-1-4939-2110-2_27

Fig. 27.1 Anatomy of the knee and its innervation

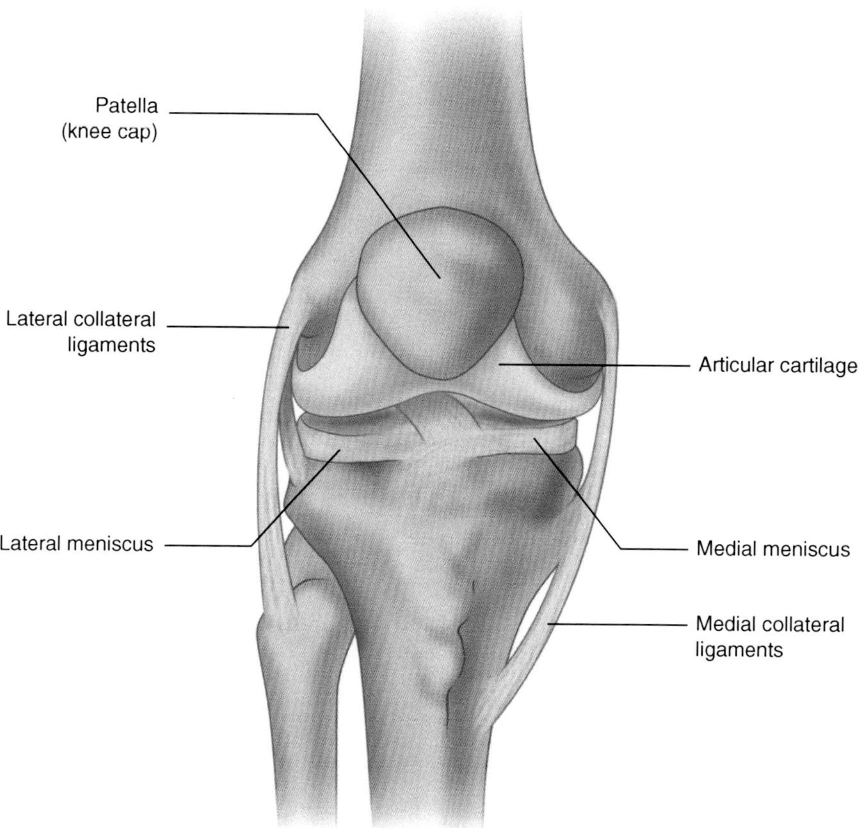

The right knee

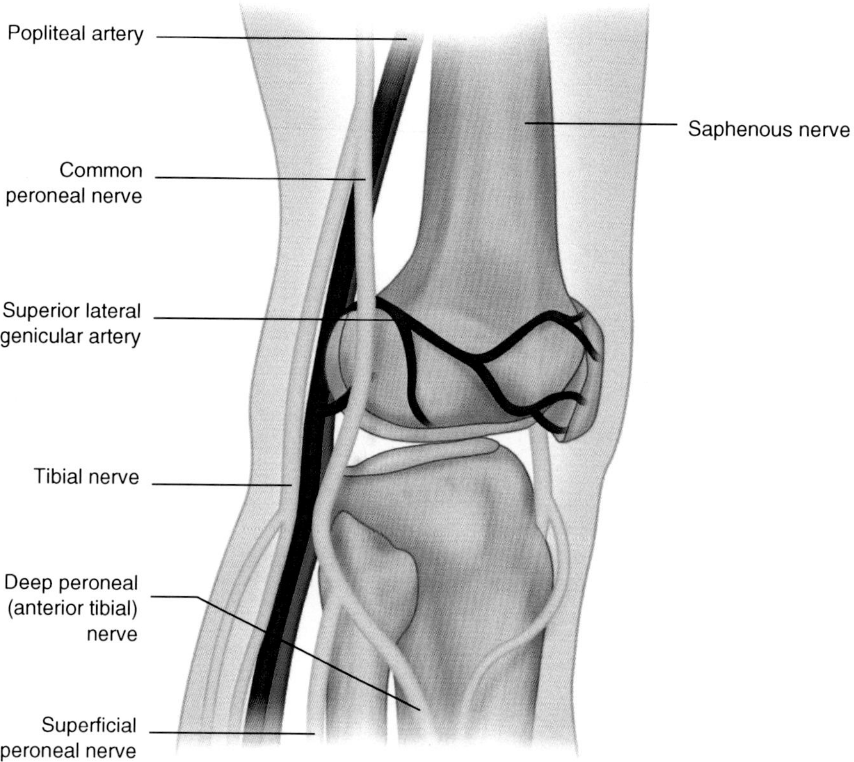

27.3 Patient Selection

The ideal patient for consideration of PNS to treat knee pain can be identified by several characteristics. The patient should complain of burning knee pain in the distribution of a definable nerve or nerve branch. The examination should demonstrate evidence of abnormal nerve function, either nerve hypersensitivity or a loss of sensation. Attempts to treat the pain with physical medicine, reasonable oral and topical medications, and other conservative measures should be unsuccessful or unacceptable. The predictive ability of a nerve block to determine a proper candidate has not been proven in any prospective study, but algorithms exist (Fig. 27.2). The patient should not have any definable contraindications to PNS. (The use of PNS may be possible in some patients who are not candidates for spinal cord stimulation because of comorbidities or increased risks.)

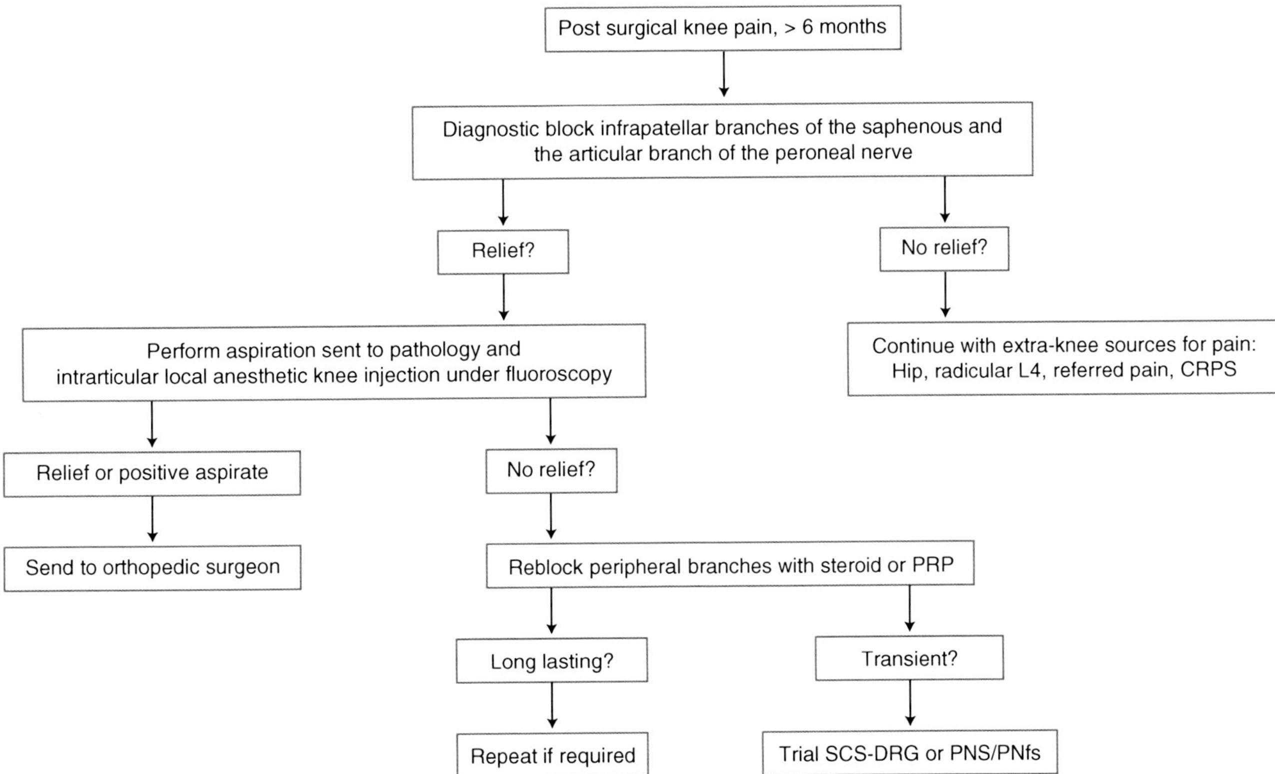

Fig. 27.2 Postsurgical knee pain work-up algorithm using a diagnostic nerve block. *CRPS* complex regional pain syndrome, *PNfs* peripheral nerve field stimulation, *PRP* platelet rich plasma

27.4 Technical Overview

The patient should undergo normal preoperative evaluation and testing. Attention should be given to hemostasis and infection risks. The integrity of the skin should be considered, and the absence of open lesions should be noted. Further, the presence of infectious postoperative knee complications should be fully interrogated and patient optimization should occur.

Once the patient has been deemed an appropriate candidate for the procedure, the use of preoperative antibiotics is recommended. The patient is brought to the operating theater after carefully mapping the nerve and pain distribution. If a conventional or new experimental trial is considered with PNS leads and no implantable programmable generator (IPG), attention is given only to the area of the limb having pain. The spacing, size, and number of leads should match the patient's painful area appropriately.

In patients who have already undergone a trial, the planning of IPG placement is essential during this time of education and discussion. Common places are the medial or lateral thigh within the subcutaneous adipose tissue.

27.4.1 Lead Placement

In the early days of PNS implants, one of the authors (TRD) used the technique of lead placement on the diseased or targeted nerve. This laborious approach involved making a surgical dissection to the nerve and then placing a unidirectional paddle lead over the nerve. Prior to implanting the lead, the surgeon had to create a fascial graft to insulate the nerve. This approach led to an initial good outcome in most patients, but unfortunately, over time the nerve would become hypersensitive and the lead would become unusable. In modern PNS placement, advancements in programming have allowed a much less invasive approach. This method involves using a styletted needle to place a lead percutaneously close to the vicinity of the nerve, with fluoroscopic landmarks or ultrasound guidance. Once the lead is in place, intra-operative computer testing using various pulse-width, frequency, and electrode combinations are used to confirm appropriate nerve activation. The lead is sutured to the skin close to the entry point to enable evaluation of pain relief and functional improvement over a trial lasting 3–14 days.

27.4.2 Permanent Implant

A successful trial, characterized by a reduction in pain scores greater than 50 %, is usually followed by scheduling of the patient for a permanent implant. The lead placement for the permanent implant is performed in the same fashion as the trial. The lead position is determined by the hard-copy x-ray saved after trial placement. In some cases, the final lead placement may be modified based on feedback from the trial paresthesia. Once the lead is placed, hand-held programming is performed to document appropriate coverage. When the final lead position is determined, a cut-down is made in the area proximal to the electrodes. In this incision, the physician must use blunt dissection to identify fascia, which will be the point of anchoring for the suture to secure the lead. Anchoring can be performed with a nonabsorbable suture directly to the fascia and lead, or a commercial Silastic anchor can be used. If an anchor is used, the implanter must pay careful attention to the skin quality and tissue depth to ensure that adequate tissue covers the anchor, as the risk of an anchor is skin erosion. Once the lead is anchored, a strain relief loop is made with the lead, and the lead is tunneled to the pocket. Current devices require an IPG, so careful planning is needed to reduce the tunneling distance from the implant. Once the lead and generator are connected, a sterile hand-held programmer can be used to retest the paresthesia coverage and impedance. Impedance numbers less than 1500 are normally associated with acceptable tissue contact. When testing is concluded, the wound is vigorously irrigated and good hemostasis is established. At this time, a two-layer or three-layer closure should be performed and proper dressings placed (Figs. 27.3, 27.4, 27.5, and 27.6).

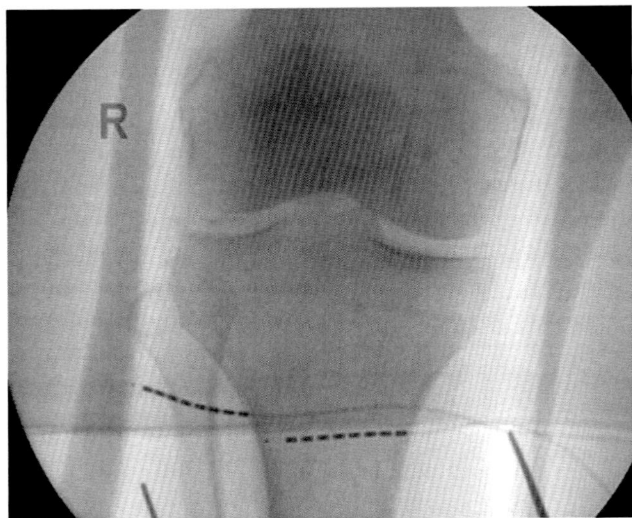

Fig. 27.3 Knee innervation with eight contact leads placed at possible locations

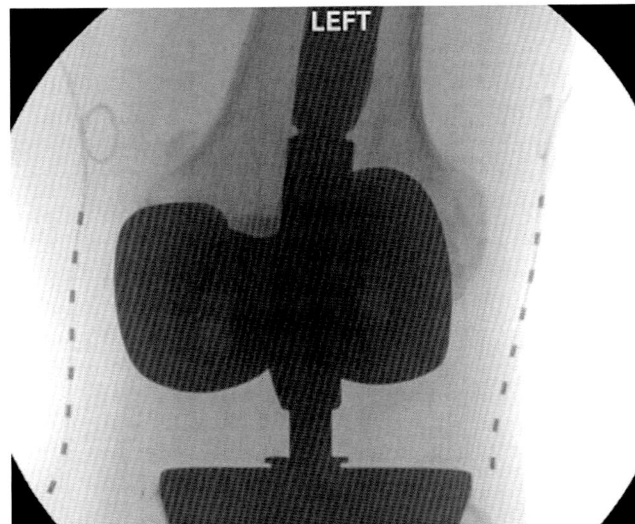

Fig. 27.4 Radiograph of lead placement (Courtesy of Paul Verrills)

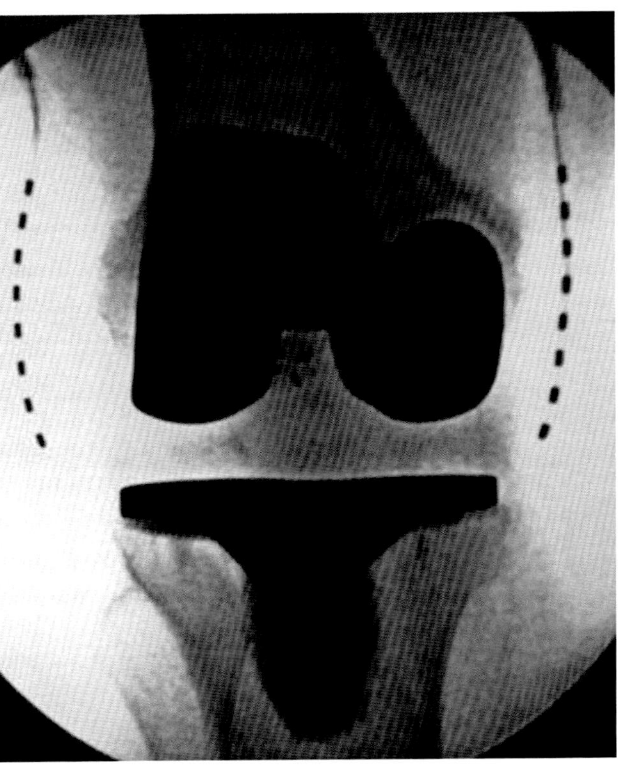

Fig. 27.5 Radiograph of lead placement (Courtesy of Jason Pope)

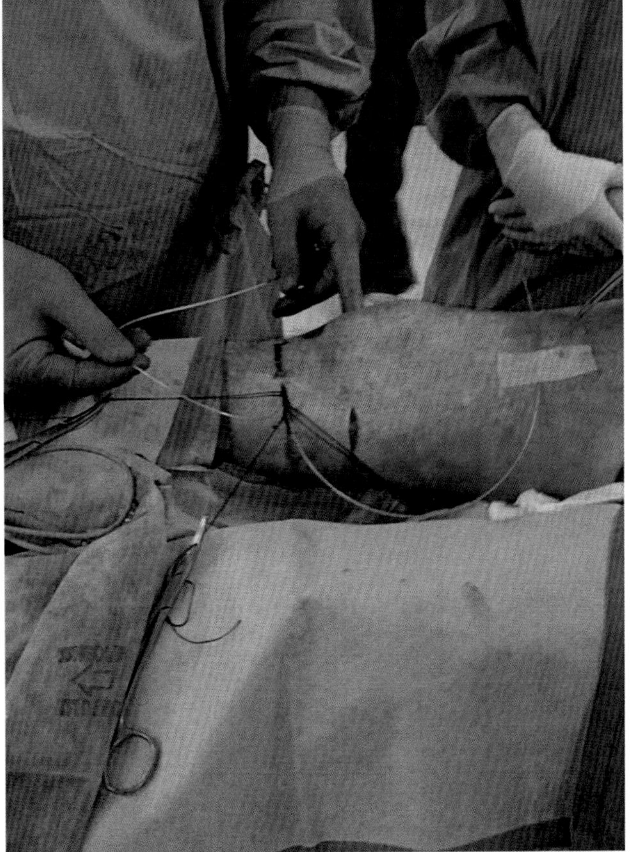

Fig. 27.6 Intraoperative view of lead placement with anchoring of leads and planned IPG placement (Courtesy of Richard Bowman and Timothy Deer)

27.5 Risk Assessment

A number of risks related to the implantation of the PNS system can result in failures and complications:

- This procedure is indicated in patients with nerve trauma in the knee. In patients with recent surgery, the possibility of an underlying infection or unstable joint should be considered before placing an implant.
- Skin integrity is very important in the area of the lead implant, tunneling, and pocketing. Poor quality of the skin or the presence of infection or disease can lead to a failed implant.
- Bleeding can occur in patients taking medications that impact clotting or those who have diseases that change hemostasis.
- Placing a pocket in the medial thigh is often a good choice because of body fat distribution, but the patient's gait, clothing choices, and cosmesis should be considered.
- A pocket that is too small may lead to pain, tissue necrosis, and erosion of the metal through the skin.
- Failure to anchor the IPG to the fascia can lead to flipping, may create difficulty in programming or recharging, and could move the lead.
- Poor anchoring of the lead can cause migration. Poor anchoring can occur when fascia is not identified in the dissection. In some patients, however, poor tissue quality related to poor nutrition, smoking, or diabetes also can result in lead migration.

27.6 Risk Avoidance

Steps taken before and during the implantation of the PNS system can help in avoiding failures and complications from the known risks:

- Before receiving a PNS implant, reasonable conservative treatments should have failed or have been unacceptable.
- The knee should be evaluated for underlying infection or an unstable prosthetic joint.
- Proper management of clotting and bleeding risks, including attention to medications and disease modification, should be addressed in the preoperative period.
- The avoidance of pocket bleeding can be achieved by attention to preoperative clotting indices, careful handling of the tissue during dissection, and hemostasis by electrocautery, suturing of vessels, and tissue pressure to clot small bleeding vessels that may not be initially obvious.
- Seroma cannot always be avoided, but the likelihood of this problem can be reduced by careful attention to detail when dissecting the pocket. The tissue should be handled carefully, electrocautery should be used judiciously, and bleeding vessels should be controlled prior to wound closure. It is also important to size the pocket properly for the device. Tissue pressure in the postoperative period may be helpful in reducing seroma. Elevating the limb also may be helpful in reducing swelling and possible fluid in the pocket.
- The lead should be anchored securely to the fascia with or without the use of a commercial anchor.
- The IPG should be anchored to fascia and oriented to reduce the possibility of skin irritation from edges or ridges in the device or header.

Conclusions

The treatment of neuropathic knee pain can be achieved by conventional spinal cord stimulation, DRG-SCS, or high-frequency stimulation, but in some patients, the option of treating this pain in the periphery is more attractive. If the pain can be mapped to a nerve distribution, or if invasion of the neuraxis is deemed too risky, the use of PNS can be a very helpful technique. New devices that are self-contained and do not require an IPG may be attractive choices going forward.

Suggested Reading

Barolat G. Subcutaneous peripheral nerve field stimulation for intractable pain. In: Krames E, Peckham PH, Rezai AR, editors. Neuromodulation. Amsterdam: Elsevier; 2009.

Deer TR, Pope JE. A novel method of peripheral nerve stimulation: the tripole technique for treatment of refractory chronic intercostal nerve pain. Pain Med News. 2012;10:8–10.

McRoberts WP, Roche M. Novel approach for peripheral subcutaneous field stimulation for the treatment of severe, chronic knee joint pain after total knee arthroplasty. Neuromodulation. 2010;13(2):131–6.

Pope JE, Deer TR, Grigsby EJ, Kim PS. Stimulation of the peripheral nerve and field. In: Deer TR, Leong MS, Buvanendran A, Gordin V, Kim PS, Panchal SJ, Ray AL, editors. Comprehensive treatment of chronic pain by medical, interventional and integrative approaches. New York: Springer; 2013.

28 Neurostimulation of the Upper Extremity by Conventional Peripheral Nerve Stimulation

Nameer R. Haider and Timothy R. Deer

28.1 Introduction

The etiology of upper extremity pain is complex and includes numerous disease processes. The presence of burning, shooting, or lancinating pain is more consistent with neuropathic pain and greatly focuses the differential diagnosis and potential treatment. Neuropathic pain is often function limiting and is usually exacerbated in the evening hours, which may limit sleep. The pain algorithm for these conditions includes oral and topical agents, physical medicine, and surgical nerve release. In many cases these innervations fail and the need to consider neurostimulation should be on the physician's radar.

This intractable neuropathic pain of the upper limb may be caused by peripheral neuropathy, nerve entrapment, peripheral nerve trauma, spinal nerve root injury, or complex regional pain syndrome. Any chronic peripheral nerve entrapment such as carpal tunnel syndrome, radial nerve injury after humeral neck fracture, or ulnar nerve entrapment may cause this condition. Postsurgical adhesions or scars resulting from ulnar transposition or carpal tunnel surgery can be causes of these issues and are often worsened by repeat surgical exploration. Chronic shoulder pain may occur after dislocation, shoulder surgery, or poststroke shoulder subluxation or as a result of adhesive capsulitis and chronic rotator cuff syndrome.

The consideration of neurostimulation often involves conventional spinal cord stimulation (SCS) at levels that range from C2 to T1. New technology in Europe and Australia has involved SCS at the dorsal root ganglion. This method may become the chosen method of upper extremity neuromodulation in the future because of the ability to stimulate discrete areas of nerve pain without unwanted parasthesias in other areas of the limb. In addition to spinal-based systems, the use of peripheral nerve stimulation (PNS) is increasing. The advantage of PNS is the reduction in risks by avoiding the need to invade the spine. The disadvantage is the limits of stimulating only specific nerves, which may not be successful when pain is outside the nerve distribution. This chapter is a demonstrative, focused discussion of placing the leads on select common peripheral nerve targets in the upper extremity.

N.R. Haider, MD
Minimally Invasive Pain Institute, Washington, DC, USA

T.R. Deer, MD (✉)
The Center for Pain Relief, 400 Court Street, Suite 100, Charleston, WV 25301, USA
e-mail: DocTDeer@aol.com

T.R. Deer, J.E. Pope (eds.), *Atlas of Implantable Therapies for Pain Management*, DOI 10.1007/978-1-4939-2110-2_28

28.2 Technical Overview

The most important parts of performing PNS of the upper extremity are critical to good success and include (1) knowing the anatomy of the upper extremity; (2) understanding patient selection; (3) learning the techniques of both surgical and percutaneous nerve implantation and the value and selection of each method; and (4) understanding the proper technique in placing the lead in the desired location.

In this brief chapter we have chosen to show the best methods for lead placement for the most utilized surgical techniques.

28.2.1 The Method of Peripheral Ulnar, Radial, and Median Nerve Stimulation

The most common causes of pain in the hand from peripheral nerve disease arise from postsurgical nerve entrapment or direct trauma to a nerve. The median and ulnar nerves are the most commonly involved structures (Fig. 28.1). PNS can be performed by either a surgically placed cuff lead or a peripherally placed lead adjacent to the nerve. Placement should be based on pain distribution, but selection can be enhanced by electromyelogram and nerve conduction studies.

A possible location for stimulation of radial and median nerves in the forearm for treatment of hand pain is shown in Fig. 28.2.

28.2.2 The Method of Suprascapular Nerve Stimulation for Treatment of Chronic Shoulder Pain

The suprascapular nerve can be a major factor in treating many painful shoulder conditions. The implanter must understand the bony anatomy of the shoulder and the nerve course. Fluoroscopic- or ultrasound-guided imaging is used to locate the suprascapular notch. The suprascapular nerve is located beneath the transverse scapular ligament in the scapular notch. Using a medial to lateral approach, the lead is placed entering over the medial scapula lateral to the upper thoracic spinous processes, traveling just superior and anterior to the spine of scapula, with electrode contacts overlying the suprascapular nerve in the scapular notch and supraspinous fossa (Fig. 28.3).

The axillary nerve has a mixed purpose of both motor and sensory function (Fig. 28.4). In recent years implant of a PNS system to treat both shoulder motor dysfunction from stroke and pain from humeral head trauma has been described.

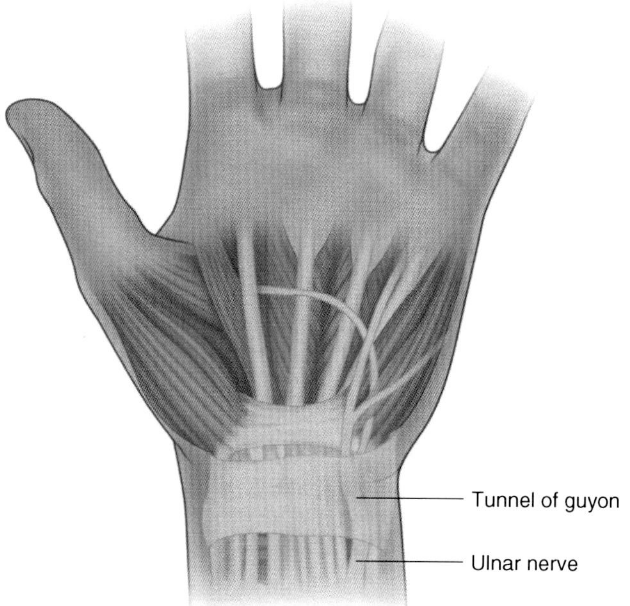

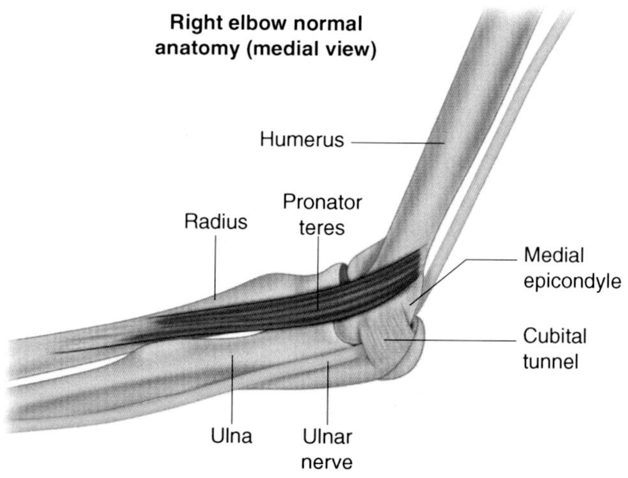

Fig. 28.1 Ulnar nerve course in the distal and proximal upper extremity

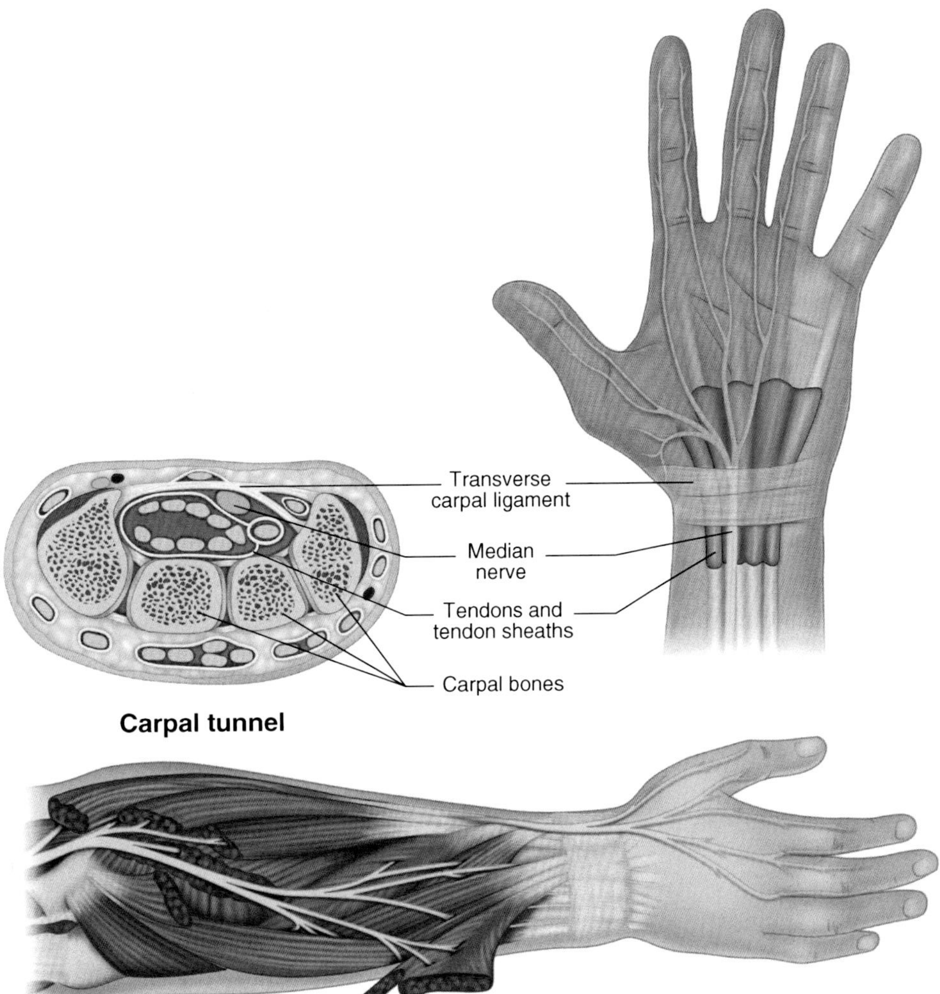

Fig. 28.2 Median nerve and radial nerve distribution

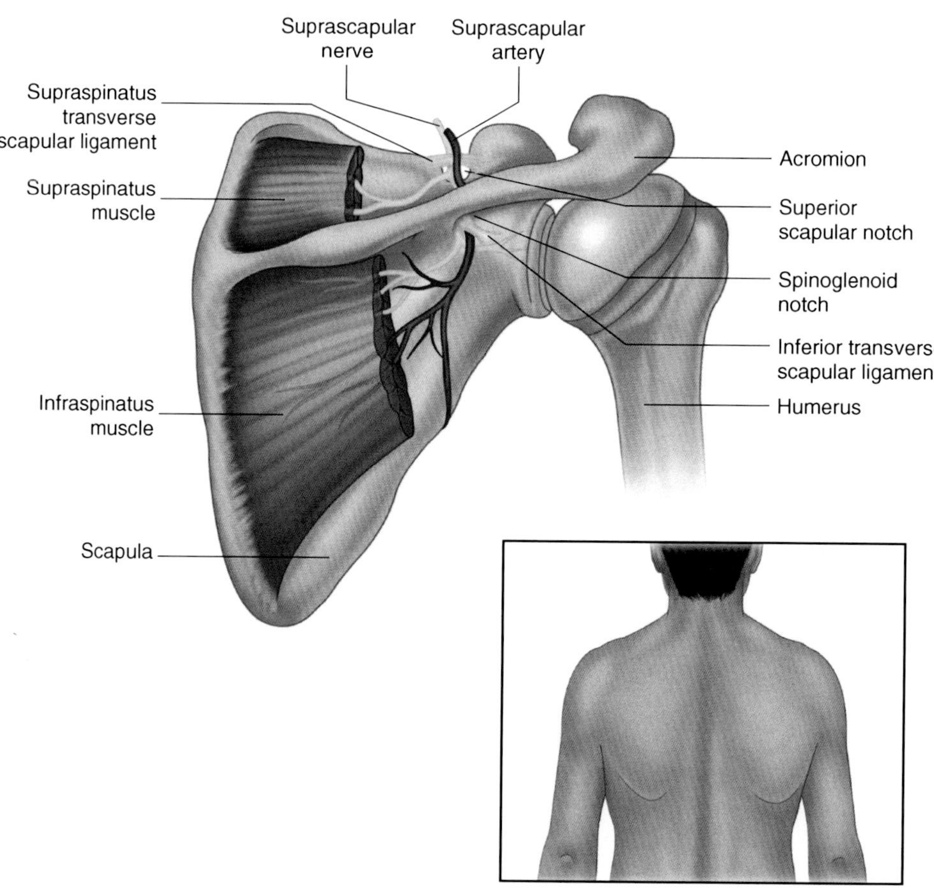

Fig. 28.3 Suprascapular nerve

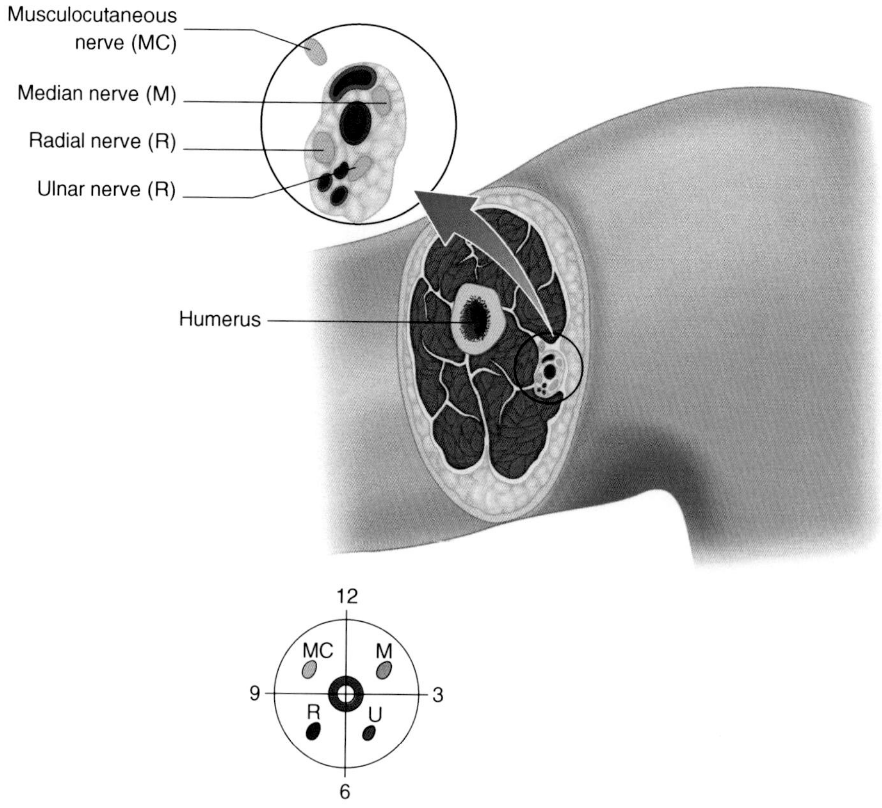

Fig. 28.4 Axillary nerve

28.3 Risk Assessment

1. The patient with a high risk for epidural lead placement or major neurosurgical interventions may be a candidate for peripheral nerve placement in the upper extremity. In some disease states the implant of any lead, even in the periphery, may be too high risk.
2. Skin infection is the most common problem with PNS. The skin condition in the area of the implant should be examined.
3. Nerve injury of the peripheral nerve or its fibers is a possible complication of PNS lead placement.
4. Injury to vascular structures is possible and may lead to critical limb ischemia.
5. Skin erosion may occur when the lead, anchor, or generator causes skin inflammation and breakdown. The skin health and tissue integrity are key factors in the preoperative evaluation.
6. Pain from device components may cause a need for device revision.
7. It may be difficult to implant the internal pulse generator in the upper extremity owing to the size of generator and the small size of the extremity and lack of body fat in that region.

28.4 Risk Avoidance

1. PNS leads can be placed percutaneously in the vicinity of the nerve to avoid direct nerve contact that in some cases can reduce the impact of scar. In cases in which the lead must be placed directly on the nerve a fascial graft may be helpful in stabilizing the stimulation pattern, although this technique is difficult to perform and has questionable long-term outcomes.
2. The risks of peripheral nerve stimulation (PNF) and peripheral nerve field stimulation (PNFS) are limited; however, it is still important to evaluate comorbidities prior to moving forward with the implantation of a device. Comorbidities such as diabetes and those involving the skin should be optimized prior to moving forward.
3. The patient should be alert and awake during the placement, and the needle and lead should be redirected if the patient complains of paresthesia. Only the entry site should be anesthetized, and the area where the lead is to be implanted adjacent to the nerve should not be anesthetized in order to prevent injury.
4. The lead should be placed into the subcutaneous tissue at a level below the dermis. The use of needle with a plastic stylet may improve the ability to direct the lead in a curvilinear fashion adjacent to the peripheral nerves.
5. The use of ultrasound guidance may enable easier tissue plane identification and optimal lead placement.
6. A loop of nonabsorbable suture may be used for the anchoring instead of traditional spinal anchors, which may erode adjacent structures and skin.
7. Carefully examine the bony structure prior to device implantation. The implantable programmable generator (IPG) pocket should be in a location that receives the least amount of tissue pressure or movement during the patient's daily activities. If pain persists after implantation, options include the use of topical anesthetics, topical patches, compounded pain creams, padding, and surgical revision.

Conclusions

A successful outcome with patients suffering from arm and shoulder pain can be achieved with SCS and PNS. The method of lead placement, pain target, generator placement, and lead programming may all play a critical role in the long-term efficacy of the device. The clinician must be an active problem solver in these situations and must actively adapt to the patient's response.

Suggested Reading

Huntoon MA, Hoelzer BC, Burgher AH, Hurdle MF, Huntoon EA. Feasibility of ultrasound-guided percutaneous placement of peripheral nerve stimulation electrodes and anchoring during simulated movement: part two, upper extremity. Reg Anesth Pain Med. 2008a;33(6):558–65.

Huntoon MA, Huntoon EA, Obray JB, Lamer TJ. Feasibility of ultrasound-guided percutaneous placement of peripheral nerve stimulation electrodes in a cadaver model: part one, lower extremity. Reg Anesth Pain Med. 2008b;33(6):551–7.

McRoberts WP, Cairns KD, Deer T. Stimulation of the peripheral nervous system for the painful extremity. In: Slavin KV, editor. Peripheral nerve stimulation. Basel: Karger; 2011. p. 156–70.

29 Ultrasound Guidance for the Placement of Peripheral Nerve Stimulation Devices

Mayank Gupta and Timothy R. Deer

Placement of implantable devices in the spine has become an integral part of the pain care algorithm for those suffering with neuropathic pain. In some settings, the use of a device in the spine is not the initial choice for neuromodulation. Using a spinal cord stimulation device to treat specific peripheral nerve–related conditions raises two issues: (1) Some regions of the body, such as the occipital nerve and the intercostal nerve, are very difficult to stimulate with a central target. (2) The risks of central neuraxis injury should be considered in the analysis of benefits versus adverse events. These two issues have led many implanters to prefer placing the lead in the direct vicinity of the nerve involved in the pain pattern distribution. This technique can be achieved using landmarks, nerve stimulation, or ultrasound-guided placement. This chapter will focus on ultrasound guidance of peripheral lead placement.

M. Gupta
Overland Park Regional Medical Center, Overland Park, KS, USA

T.R. Deer, MD (✉)
The Center for Pain Relief, 400 Court Street, Suite 100, Charleston, WV 25301, USA
e-mail: DocTDeer@aol.com

T.R. Deer, J.E. Pope (eds.), *Atlas of Implantable Therapies for Pain Management*, DOI 10.1007/978-1-4939-2110-2_29

29.1 History

Peripheral nerve stimulation (PNS) began as a very invasive method. The implanter would make an incision, dissect to the nerve, harvest a piece of fascia, and wrap the nerve in fascia prior to placing the lead just above the nerve (Fig. 29.1a). This invasive technique led to tissue trauma, and in many cases scar tissue formed and led to increased sensitivity or high impedance and lack of paresthesia (Fig 29.1b). Over time, the placement of PNS devices evolved to placement based on landmarks. Ultrasound-guided PNS grew out of the use of this technology to place nerve blocks in the operating room. The logical progression was to bring this pinpoint method to placing catheters for chronic pain and eventually placing PNS leads. Ultrasound guidance thus is important because it makes it possible to reduce the invasiveness of the procedure.

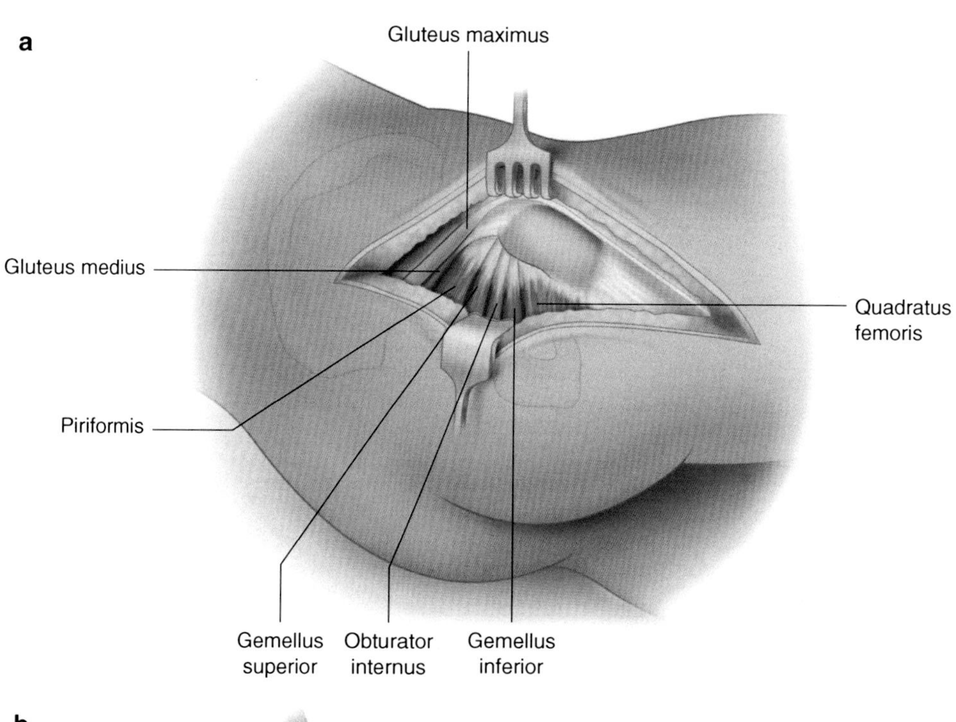

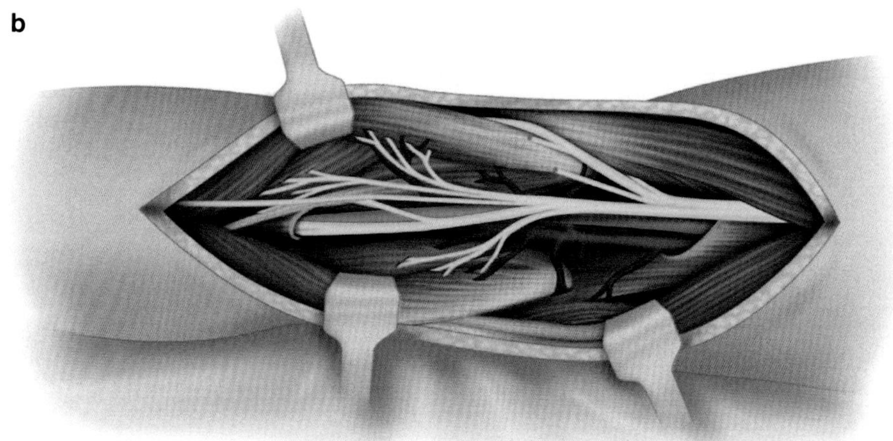

Fig. 29.1 (**a**) Dissection of muscles in the buttock. (**b**) Dissection to the popliteal nerve for open technique nerve placement

29.2 Technical Overview

Ultrasound guidance technology can be used for many peripheral nerve targets, including the occipital nerve, ilioinguinal nerve, intercostal nerve, axillary nerve, median nerve, ulnar nerve, sciatic nerve, posterior tibial nerve, common peroneal nerve, and saphenous nerve. The basic principal is the same: First, the nerve location is identified under ultrasound guidance and then a peripheral electrode is placed in closed proximity. It has most often been observed that best stimulation is achieved by placing the electrode perpendicular to the course of the nerve. Initially, a three and one half–inch 22G spinal needle is used to visualize the path, and then a 14G needle should be placed in the same direction under ultrasound guidance. The 22G needle is used as a safety precaution in the event of invasion of the nerve or a blood vessel.

29.3 Technique Examples

Ultrasound guidance is especially helpful for initial placement of the PNS lead, as illustrated by the following examples.

29.3.1 Occipital Nerve Stimulation

The patient is placed in the prone position. The ultrasound probe is placed just lateral to the occipital protuberance bilaterally. The probe is gradually moved laterally to visualize the pulsation of the greater and lesser occipital artery. The nerve is in close proximity to artery pulsation and on the medial aspect in most patients. In the plane approach, the lead is placed perpendicular to the course of the occipital nerve (Fig. 29.2).

29.3.2 Ilioinguinal Nerve Stimulation

The patient is placed in the supine position. The ultrasound probe is placed 2 cm medial and 2 cm inferior to the anterior superior iliac spine. Under ultrasound guidance, the plane between the internal oblique muscle and the transverse abdominis muscle is visualized and its depth is gauged and marked. At the same depth, the lead is passed under ultrasound guidance in the same plane and perpendicular to the inguinal ligament (Fig. 29.3).

29.3.3 Common Peroneal and Posterior tibial Nerves

The patient is placed in the prone position. The ultrasound probe is placed about 5 cm proximal to the popliteal crease. The popliteal artery pulsation is visualized and its depth is gauged. Both the common peroneal nerve and posterior tibial nerves are superficial to the artery. The lead is placed more medial for individual stimulation of the posterior tibial nerve, and more lateral for the common peroneal nerve. If the ultrasound probe is moved more proximally, the common peroneal nerve can be visualized joining the posterior tibial nerve and forming the sciatic nerve (Fig. 29.4).

29.3.4 Saphenous Nerve

The patient is placed in the prone position. The ultrasound probe is placed about 5 cm proximal to the popliteal crease on the medial aspect. The sartorius muscle is visualized. The lead is placed adjacent to the sartorius muscle, perpendicular to the course of the muscle (Fig. 29.5).

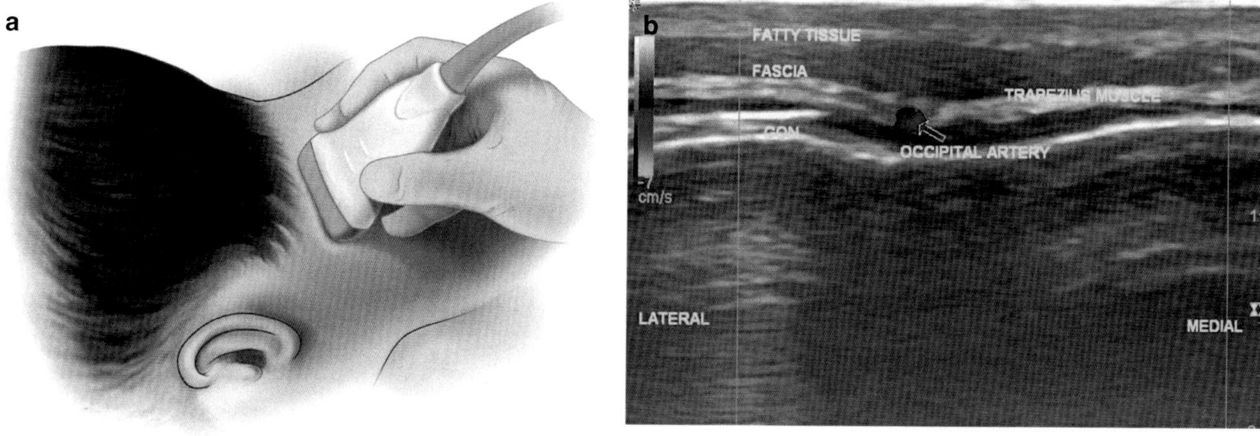

Fig. 29.2 (**a**) Out of plane position of transducer to locate the occipital nerve. (**b**) Highlighted US image of greater occipital nerve, and the surrounding anatomy

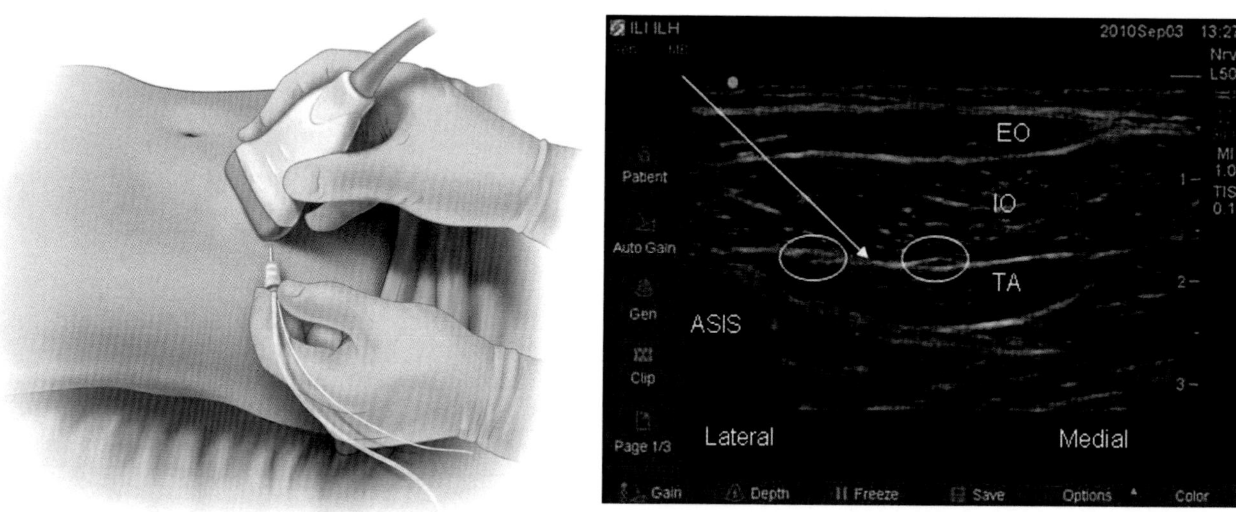

Fig. 29.3 Transducer approach and US image of ilioinguinal anatomy

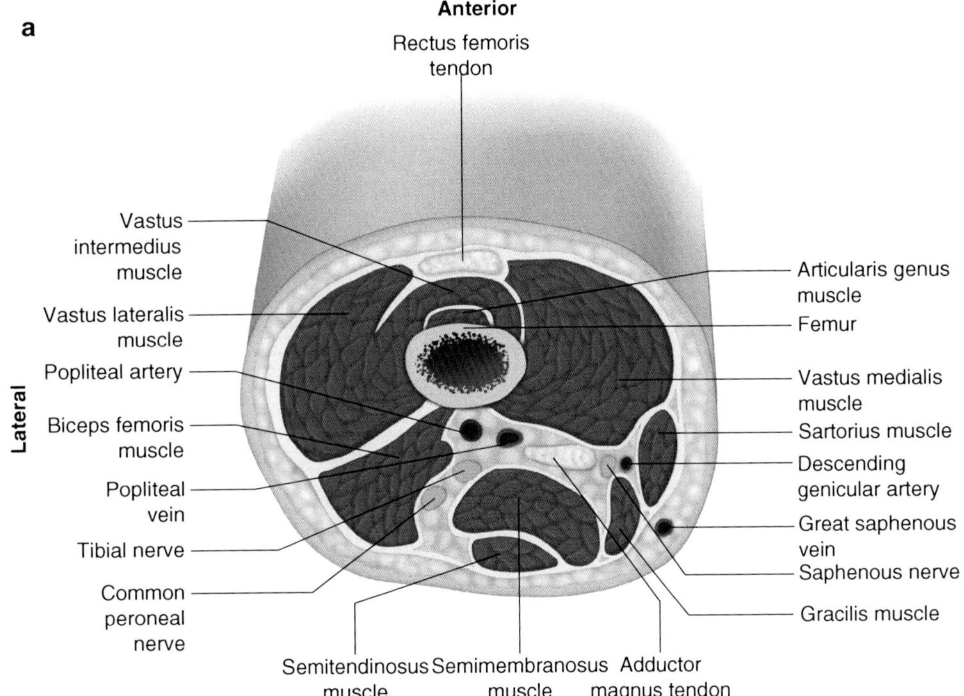

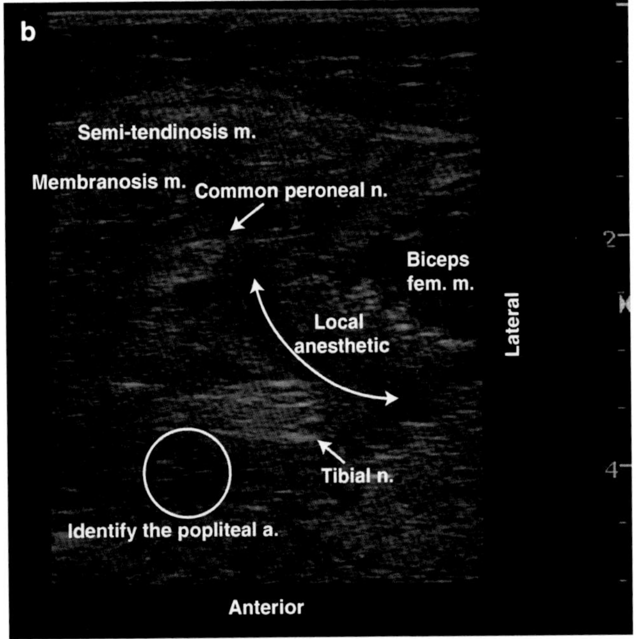

Fig. 29.4 (**a**) Axial slice of right LE 8 cm above the knee. (**b**, **c**) US-guided image and figure representation of ultrasound probe orientation

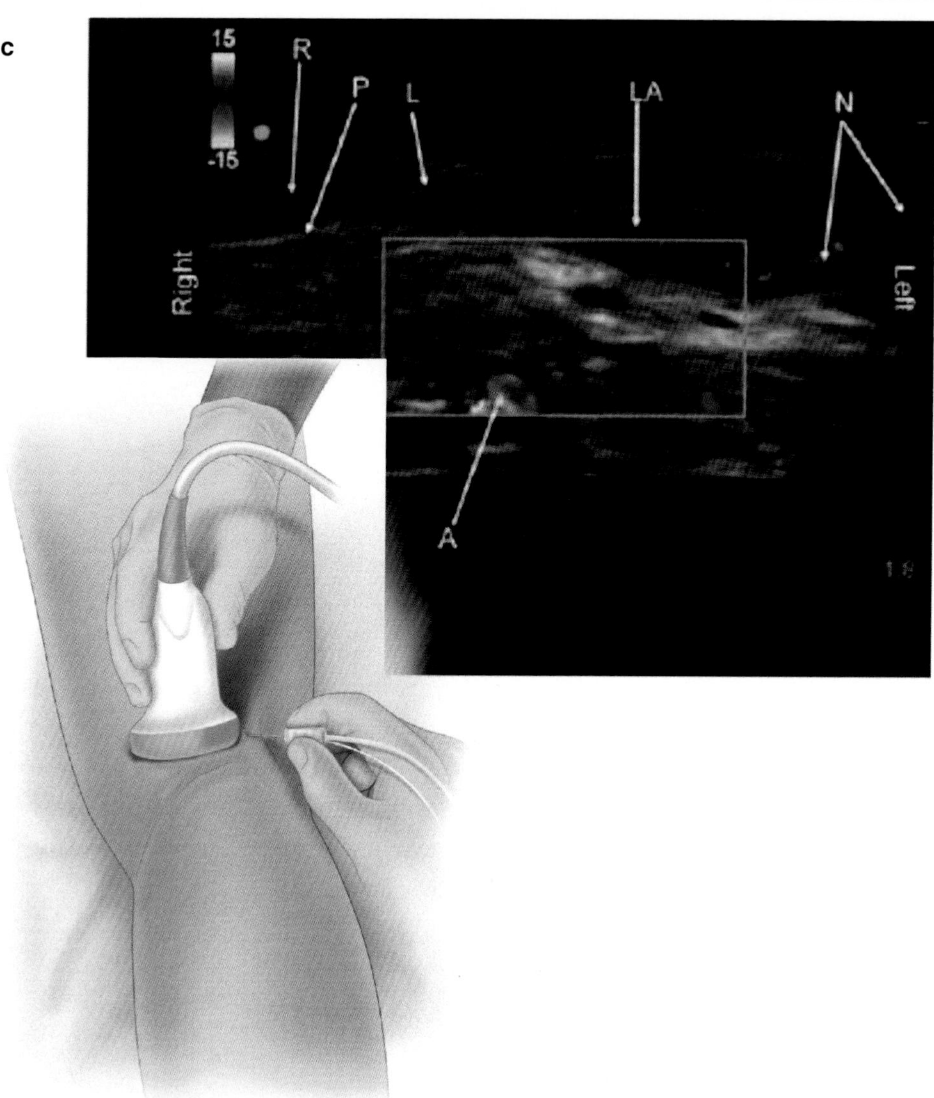

Fig. 29.4 (continued)

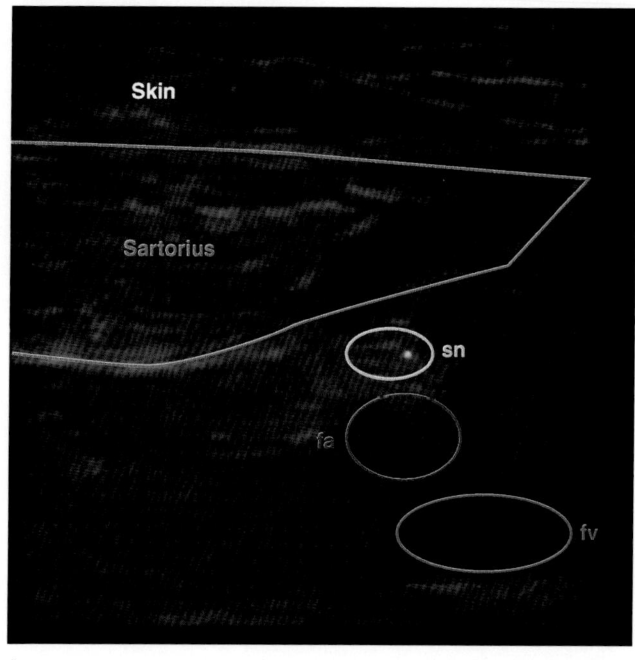

Fig. 29.5 US image of anatomy surrounding saphenous nerve

29.4 Electrode Positioning and Permanent Device Implantation

Once the lead is placed as described above for the applicable nerve, minor changes can be made in electrode position based on stimulation pattern. For permanent implantation, a small incision is made at the needle entry site and the fascia is exposed. The lead is anchored to the fascia using nonabsorbable suture. In most settings, an anchor is not used, because of the risk of tissue erosion. The internal programmable generator site varies, based on patient choice, the area of the body, and physician preference. Commonly used pocket sites for battery placement are the upper thoracic area and low back for occipital nerve stimulation, the anterior abdomen for the ilioinguinal nerve, and the posterior thigh or buttock for the sciatic and saphenous nerves.

29.5 Risk Assessment

Ultrasound-guided PNS is still new in the field of modern pain management. No major complications specific to the use of ultrasound guidance have yet been reported. The risk of complications for PNS is similar to that of other peripheral implants, but it is likely that the risk of nerve injury or bleeding is less with ultrasound guidance, particularly using Doppler technology to identify blood vessels. As with any implant, the risk of infection should be considered.

29.6 Risk Avoidance

Prior to implantation, the physician should evaluate the integrity of the skin in the local area and rule out infection or skin breakdown. As with other surgical techniques, intravenous antibiotics should be given within the hour prior to skin invasion. The clinician should have proper training and acceptable operating skill prior to placing the implant, and the physician should be especially familiar with the anatomy of the implant area. Vessel depth and nerve anatomy should be identified prior to lead placement. Seeker needles are helpful in reducing the risk of needle trauma prior to implantation. A conversant patient is helpful in improving safety in these cases, as injury to a peripheral nerve will cause a paresthesia.

Conclusion

The introduction of ultrasound enables individual peripheral nerves to be stimulated in a safe, effective, and minimally invasive way. With improving technology, ultrasound guidance will become a more common method of providing this important implantation technique.

Suggested Reading

Chan I, Brown AR, Park K, Winfree CJ. Ultrasound-guided, percutaneous peripheral nerve stimulation: technical note. Neurosurgery. 2010;67:136–9.

Huntoon MA, Huntoon EA, Obray JB, Lamer TJ. Feasibiility of ultrasound-guided percutaneous placement of peripheral nerve stimulation electrodes in a cadaver model: part one, lower extremity. Reg Anesth Pain Med. 2008;33:551–7.

Kent M, Upp J, Spevak C, Shannon C, Buckenmaier 3rd C. Ultrasound-guided peripheral nerve stimulator placement in two soldiers with acute battlefield neuropathic pain. Anesth Analg. 2012;114: 875–8.

Peng P. Peripheral applications of ultrasound for chronic pain. In: Huntoon M, Benzon H, Nauroze S, editors. Spinal injections and peripheral nerve blocks, Interventional and neuromodulatory techniques for pain management, vol. 4. Philadelphia: Elsevier Saunders; 2012.

High-Frequency Electric Nerve Block to Treat Postamputation Pain

30

Amol Soin, Zi-Ping Fang, Jonathan Velasco, and Timothy R. Deer

The use of peripheral nerve stimulation (PNS) has been a part of neuromodulation for over three decades. Initially, the therapy was offered by a very invasive method involving a cut down to the nerve and the placement of a large paddle lead directly adjacent to the nerve fibers. This method fell out of favor, as the low-frequency stimulation sometimes caused pain with nerve activation, or a lack of stimulation occurred secondary to increasing impedance. In recent years, the use of PNS with percutaneous leads has changed the situation: With the advent of improved programming and platforms, the implanting doctor can create pain relief by placing a lead in the area near the nerve by landmarks, ultrasound, or nerve stimulation. This method has been more successful, but new solutions are still needed to treat patients with severe pain of the limb after trauma. This chapter illustrates an option to treat postamputation pain using high-frequency (10 kHz) electrical nerve block via a surgically implanted, minimally invasive peripheral nerve cuff electrode.

A. Soin, MD, MBA
Greene Memorial Hospital,
Wright State University School of Medicine,
8934 Kingsridge Drive Suite 101, Centerville, OH 45458, USA
e-mail: drsoin@gmail.com

Z.-P. Fang
Neuros Medical, Inc., 35010 Chardon Road, Suite 210,
Willoughby Hills, OH 44094, USA
e-mail: zpfang@neurosmedical.com

J. Velasco
Dayton Surgeons Inc.,
1 Elizabeth Place #10A, Dayton, OH 45417, USA
e-mail: jj.velasco@rocketmail.com

T.R. Deer, MD (✉)
The Center for Pain Relief, 400 Court Street, Suite 100,
Charleston, WV 25301, USA
e-mail: DocTDeer@aol.com

30.1 Introduction and Scope of the Problem

Currently, about 2,000,000 patients in the United States have major limb amputations, and approximately 185,000 new amputations are performed annually [1]. After amputation of a major limb, many patients develop debilitating, chronic pain disorders such as residual limb or phantom limb pain. It is been estimated that residual limb pain is experienced by up to 76 % of major limb amputees [2]. These disabling conditions have proven difficult to treat despite many modern advancements in medicine.

The algorithm to treat residual limb pain includes opioid analgesics, anticonvulsants, NSAIDs, physical therapy, spinal cord stimulation, pulsed radiofrequency of the dorsal root ganglion, dorsal root ganglion spinal cord stimulation, intrathecal drug delivery, and dorsal root entry zone (DREZ) lesioning. Patients may also undergo amputation revision surgeries or neurectomy to remove painful neuromas, procedures that have shown limited and inconsistent results.

30.2 Pathophysiology

Postamputation pain is usually divided into two different types of painful conditions: phantom limb pain and residual limb pain, which presents at the end of the stump. After an amputation, a neuroma forms at the distal end of the severed nerve. This neuroma may fire abnormal action potentials, which cause unpleasant sensations such as phantom or residual limb pain [3]. Residual limb pain may be exacerbated with palpation or pressure placed directly on a neuroma—such as when patients use their prosthetic devices—which can limit the patient's ability to maintain activities of daily living.

Spinal or central nervous system mechanisms also may influence residual limb or phantom pain. Neuromas or damaged peripheral nerve tissue can lead to degeneration of C fibers in the dorsal horn of the spinal cord and terminating A

T.R. Deer, J.E. Pope (eds.), *Atlas of Implantable Therapies for Pain Management*, DOI 10.1007/978-1-4939-2110-2_30

fibers, which may subsequently branch into the same lamina. The A fiber inputs may then be reported as noxious stimuli that may lead to hyperexcitability of the spinal cord, thus producing chronic pain [4]. The result can be a change in the wide dynamic range nerve fibers that makes the condition progressively more difficult to treat.

Additionally, peripheral mechanisms may influence post-amputation pain conditions. At the end of a severed peripheral nerve, a neuroma may form. On this neuroma, there is often a proliferation of sodium channels, which can transmit significant abnormal and unwanted action potentials that can be perceived as a painful sensation. If these action potentials could somehow be blocked, then the painful condition could be eliminated. This is the established mechanism of action for high-frequency electric nerve block in the periphery to achieve pain reduction. The cuff electrode is attached to a targeted nerve proximal to a neuroma located near the amputation stump to block the pain signals originating in the residual limb. Unlike other forms of PNS, this high-frequency method leads to a major change in the nerve signal.

30.3 High-Frequency Electric Conduction Block: Mechanism of Action

By placing a nerve cuff electrode around a severed peripheral nerve proximal to a neuroma and administering high-frequency alternating current (HFAC), it is possible to block unwanted painful action potentials and prevent neurotransmission of the unpleasant stimuli [5–11].

Drs. Kevin Kilgore and Niloy Bhadra from Case Western Reserve University showed that HFAC using sinusoidal waveforms could be used to block peripheral motor activity in an in vivo mammalian model [12]. The block threshold amplitudes showed a linear relationship with frequency, the lowest threshold being at 5 kHz. These pioneering scientists showed that HFAC block has three phases: an onset phase, a period of asynchronous firing, and then a period of steady-state complete nerve block. The onset response and the asynchronous firing can be minimized by using an optimal frequency-amplitude combination [13].

HFAC block creates a complete depolarizing nerve block around the targeted peripheral nerve. Its mechanism of action is very similar to that of amide local anesthetics, in that HFAC also blocks action potentials. Therefore, the mechanism of action of HFAC electrical nerve block is different from that of spinal cord stimulation or traditional peripheral nerve stimulation modalities. Also, unlike spinal cord stimulation and traditional peripheral nerve stimulation techniques, the patient feels no paresthesia. The sensation felt by the patient after HFAC block is similar to that felt after a peripheral nerve block with local anesthetic.

With this mechanism of action, HFAC block has been applied in humans with amputation stump pain to achieve a complete nerve block and prevent neurotransmission of pain signals. The result is a blunting of many of the central neuroplastic mechanisms discussed above, which may result in significant pain reduction, improved function, and improved quality of life in the properly selected patient.

30.4 Feasibility Study

30.4.1 Patient Selection

Following Investigational Device Exemption (IDE) approval by the US Food and Drug Administration (FDA) and protocol approval by our designated institutional review board, we conducted a study to determine the feasibility of using HFAC block to achieve consistent and reproducible pain reduction in patients with postamputation pain. The eligibility criteria for inclusion are listed on Table 30.1. Since amide local anesthetics (such as 1 % lidocaine without epinephrine) block action potentials [14], patients underwent screening using local anesthetic nerve blocks proximal to the neuroma as a "trial" prior to surgical implantation of the nerve cuff electrode (Fig. 30.1).

Table 30.1 Eligibility criteria for study of high-frequency electric conduction block

Inclusion criteria
Amputation of lower or upper limb
Chronic pain from amputation for ≥6 months
Pain refractory to conventional medical management
Severe pain in an amputated limb (worst pain intensity ≥7 on 0–10 Numerical Rating Scale [NRS])
Frequent occurrence of severe pain (≥2 episodes/week on average by recall, confirmed by screening diary of 2–4 weeks)
Significant pain reduction (≥50 % on NRS) after local anesthetic injection for temporary nerve block; no significant pain reduction after saline injection as a placebo injected prior to the anesthetic
Exclusion criteria
Pacemaker or other implanted devices
Debilitating pain other than pain in amputated limb
Pregnancy
Inability to accurately and consistently report pain intensity and related information
High risk of infection due to comorbidity or compromised immune state (e.g., chemotherapy)
High risk of mortality for general anesthesia (e.g., severe cardiopulmonary disease)
Infectious etiology for amputation (e.g., osteomyelitis, cellulitis)
Uncontrolled diabetic vascular disease or neuropathy
Skin graft or severe scarring over targeted implant site

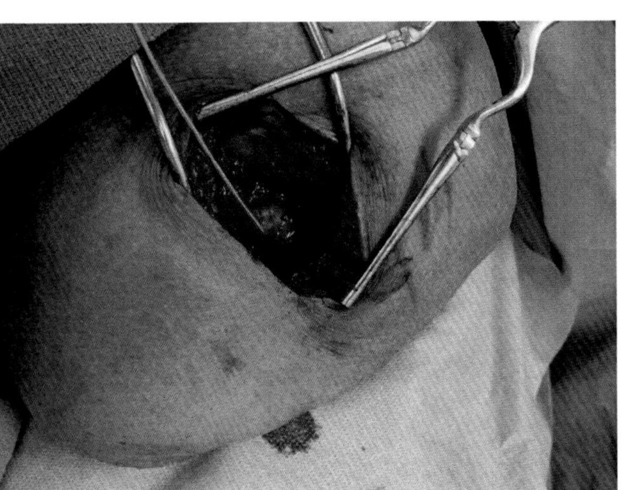

Fig. 30.1 The stimulating nerve cuff placed around the sciatic nerve in an above-the-knee amputee

30.4.2 Preimplant Testing

In our first-in-human and pilot studies, the screening local anesthetic peripheral nerve blocks used as a trial for HFAC block were done under ultrasound guidance. This method allowed the practitioner to visualize the neuroma at the end of the severed nerve and allowed identification of the location, depth, and diameter of the targeted nerve, to help facilitate surgical placement of a peripheral nerve cuff (Fig. 30.2). Other traditional peripheral nerve block modalities would also be acceptable ways to complete the "trial" local anesthetic block, however. These could include direct infiltration of local anesthetic proximal to the neuroma via palpation technique, or the use of a Stimuplex® needle (B. Braun Medical; Bethlehem, PA) to complete the peripheral nerve block.

The location and placement of the cuff electrode depends on which of the severed peripheral nerves are transmitting the pain signals. Local anesthetic peripheral nerve blocks help to identify which nerves are involved in pain transmission. Once the practitioner achieves significant pain reduction after local anesthetic blocks to a nerve or group of nerves, he or she has a roadmap showing the nerves to which the nerve cuff electrode should be attached to achieve effective pain relief. The metric of success is pain reduction of more than 50 % after two local anesthetic peripheral nerve blocks.] Two local anesthetic blocks are recommended to help rule out a placebo effect from a single, one-time injection. It is also recommended that each block be performed on a different day, with the patient filling out a pain diary charting his or her pain reduction and duration of pain relief.

After the peripheral nerve is identified and the patient has had two successful screening injection blocks with more than 50 % pain relief, peripheral nerve cuffs are placed around the appropriate nerves. In below-the-knee amputation patients, painful neuromas typically occur near the common peroneal and tibial nerves (Fig. 30.3). In patients with above-the-knee amputations, the sciatic nerve is usually the pain generator.

For upper extremity amputations, painful neuromas typically occur around the radial, ulnar, median, or musculocutaneous nerves.

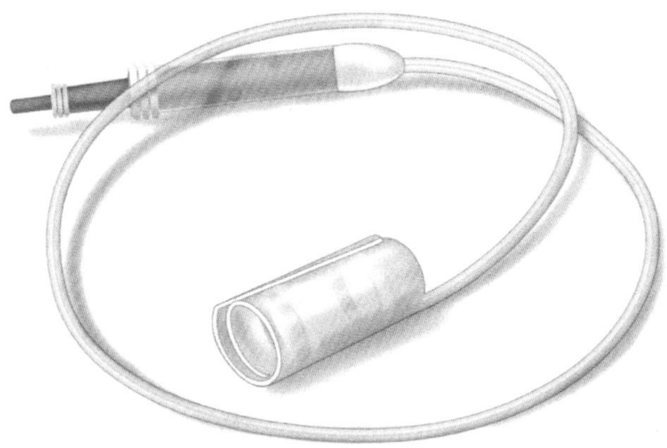

Fig. 30.2 The peripheral nerve cuff electrode

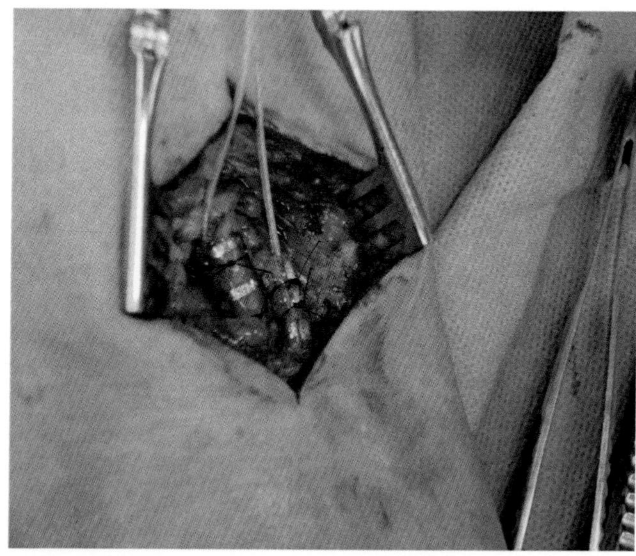

Fig. 30.3 Peripheral nerve cuffs placed around the common peroneal and tibial nerves in a below-the-knee amputee

30.4.3 Implantation Technique

The implantation of the high-frequency PNS device requires specialized training in the field of neuromodulation so that implantation can be achieved in a timely and minimally invasive fashion. The electrode implantation is achieved via surgical dissection to adequately place the nerve cuff electrode around the peripheral nerve(s). Meticulous attention is required in this surgical dissection to ensure that vascular or adjacent nerve structures are not damaged when placing the peripheral nerve cuff. These risks can potentially be decreased by perioperative ultrasound mapping of the patient's vascular and nerve structures. In clinical studies, a preoperative ultrasound was completed in the preoperative holding area to mark the location and depth of the targeted nerves. This technique allowed faster and more efficient cuff placement, providing the implanting physician with accurate knowledge of the nerve depth and location prior to incision. Additionally, during the preoperative ultrasound mapping, the surgeon can choose to inject 0.1 mL of methylene blue near the targeted nerve so that, after the incision is made and dissection is carried out to the desired depth, the surgeon can see the methylene blue surrounding the targeted nerve. These techniques allow for not only more rapid nerve exposure (average time for exposure of the targeted nerve was less than 10 min) but also a smaller incision (Fig. 30.4).

Upon exposure of the peripheral nerve, a cuff electrode is wrapped around the nerve. The cuff electrode is sized to fit the appropriate nerve, and the diameter of the nerve is confirmed intraoperatively by direct measurement prior to placing the nerve cuff around the desired nerve. After cuff placement, an impedance check is completed and the cuff is secured with one or two nonabsorbable sutures around the diameter of the nerve. Caution must be used to ensure that the sutures are not placed too tightly around the nerve. A tension loop is created with the lead, similar to loops used during implantation of a spinal cord stimulation lead (Fig. 30.4). The lead is then tunneled for connection with the pulse generator (Figs. 30.5 and 30.6).

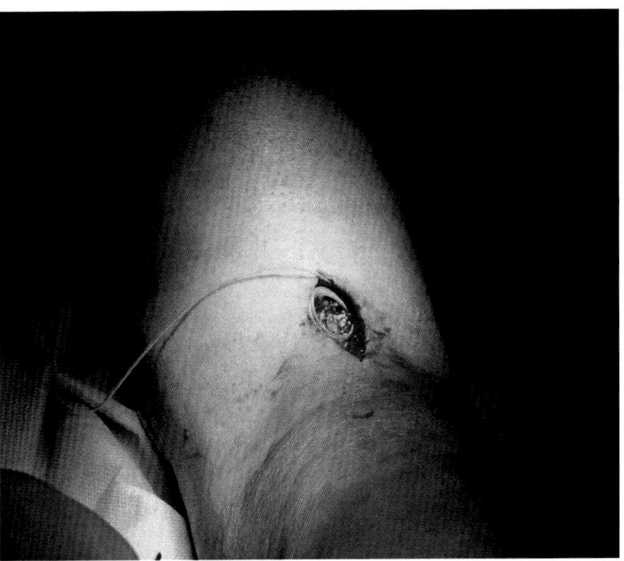

Fig. 30.4 Preoperative ultrasound mapping facilitates small incision size. Also note that a tension loop is created at the site, similar to those used with spinal cord stimulation implants

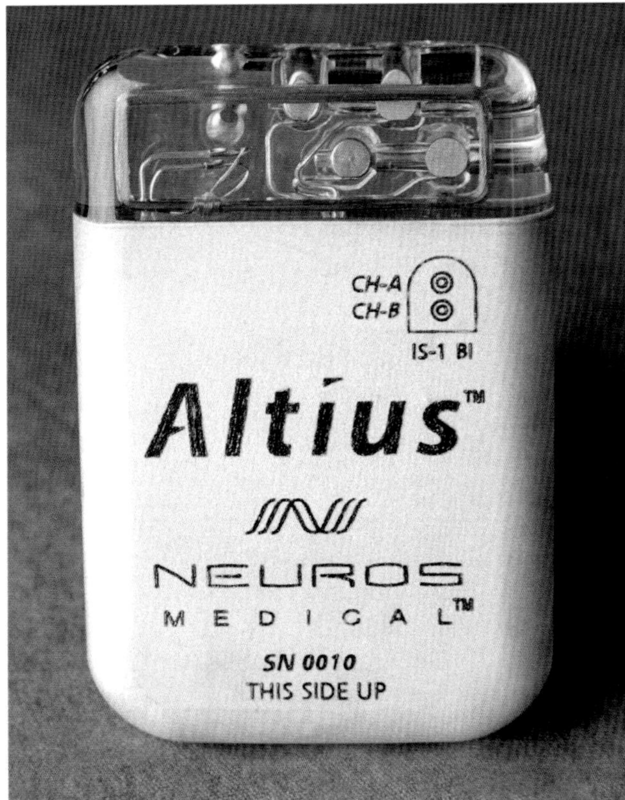

Fig. 30.5 The internal pulse generator (IPG), which allows up to two peripheral nerve cuff electrodes to be implanted in the patient

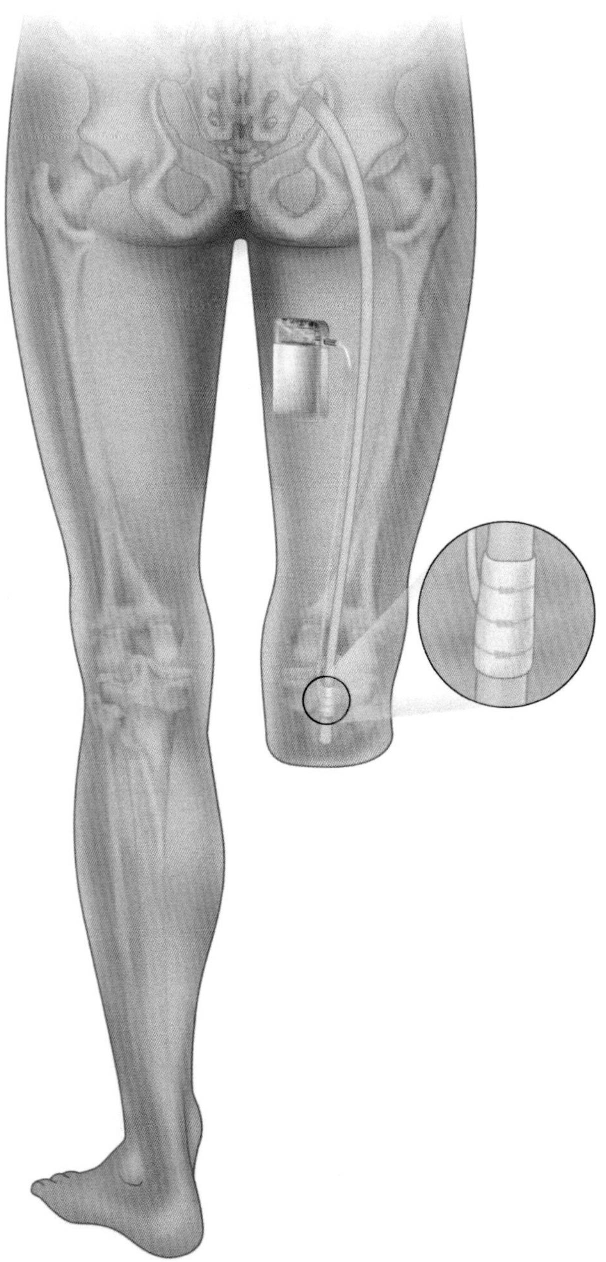

Fig. 30.6 Lead placement around a peripheral nerve attached to the IPG

30.4.4 Therapy Parameter Settings

In our studies, the therapy parameters were set approximately 1–2 weeks after implantation surgery. During the programming process, the amplitude of a 10 kHz waveform was gradually increased to achieve pain reduction without inducing a sensation of discomfort. This was achieved with a 5-min linear ramp-up followed by a 25-min plateau of stimulation, with a plateau of 2–7 V. The total therapy session time was 30 min. Pain reduction was reported within a matter of minutes after the treatment session commenced. The duration of pain relief per therapy session mirrored the results of the peripheral nerve block screening using a rapid-acting amide local anesthetic.

30.4.5 Clinical Outcomes and Conclusions

In our IDE-approved pilot study, ten patients were implanted. Nine patients received in-clinic testing, and seven patients progressed into long-term home use. The average NRS pain scale for tested patients decreased from 5.7–1.4 (out of 10) after HFAC electrical nerve block therapy, with 85 % of all testing sessions yielding a pain reduction greater than 50 %.

Also compelling was the reduction in the patients' medication dosage. Tested patients noted a very significant reduction in the use of opioid and other analgesics; several patients were able to eliminate opioids and NSAID medications completely, and all tested patients significantly decreased their daily analgesic pill counts.

Patients achieved meaningful and significant pain reduction throughout the study, and patients who had phantom pain (in addition to stump pain) that responded to local anesthetic injections also responded favorably with HFAC electrical nerve block. In that patient subset, it is thought that the phantom symptoms were peripherally generated. Each of the tested patients reported that HFAC electrical nerve block provided the most significant amount of pain reduction they had ever experienced, compared with other pain modalities tried since their amputations.

At the time of this publication, the high-frequency electric nerve block technique is currently investigational, pending FDA clearance. The next step for this modality is a pivotal trial, with the goal of having this therapy available to the mass market upon FDA clearance.

References

1. National Limb Loss Information Center. Fact sheet: pain management for the amputee. 2006. www.amputee-coalition.org/fact_sheets/painmgmt.html.
2. Ramachandran VS, Hirstein W. The perception of phantom limbs. The D. O. Hebb lecture. Brain. 1998;121:1603–30.
3. Cruz VT, Nunes B, Reis AM, Pereira JR. Cortical remapping in amputees and dysmelic patients: a functional MRI study. NeuroRehabilitation. 2003;18:299–305.
4. Karl A, Birbaumer N, Lutzenberger W, Cohen LG, Flor H. Reorganization of motor and somatosensory cortex in upper extremity amputees with phantom limb pain. J Neurosci. 2001; 21:3609–18.
5. Peng CW, Chen JJ, Lin CC, Poon PW, Liang CK, Lin KP. High frequency block of selected axons using an implantable microstimulator. J Neurosci Methods. 2004;134:81–90.
6. Baratta R, Ichie M, Hwang SK, Solomonow M. Orderly stimulation of skeletal muscle motor units with tripolar nerve cuff electrode. IEEE Trans Biomed Eng. 1989;36:836–43.
7. Tanner JA. Reversible blocking of nerve conduction by alternating current excitation. Nature. 1962;195:712–3.
8. Abdel-Gawad M, Boyer S, Sawan M, Elhilali MM. Reduction of bladder outlet resistance by selective stimulation of the ventral sacral root using high frequency blockade: a chronic study in spinal cord transected dogs. J Urol. 2001;166:728–33.
9. Cattel M, Gerard RW. The "inhibitory" effect of high-frequency stimulation and the excitation state of nerve. J Physiol. 1935;83:407–15.
10. Woo MY, Campbell B. Asynchronous firing and block of peripheral nerve conduction by 20 Kc alternating current. Bull Los Angel Neuro Soc. 1964;29:87–94.
11. Ishigooka M, Hashimoto T, Sasagawa I, Izumiya K, Nakada T. Modulation of the urethral pressure by high-frequency block stimulus in dogs. Eur Urol. 1994;25:334–7.
12. Kilgore KL, Bhadra N. Nerve conduction block utilizing high frequency alternating current. Med Biol Eng Comput. 2004;42: 394–406.
13. Gerges M, Foldes EL, Ackermann DM, Bhadra N, Bhadra N, Kilgore KL. Frequency- and amplitude-transitioned waveforms mitigate the onset response in high-frequency nerve block. J Neural Eng. 2010;7:066003. doi:10.1088/1741-2560/7/6/066003.
14. Park JS, Jung TS, Noh YH, Kim WS, Park WI, Kim YS, et al. The effect of lidocaine HCl on the fluidity of native and model membrane lipid bilayers. Korean J Physiol Pharmacol. 2012;16:413–22.

31 Peripheral Nerve Stimulation Miniaturization

Tory McJunkin, Paul Lynch, and Timothy R. Deer

31.1 Introduction

As new devices and technologies specifically designed for peripheral nerve stimulation (PNS) emerge, they promise a number of potential advantages over current PNS devices or spinal cord stimulation (SCS) devices currently used for PNS applications. One emerging trend is the miniaturization of the PNS system itself. Such devices present several advantages over larger devices, such as decreased trauma from surgery; easier, less invasive placement; the lack of extensive tunneling in some patients; and reduced discomfort from the size and weight of the internal pulse generator (IPG) once it has been implanted. The miniaturization of the device may also make it possible to treat conditions that have been untreated up to the present time because of the disadvantages or difficulties using existing systems. PNS devices are also currently being tested that use leads made from more flexible materials than traditional neurostimulation leads. Lead flexibility may decrease the chance of lead fracture or migration.

Several advances in PNS miniaturization or PNS technology have been investigated or are currently being investigated. Some of these include the Bion implantable neurostimulator device, the Bioness StimRouter, the Neuros Altius system, and even nonimplantable transcutaneous PNS devices like the Electrocore system. On the horizon are devices from new thought leaders such as Axionics that combine the advances of current stimulator technology that are at present available with smaller generators and more flexible leads.

T. McJunkin • P. Lynch
Arizona Pain Specialists,
9787 North 91st Street, Scottsdale, AZ 85258, USA

T.R. Deer, MD (✉)
The Center for Pain Relief, 400 Court Street, Suite 100,
Charleston, WV 25301, USA
e-mail: DocTDeer@aol.com

T.R. Deer, J.E. Pope (eds.), *Atlas of Implantable Therapies for Pain Management*, DOI 10.1007/978-1-4939-2110-2_31

31.2 Boston Scientific Bion Implantable Neurostimulator Device

The Boston Scientific Bion is a small cylindrical (27.5 mm long × 3.2 mm wide) implantable neurostimulator (Fig. 31.1) [1]. The Bion has been studied in clinical trials as a potential PNS neurostimulation device. This device contains an electrode and a rechargeable lithium ion battery. This device was implanted in the occipital region of nine patients experiencing chronic cluster headache (CCH) that was not adequately relieved by preventive medications (Fig. 31.2). Of these patients, three completed long-term follow-up, with two experiencing a reduction of at least 50 % in the frequency of cluster headaches at 6 months. The three patients followed up continued to experience benefits 58–67 months after implantation.

In another study, nine patients had the Bion implanted in the occipital region for chronic migraine, hemicranias continua, or cluster headaches [2]. Of these patients, eight completed the 12-month follow-up with seven of eight obtaining fair or better results (at least a 25 % reduction) in reducing their disability. Six patients suffering from hemicrania continua (HC) had the Bion implanted in a crossover study [3]. In long-term follow-up, four of six patients reported substantial (≥80 %) reduction in pain severity and another reported a 30 % reduction. One patient reported a 20 % increase in pain. Although these studies examine small numbers of patients without randomization, they appear to demonstrate some promise of small implantable neurostimulators for treating pain, particularly in chronic headache disorders. In addition to evidence of its efficacy, these studies found the Bion to generally be safe.

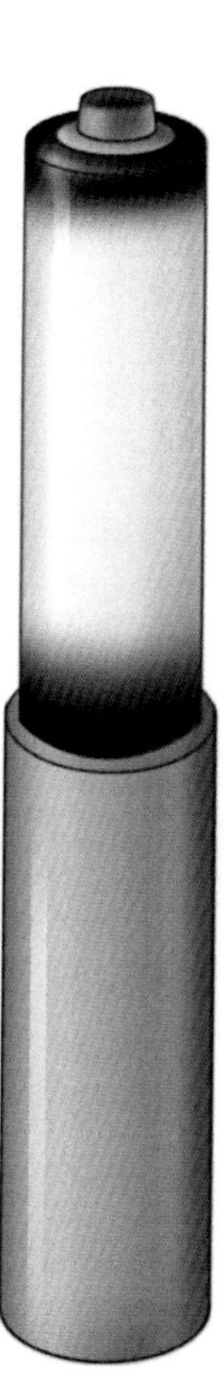

Fig. 31.1 The Bion implantable neurostimulator device. For investigational use only. Not approved for sale in the United States

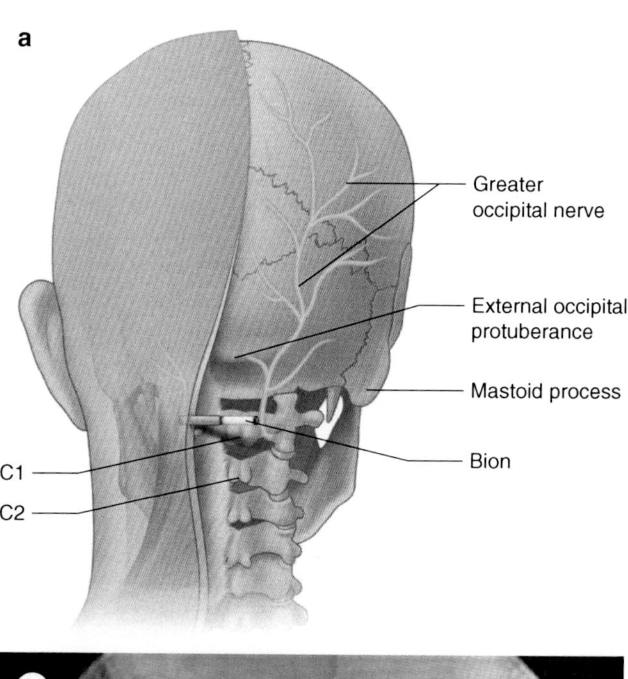

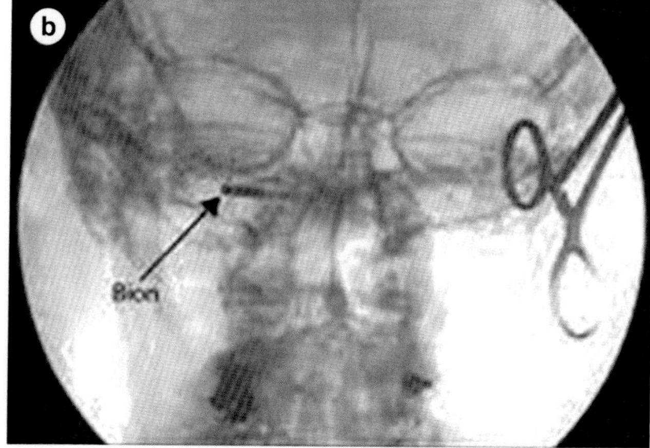

Fig. 31.2 (a) The implant location of the Bion in the occipital region for the treatment of chronic headaches. (b) AP radiograph of an implanted Bion device

31.3 Bioness StimRouter

The Bioness StimRouter is a single percutaneously inserted lead that has three tightly spaced contacts on its head and a radiofrequency receiver on its tail [4]. This device is currently being studied in a clinical trial for post-traumatic or postsurgical neuropathic pain of a single peripheral nerve. A patient wears an external patch that acts as the generator and transmits radiofrequency energy transcutaneously to power the device. The system offers several advantages over existing PNS devices. The device implantation is simple and minimally invasive. The device's small size avoids the discomfort to the patient of a larger implanted device. The external pulse transmitter avoids the need for an implanted battery and subsequent surgical procedures for battery replacement. Disadvantages may include the relatively small surface area of the active contacts on its head, the fact that a patient must wear an external patch whenever she or he want the device to be operational, and the possibility of skin erosion from the adhesive of the patch.

The StimRouter was tested in an open-label study with eight patients suffering from carpal tunnel syndrome and chronic pain despite carpal tunnel release and medication [5]. The StimRouter was implanted along the median nerve of eight patients (six patients receiving a single StimRouter and two receiving bilateral device implantations). Patients received 5 days of stimulation with the device, experiencing a mean pain reduction of 37 % from baseline on day 5 and reduced their oral opioid medication use while receiving stimulation. No adverse events were reported.

31.3.1 Lead

The StimRouter consists of a single 15-cm lead with a body diameter of 1.2 mm. The lead is made from a platinum-iridium alloy covered in silicone tubing. One end of the lead contains a single receiver; the other end contains three stimulating electrodes. The stimulating end also has a four-pronged polypropylene anchor. This anchor helps ensure that the lead stays in place once the device has been implanted. The lead is flexible, making lead migration and fracture less likely.

31.3.2 External Pulse Transmitter

The StimRouter lacks an IPG. Instead the device is powered by an external pulse transmitter (EPT). This EPT connects to a disposable patch with an adhesive electrode hydrogel. This user patch must be replaced every 2–3 days. The EPT and patch are placed on the skin over the implanted lead. The EPT and user patch transmit transdermal electrical stimulation that is picked up by the lead's receiver electrode and transmitted through the stimulation electrodes to the target nerve. A rechargeable battery built into the EPT's case provides power.

31.3.3 Patient Programmer

The StimRouter can be turned on or off and the device settings adjusted with a patient programmer. This programmer wirelessly communicates with the EPT. During office visits a clinician programmer is used to set device parameters for delivering effective stimulation. The patient programmer allows the patient to make finer adjustments to the intensity of the stimulation and to switch among up to eight stimulation programs.

31.3.4 Target Patients for the StimRouter

The StimRouter is intended to treat patients with peripheral mononeuropathies. These include post-traumatic neuropathies, postsurgical neuropathies, and other neuropathies. Patients who experience moderate to severe chronic pain limited to a single peripheral nerve may be good candidates for this treatment. Patients with appropriate neuropathies may be identified by electromyography (EMG) testing or diagnostic nerve blocks using local anesthetic. Patients who receive significant temporary relief from a nerve block of a single peripheral nerve may get relief from a PNS such as the StimRouter (Fig. 31.3).

Possible target nerves for PNSs include:

Arms: axillary, radial, ulnar, median, digital

Legs: femoral, sciatic, saphenous, tibial, sural, deep peroneal, common peroneal, superficial peroneal, lateral cutaneous, posterior cutaneous

Trunk: suprascapular, thoracic, intercostal, ilioinguinal, iliohypogastric, gluteal

31.3.5 Lead Implantation

The StimRouter lead is implanted in a 30- to 45-min outpatient procedure. Conscious sedation is generally used during this procedure.

1. Inserting the stimulation probe (Fig. 31.4). An initial 1-cm incision is made approximately 8–10 cm from the target nerve under local anesthetic. A stimulation probe is inserted into the incision and guided to the nerve. This can be performed under ultrasound guidance. Electrical stimulation is sent through the stimulation probe to test for paresthesia in the area of the patient's typical pain.

2. Inserting the loader (Fig. 31.5). Once paresthesia is achieved the target area, a loader is inserted over the stimulation probe.
3. Inserting the lead into the loader (Fig. 31.6). The probe is then removed and the lead is placed inside the loader. The rubber ring on the reed containing the lead is rolled back to expose the electrodes on the lead. The lead is then used to deliver stimulation.
4. Deploying the lead anchor (Fig. 31.7). Once paresthesia is achieved with the lead, it is ready to be deployed. The reed covering the lead is pulled back, exposing the anchor. The stimulating end of the lead is now anchored. The loader is then removed while applying pressure to the skin over the stimulating end of the lead to prevent it from moving as the loader is withdrawn. Stimulation can be tested again at this point. If paresthesia has been lost, the lead must be removed and implantation must begin with a new lead.
5. Inserting the tunneling device (Fig. 31.8). With the stimulating end of the lead anchored in place, a second 1-cm incision is made approximately 10–15 cm away from the first incision. This incision will determine the subsequent placement of the EPT, so the location should be based on consideration for the patient's anatomy and comfort. Local anesthetic is applied to the path between the two incisions, and the tunneling device is inserted through the second incision to the first incision. The receiving end of the lead is placed in the end of the tunneling device and pulled through into place.
6. Skin closure (Fig. 31.9). Once the receiving end is in place, the incisions can be sealed with Steri-Strips or sutures.

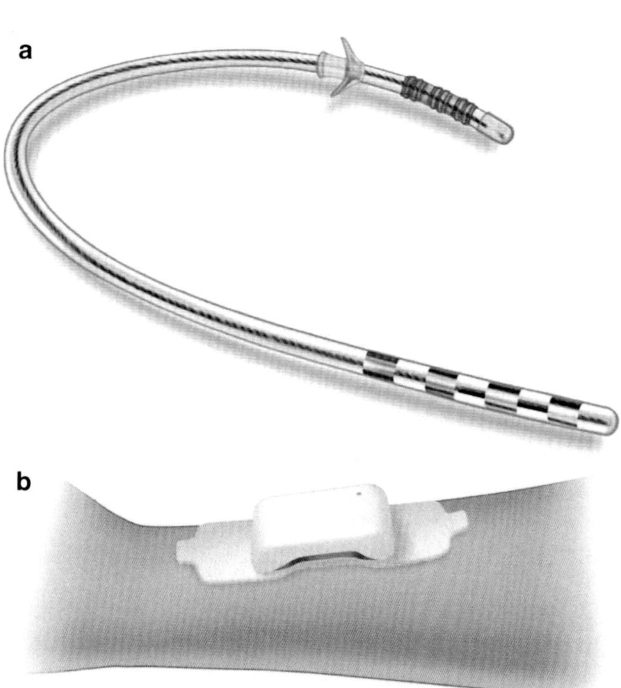

Fig. 31.3 (**a**) The Bioness StimRouter peripheral neurostimulator lead. For investigational use only. Not approved for sale in the United States. (**b**) The Bioness StimRouter peripheral neurostimulator EPT and electrode patch. For investigational use only. Not approved for sale in the United States

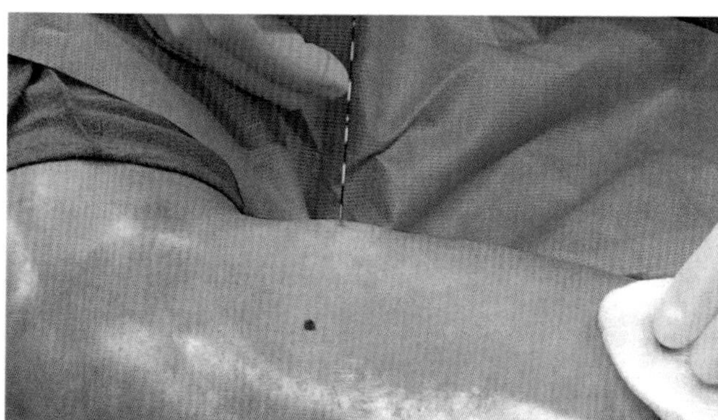

Fig. 31.4 Inserting the stimulation probe for Bioness StimRouter placement

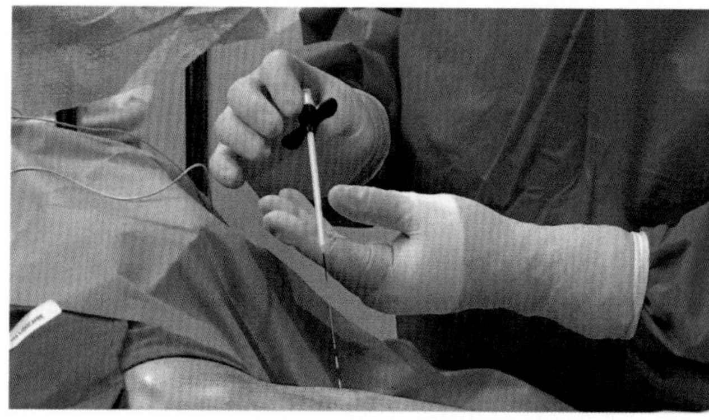

Fig. 31.5 Inserting the loader for Bioness StimRouter placement

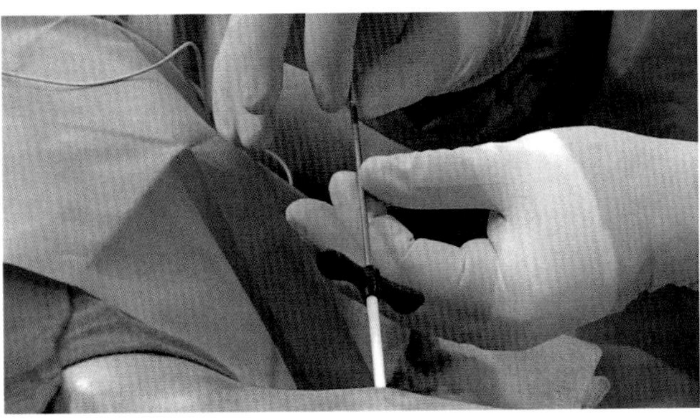

Fig. 31.6 Inserting the lead into loader for Bioness StimRouter placement

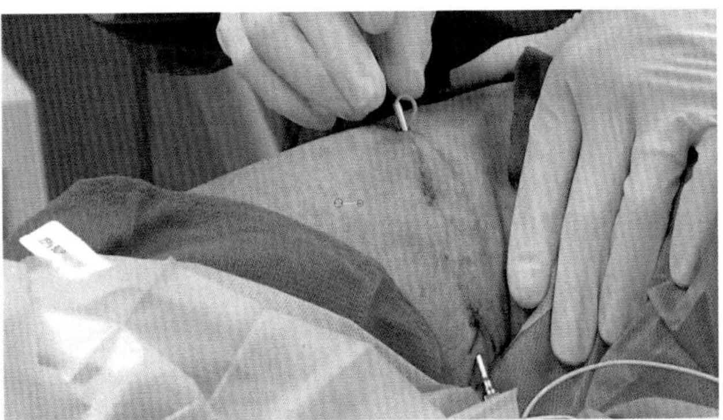

Fig. 31.8 Inserting tunneling device for Bioness Stimrouter placement

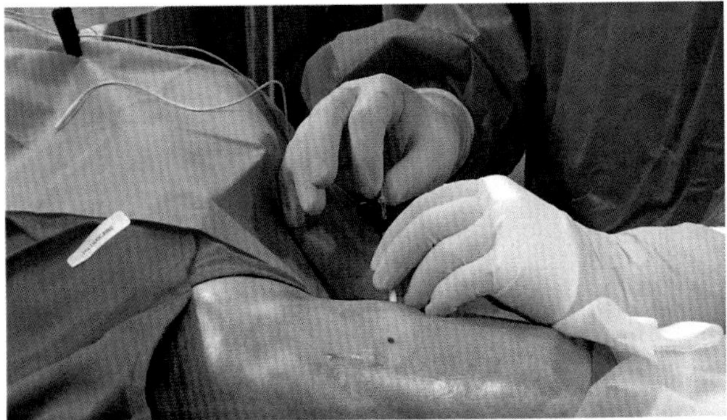

Fig. 31.7 Deploying lead anchor for Bioness Stimrouter placement

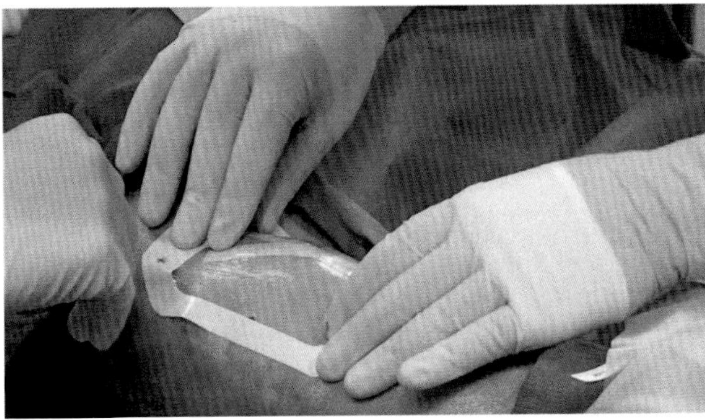

Fig. 31.9 Skin closure for Bioness StimRouter placement

31.4 Neuros Altius

The Neuros Altius is a peripheral neurostimulation device that uses high-frequency alternating current (HFAC) to block nerve conduction. This device is currently being studied in clinical trials. Unlike other electrical stimulation techniques for pain relief, HFAC affects different nerve mechanisms. Specifically a cuff electrode with a diameter from 5 to 12 mm is placed around a peripheral nerve (e.g., sciatic nerve, common peroneal nerve; Fig. 31.3). The first application of this device is in the treatment of intractable postamputation nerve pain. The cuff is placed proximal to the neuroma (Fig. 31.10). Whereas conventional PNS relies on the interaction of sensory nerve stimulation with pain signals in the central nervous system, HFAC stimulation is more predictable because it directly blocks conduction of pain signals within the peripheral nervous system [6]. Preclinical studies in animal models (e.g., rats) have demonstrated the efficacy of HFAC for relieving pain [7].

In a study of ten lower limb amputees with chronic severe pain in the amputated limb, the Neuros Altius was placed on the sciatic nerve (for above-knee amputees) or tibial and common peroneal nerves (for below-knee amputees; Fig. 31.11) [8]. Patients completed an average of four sessions of neurostimulation per week over a period of 3–12 months. Patients experienced at least 50 % pain relief during 92 % of the stimulation sessions. Four patients were able to discontinue pain medications. The pain relief produced from brief (10–30 min) HFAC stimulation resulted in relief extending for minutes or hours after use. No safety issues were reported. Although randomized clinical trial data are required to draw firm conclusions regarding efficacy the efficacy of HFAC neurostimulation, devices such as the Neuros Altius appear promising for relieving some types of nerve pain (Fig. 31.12).

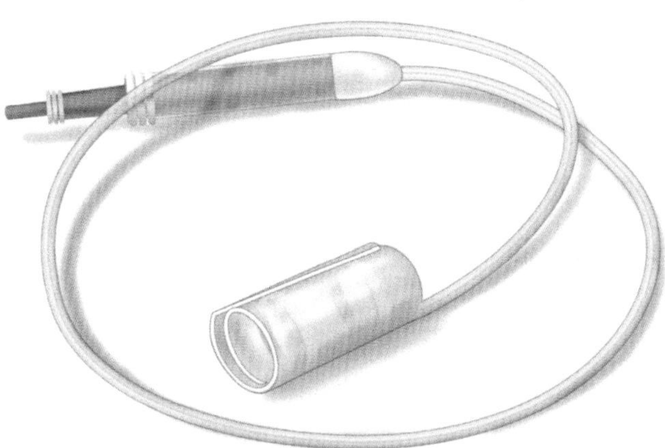

Fig. 31.10 The Neuros Altius cuff electrode

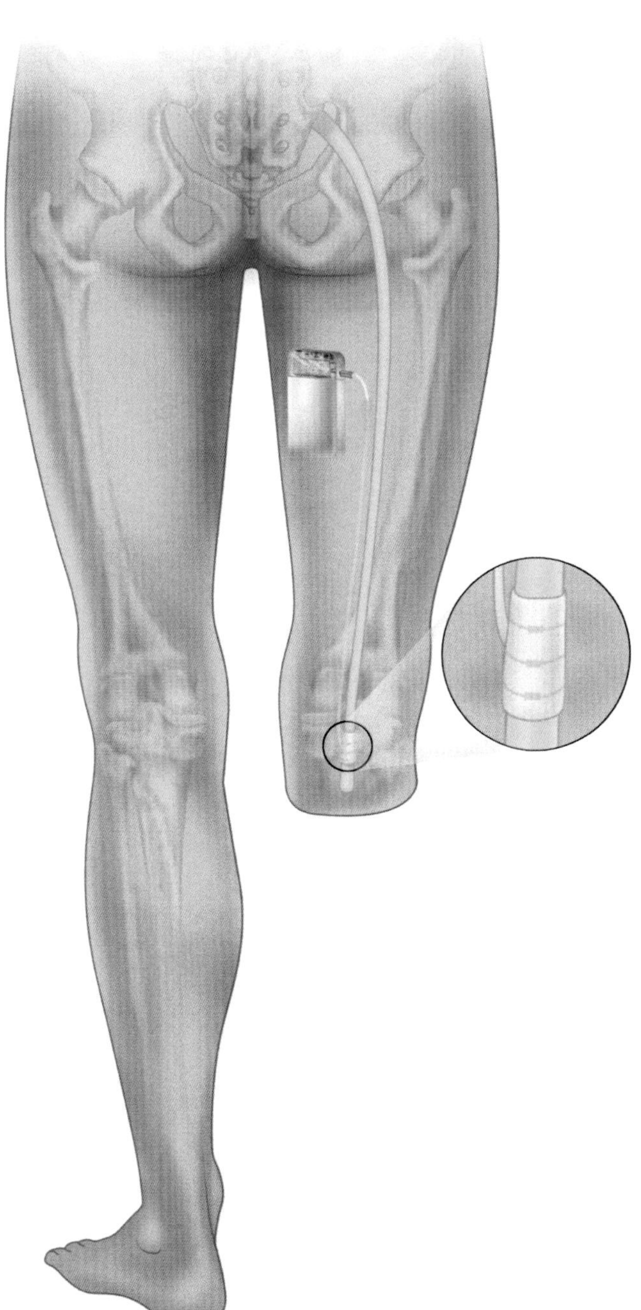

Fig. 31.11 The Neuros Altius implant placement in a below-knee amputee

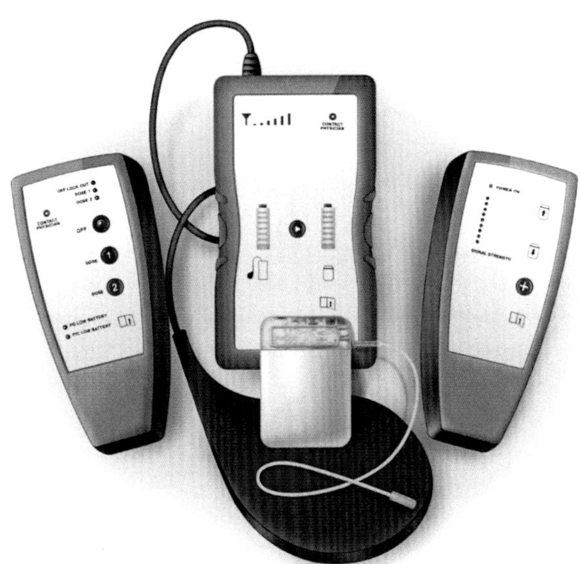

Fig. 31.12 The Neuros Altius HFAC stimulator

31.5 Other Advances

Many other recent neurostimulation devices have undergone similar miniaturization and changes to become less invasive. Although it does not target a conventional peripheral nerve, ElectroCore's gammaCore is a noninvasive vagus nerve stimulator (nVNS; Fig. 31.13). This device delivers electrical signals to the vagus nerve to treat primary headache [9]. A microwave-powered neural transmitter small enough to be injected via syringe has been tested in animal studies [10]. This device consists of a 1-cm dipole antenna, 0.8 mm thick, with 1-mm platinum balls at each end. A microwave transmitter can deliver stimulation to these electrodes from outside the body. This device has been found capable of activating motor nerves through over 5 cm of tissue.

Other advancements in PNS treatment may come from other therapies used in conjunction with PNS. For example, the use of regenerative treatments, such as stem cell therapy, in combination with PNS device implantation may offer advantages for certain patients. Recent research suggests that pulses of electrical stimulation can improve the viability of oligodendrocytes [11]. The use of neurostimulation after the transplantation of mesenchymal stem cells led to greater functional improvement in patients with spinal cord injury than stem cell therapy alone [12, 13]. In addition, autologous injections of platelet-rich plasma (PRP) have been found to reduce the risk of infections when injected during spinal implant surgeries [14]. This may be due to the fact that, in addition to its potential healing properties, the platelets concentrated in PRP also contain antimicrobial proteins (e.g., β-lysin) [15]. Given the potentially serious consequences of infections during procedures such as device implantation, the use of PRP during implantation may be helpful for patients at greater risk of infection during PNS device implantation.

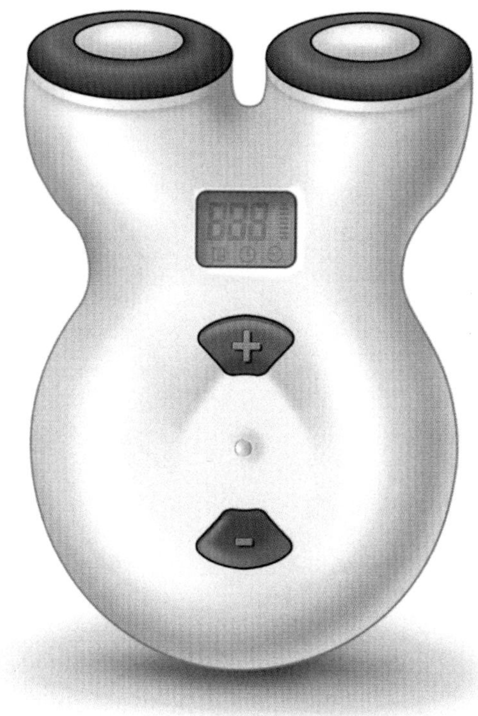

Fig. 31.13 ElectroCore gammaCore nVNS

Conclusion

Although current PNS devices can be effective in relieving pain, these devices face various limitations based on the size and weight of the implanted device and the need for invasive procedures to replace device components. Ongoing advancements in PNS devices, such as miniaturization, external device components, and new modes of stimulation (e.g., HFAC) will further enhance the benefits provided by PNS. Smaller devices can be implanted through less invasive procedures, reducing the risk of infection and other complications as well as the time required for implantation. Some implantable devices and those that remotely power the device may allow the treatment of pain in harder to treat areas, such as the head. The miniaturization of PNS devices can reduce recovery time and the discomfort caused by the device. New lead materials and designs, such as flexible leads, can reduce the risks of lead fracture or migration. Taken together, ongoing advancements in PNS devices have the potential to improve the safety, comfort, applicability, widespread use, and efficacy of PNS treatment.

References

1. Strand NH, Trentman TL, Vargas BB, Dodick DW. Occipital nerve stimulation with the Bion microstimulator for the treatment of medically refractory chronic cluster headache. Pain Physician. 2011;14:435–40.
2. Trentman TL, Rosenfeld DM, Vargas BB, Schwedt TJ, Zimmerman RS, Dodick DW. Greater occipital nerve stimulation via the Bion microstimulator: implantation technique and stimulation parameters. Pain Physician. 2009;12:621–8.
3. Burns B, Watkins L, Goadsby PJ. Treatment of hemicranias continua by occipital nerve stimulation with a Bion device: long-term follow-up of a crossover study. Lancet Neurol. 2008;7:1001–12.
4. Deer TR, Pope JE, Kaplan M. A novel method of neurostimulation of the peripheral nervous system: the StimRouter implantable device. Tech Reg Anesth Pain Manag. 2012;16:113–7.
5. Deer TR, Levy RM, Rosenfeld EL. Prospective clinical study of a new implantable peripheral nerve stimulation device to treat chronic pain. Clin J Pain. 2010;26:359–72.
6. Hsu E, Cohen SP. Postamputation pain: epidemiology, mechanisms, and treatment. J Pain Res. 2013;6:121–36.
7. Bhadra N, Kilgore KL. High-frequency electrical conduction block of mammalian peripheral motor nerve. Muscle Nerve. 2005;32:782–90.
8. Soin A, Shah NS, Fang ZP. Update of pilot study on high-frequency nerve block for post-amputation pain. Paper presented at 19th annual Napa pain conference, 24 Aug 2013, Napa.
9. Goadsby P, et al. Non-invasive vagus nerve stimulation (nVNS) for acute treatment of migraine: an open-label pilot study. In: Submitted to the 2013 AAN meeting.
10. Towe BC, Larson PJ, Gulick DW. A microwave powered injectable neural stimulator. Conf Proc IEEE Eng Med Biol Soc. 2012;2012:5006–9.
11. Gary DS, Malone M, Capestany P, Houdayer T, McDonald JW. Electrical stimulation promotes the survival of oligodendrocytes in mixed cortical cultures. J Neurosci Res. 2012;90:72–83.
12. Liu H, Yang K, Xin T, Wu W, Chen Y. Implanted electro-acupuncture electric stimulation improves outcome of stem cell's transplantation in spinal cord injury. Artif Cells Blood Substit Immobil Biotechnol. 2012;40:331–7.
13. Wu W, Zhao H, Xie B, et al. Implanted spike wave electric stimulation promotes survival of the bone marrow mesenchymal stem cells and functional recovery in the spinal cord injured rats. Neurosci Lett. 2011;491:73–8.
14. Li H, Hamza T, Tidwell JE, Clovis N, Li B. Unique antimicrobial effects of platelet-rich plasma and its efficacy as a prophylaxis to prevent implant-associated spinal infection. Adv Healthc Mater. 2013;2:1277–84.
15. Donaldson DM, Tew JG. Beta-lysin of platelet origin. Bacteriol Rev. 1977;41:501–3.

Part III

Neurostimulation: The Cranium and the Head

32 Neurostimulation: Stimulation of the Cranium and Head: Stimulation of the Deep Brain for the Treatment of Chronic Pain

Shivanand P. Lad, Erika A. Petersen, Andrew Marky, Timothy R. Deer, and Robert M. Levy

32.1 Introduction

Deep brain stimulation (DBS) is a therapy that has been used for more than half a century to treat chronic pain. The first use of these treatments occurred in the 1950s when neurosurgeons stimulated the septal region nuclei in patients with psychiatric diseases who also suffered from chronic pain. Over the next 20 years, the therapy evolved to include the sensory thalamic nuclei to treat pain of neuropathic origin. Stimulation of the periventricular grey matter (PVG) has generally been recommended for the treatment of nociceptive pain, whereas the sensory thalamus (ST) remains the preferred stimulation site for neuropathic pain. Currently several new targets are under investigation. Outcomes for both facial and extremity pain have been positive with appropriate patient and target selection. The use of DBS in the neuromodulation algorithm is increasingly helpful to those who have severe pain. Because of its invasiveness and the risks associated with DBS, it is restricted to a selected group of patients in whom conservative treatment of chronic pain syndromes has been ineffective.

Effective application of DBS requires a thorough knowledge of the theory of modulating the central pain matrix including neuroanatomy, neural circuits, and individual targets involved in pain processing. Many patients have mixed pain syndromes of neuropathic and nociceptive character. It is now thought that white matter pathways passing through the PVG may be involved in stimulation-induced pain relief. Increased activation of the medial dorsal nucleus of the thalamus, an area associated with the limbic system including the amygdala and cingulate cortex, has been observed during PVG stimulation. Thus, in addition to activating the descending opioid system, stimulation of the PVG may also modify the patient's emotional response to pain. The mechanism of analgesia elicited by electrical stimulation of the ST is similarly incompletely understood. Its effect may be mediated by activation of the inhibitory corticofugal fibers that prevent the pathological spread of painful stimuli.

S.P. Lad • A. Marky
Division of Neurosurgery, Department of Surgery, Duke University Medical Center, Durham, NC, USA

E.A. Petersen
Department of Neurosurgery, University of Arkansas for Medical Sciences, Little Rock, AR, USA

T.R. Deer, MD (✉)
The Center for Pain Relief, 400 Court Street, Suite 100, Charleston, WV 25301, USA
e-mail: DocTDeer@aol.com

R.M. Levy
Harvey Sandler Department of Neurosurgery, Marcus Neuroscience Institute, Boca Raton, FL, USA

T.R. Deer, J.E. Pope (eds.), *Atlas of Implantable Therapies for Pain Management*, DOI 10.1007/978-1-4939-2110-2_32

32.2 Technical Overview

DBS electrodes are implanted to the desired target using either a frame-based or a frameless stereotactic approach. Numerous variations in surgical technique—general anesthesia versus local anesthesia with or without sedation, use of microelectrode recording, use of intraoperative imaging, and staging of implantation of electrodes and pulse generators—exist, often determined by surgeon preference and the circumstances of the individual patient. A preoperative high-resolution stereotactic magnetic resonance imaging (MRI) and/or computed tomography (CT) scan is obtained (Fig. 32.1). After completion of the imaging and planning, the patient is brought to the operating room, where she or he is carefully positioned on the operating table and local anesthesia along with mild intravenous sedation is administered.

Stereotactic localization of bilateral entry points is performed and these areas are then marked. The head is shaved, prepared, and draped in the standard sterile fashion. Incisions are opened and meticulous hemostasis achieved. Two 14-mm bur holes are then drilled bilaterally centered over the prior stereotactic localization points. A number of frame, mini-frame, or frameless systems are now available; however, the general principles are similar. Registration is performed with the intraoperative navigation station and less than 0.5 mm error is preferred.

Once exposure is achieved, physiological microelectrode recording is performed to achieve optimal electrode positioning. It is a key point to remember that the stereotactic coordinates represent the starting point for target identification, but that the end target is identified in the operating room.

The dura, pia, and cortical surface are coagulated and incised on one side, beginning contralateral to the patient's worst symptoms. The trajectory is aligned using the previous target and entry projection. Initial depth is commonly set to 10 mm above target, ensuring that the patient's blood pressure is normotensive. Electrophysiological activity is typically used to identify exact targets. This is done by microelectrode recording and microelectrode stimulation followed by macrostimulation. The microelectrode is advanced in a stepwise fashion, continuously recording. A DBS electrode is then measured to the appropriate length and introduced to the target point (Fig. 32.2). Test stimulation is carried out with the goal of minimal adverse effects with good therapeutic benefit. Once the lead position has been confirmed, the outer cannula is withdrawn and a skull fixation device is fastened to ensure that the electrode is held firmly in place. The leads are connected to temporary externalized extensions for a trial phase of stimulation.

In the postoperative period, close attention to blood pressure control is performed and the postoperative CT or MRI performed to confirm accurate electrode placement and to rule out any evidence of intracranial hemorrhage. In general, combined stimulation of periventricular gray (PVG) and ventral posterior lateral thalamus (VPL) has been superior to single-lead stimulation. In most patients a certain subperception threshold is needed to produce a pain-relieving effect. If appropriate and acceptable pain relief is achieved, the patient is brought back to the operating room, where the temporary connector is removed and a permanent extension cable is used to connect to the lead to the implanted pulse generator. A subcutaneous pocket is prepared for the internal generator and the extensions are passed through the subcutaneous tissue to connect the system. If the system fails to provide relief, the patient is not a candidate for a permanent device, and the lead is explanted.

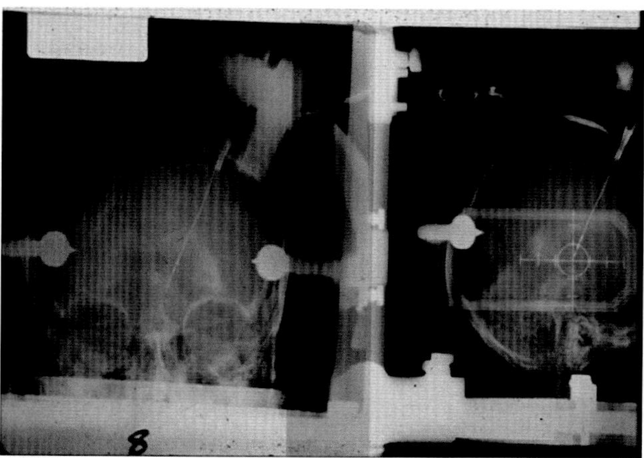

Fig. 32.1 Frame-based stereotactic guidance for deep brain lead placement (*left*). Frameless stereotactic guidance for deep brain lead placement (*right*)

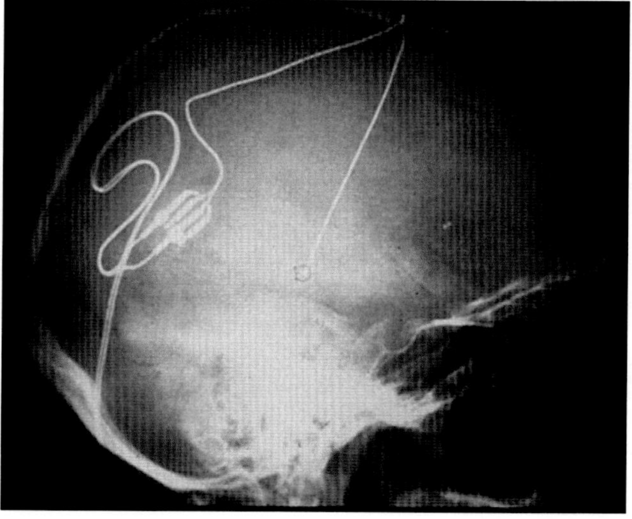

Fig. 32.2 Final lead placement for DBS target

32.3 Risk Assessment

1. Mortality from DBS is a rare complication that occurs in less than 0.4 % of patients.
2. Neurological compromise occurs in less than 1.3 % of patients on a permanent basis.
3. The most devastating risk of DBS is intracranial hemorrhage. Hemorrhages are identified in 2–5 % of patients receiving DBS and can occur at the time of implant or at the time of removal. Asymptomatic hemorrhage occurs in 1.9 % of implanted patients, where symptomatic hemorrhage occurs in 2.1 % and hemorrhage resulting in death or permanent deficit in 1.1 %. Postimplantation infarcts occur in under 1 % of patients [1].
4. Infection rates vary among institutions and have been reported between 1% and 13 %. Infectious complications can include meningitis, encephalitis, skin infection, sepsis, and death [2].
5. Hardware-related complications including lead fracture, short circuit, and electrode migration occur in under 4 % of cases. Loss of effective stimulation coupled with imaging evidence of fracture or persistent high or extremely low impedance readings across several contacts of the electrode are most indicative of a hardware failure [3].
6. Less serious but troubling complications include seizures and stimulation-related side effects such as diplopia, nausea, vertical gaze palsies, nystagmus, oscillopsia, and blurred vision depending on lead location and stimulation side effects that are often overcome with proper programming. In infrequent instances, a misplaced electrode must be surgically relocated to a more effective target site [4].

32.4 Risk Avoidance

1. Preoperative screening for DBS should be similar to screening performed for other neurosurgical procedures including preadmission testing, a focus on comorbidities, and an evaluation of current medications. Preoperative anesthesia consultation is a necessity to improve overall outcomes.
2. Prior to surgery the physician should review the patient's medications and ensure that all medical conditions are under adequate control prior to moving forward. Drugs that affect bleeding should be discussed with the proper medical specialist and discontinued when safe and advisable.
3. Preoperative and intraoperative antibiotics are recommended. Most infections with deep brain implants resolve with proper antibiotics and only if severe and refractory, require wound debridement and/or removal of all hardware.
4. It is critical to have the patient keep a good diary of the pain level and patterns prior to the implant and during the course of the trial. The patient should experience significant relief of the pain and be educated about the system prior to the permanent generator placement.
5. When tunneling the permanent system, the clinician must be careful to avoid blood vessels along the path of the extension. The carotid and jugular vessels are of particular concern.
6. The position of the generator pocket should be carefully planned to allow patient comfort and to avoid tissue irritation or skin erosion. Most of these devices are placed in the infraclavicular soft tissue superficial to the pectoralis fascia. In thinner individuals an abdominal or flank location may be considered.

Conclusions

DBS has been a treatment option for over 50 years and the therapy continues to evolve. Current studies geared toward expanding our understanding of DBS for the treatment of pain may lead to improved patient outcomes related to better matching of pain patterns with the optimal DBS target. The use of DBS offers hope to those who have failed other pain treatment modalities for severe neuropathic pain. The use of DBS should be considered a last resort when spinal cord stimulation and peripheral nerve stimulation are not reasonable options.

References

1. Zrinzo L, Foltynie T, Limousin P, Hariz MI. Reducing hemorrhagic complications in functional neurosurgery: a large case series and systematic literature review. J Neurosurg. 2012;116:84–94.
2. Falowski S, Ooi YC, Smith A, Verhargen Metman L, Bakay RA. An evaluation of hardware and surgical complications with deep brain stimulation based on diagnosis and lead location. Stereotact Funct Neurosurg. 2012;90:173–80.
3. Baizabal Carvallo JF, Mostile G, Almaguer M, Davidson A, Simpson R, Jankovic J. Deep brain stimulation hardware complications in patients with movement disorders: risk factors and clinical correlations. Stereotact Funct Neurosurg. 2012;90:300–6.
4. Coley E, Farhadi R, Lewis S, Whittle IR. The incidence of seizures following deep brain stimulating electrode implantation for movement disorders, pain and psychiatric conditions. Br J Neurosurg. 2009;23:179–83.

Suggested Reading

Abosch A, Timmermann L, Bartley S, Rietkerk HG, Whiting D, Connolly PJ, et al. An international survey of deep brain stimulation procedural steps. Stereotact Funct Neurosurg. 2013;91(1):1–11.

Boccard SG, Pereira EA, Moir L, Aziz TZ, Green AL. Long-term outcomes of deep brain stimulation for neuropathic pain. Neurosurgery. 2013;72:221–30.

Hosobuchi Y. Dorsal periaqueductal gray matter stimulation in humans. Pacing Clin Electrophysiol. 1987;10:213–6.

Kumar K, Toth C, Nath RK. Deep brain stimulation for intractable pain: a 15-year experience. Neurosurgery. 1997;40:736–46.

Kumar K, Wyant GM, Nath R. Deep brain stimulation for control of intractable pain in humans, present and future: a ten-year follow-up. Neurosurgery. 1990;26:774–82.

Levy RM, Lamb S, Adams JE. Treatment of chronic pain by deep brain stimulation: long-term follow-up and review of the literature. Neurosurgery. 1987;21:885–93.

Pool JL, Clark WD, Hudson P, Lombardo M. Hypothalamic-hypophyseal interrelationships. Springfield: Charles C. Thomas; 1956.

Rinaldi PC, Young RF, Albe-Fessard D, Chodakiewitz J. Spontaneous neuronal hyperactivity in the medial and intralaminar thalamic nuclei of patients with deafferentation pain. J Neurosurg. 1991;74:415–21.

33 Stimulation of the Motor Cortex to Treat Chronic Pain

Shivanand P. Lad, Andrew Marky, Timothy R. Deer, Robert M. Levy, and Erika A. Petersen

33.1 Introduction

Motor cortex stimulation (MCS) is a technique that allows physicians to offer treatment to many individuals who would otherwise have no treatment options. The increasing use of this modality is a reflection on the safety, perceived good outcome, and surprisingly long history of human use. This surgical technique has shown good potential in patients suffering from many severe pain conditions including trigeminal neuralgia, poststroke central pain syndromes, phantom limb pain, facial pain, pain from injury to the spinal cord, and postherpetic neuralgia.

Intracranial stimulation, which includes deep brain and MCS targets, is not a new option for patients. These techniques were first used experimentally in the deep brain in 1954 and were actually described prior to the much more accepted method of spinal cord stimulation. Although many consider MCS to be a new or novel treatment option clinically, the procedure was first reported in 1991 [1]. Their work, and that of other pioneers, showed that stimulation of the sensory cortex gave equivocal results, and was not as helpful as direct stimulation to the motor and premotor cortex. Modern outcome studies have shown success with this treatment option in more than 60 % of those suffering from poststroke pain and greater than 75 % in those with persistent trigeminal neuropathic pain refractory to other treatments [2].

Current studies are ongoing to evaluate the use of MCS for other diseases of the neurological system such as traumatic brain disorders, essential tremor, obsessive-compulsive disorder, depression, and dystonia.

S.P. Lad • A. Marky
Division of Neurosurgery, Department of Surgery, Duke University Medical Center, Durham, NC, USA

T.R. Deer, MD (✉)
The Center for Pain Relief, 400 Court Street, Suite 100, Charleston, WV 25301, USA
e-mail: DocTDeer@aol.com

R.M. Levy
Harvey Sandler Department of Neurosurgery, Marcus Neuroscience Institute, Boca Raton, FL, USA

E.A. Petersen
Department of Neurosurgery, University of Arkansas for Medical Sciences, Little Rock, AR, USA

T.R. Deer, J.E. Pope (eds.), *Atlas of Implantable Therapies for Pain Management*, DOI 10.1007/978-1-4939-2110-2_33

33.2 Technical Overview

Once the patient is identified as a candidate for the procedure, and has undergone appropriate neuropsychological screening, a functional magnetic resonance imaging (fMRI) is performed to successfully locate the site in which the motor cortex should be activated to treat the specific pain pattern. In some settings the implanter may prefer to use a conventional MRI to provide anatomical information without adding the functional component. Once these steps have been completed, the patient is taken to the operating room. The surgery is performed in two stages separated by a trial period several days long: (1) tunneled paddle trial and (2) implantation of an internal pulse generator. For the implantation of the paddle lead, choice of neuroanesthetia can range from an awake craniotomy procedure to general anesthesia with neuromonitoring, depending on surgeon preference. Careful attention is given to positioning, preparing, and draping (Fig. 33.1). The incision is planned over the contralateral motor cortex (i.e., right-sided craniotomy for left-sided facial pain) (Fig. 33.2). Stereotactic image guidance (computed tomography [CT] and/or MRI) is performed preoperatively and transferred to the neuronavigational system in the operating room. The three-dimensional images are reconstructed and coregistration is performed based on surface landmarks. This is essential for obtaining good accuracy and localization of the craniotomy (Fig. 33.3). A linear incision is mapped out over the area of the presumed motor strip based on external anatomical landmarks. The planned craniotomy is outlined and local anesthetic applied to each of the three pin sites. After a surgical time-out a linear incision is opened sharply along the frontoparietal area and carried down to the periosteum. An approximately 4 × 4 cm craniotomy is fashioned to allow adequate localization of the desired target and suturing and anchoring of leads to prevent migration. The central sulcus, motor, and premotor areas are localized on navigation to ensure that they are centered in the planned craniotomy (Fig. 33.4). Bur holes using a pneumatic drill are connected with a footplate. The bone flap is carefully detached from the dura and the dural edges are tacked in each quadrant. The neuronavigational probe is then used to define the epidural location of the motor and premotor regions (Figs. 33.5 and 33.6). The intraoperative neuromonitoring paddle electrode is placed over the navigation-mapped area of the central sulcus and motor strip to identify N20-P20 phase reversal (Fig. 33.7). The premotor and motor areas are carefully mapped out and marked on the dura.

Once the target cortex has been identified using both neuronavigation and electrocortical mapping, two 1 × 4 paddle leads are placed over the previously marked motor and premotor areas that correspond to the contralateral painful area (e.g., face area at the junction of the inferior frontal sulcus and the motor strip). The two leads are placed adjacent to one another and test stimulation is carried out with serial cycling and a slow increase in voltage. Given that no paresthesias are apparent in MCS, one relies on a combination of neurophysiology as well as patient interaction to assess adequate placement of the final electrode position. The patient is awakened from monitored anesthesia. The patient should be able to report good pain relief in the area of pain (e.g., trigeminal distribution on the contralateral side). Stimulation parameters are gradually increased to produce facial twitching and gauge of preseizure threshold, with ice saline available as needed. Once adequate position had been localized over the motor and premotor area, each of the 1 × 4 electrodes is then carefully anchored down with multiple 4-0 Nurolon sutures to the outer layer of the dura. The patient is given further anesthetic to ensure comfort for the remainder of the operation. The leads are tunneled through the posterior bur hole and bone flap is carefully reapplied with titanium plates and screws. Extension wires are then tunneled posteriorly at the level of the parietal boss and attached to two stimulator leads, clearly identifying anterior (premotor) and posterior (motor).

Once the leads are in place, the electrode is connected to trialing cables and an inpatient trial of 3–7 days is carried out. Amplitudes for stimulation vary between 0.5 and 10 V, rate varies from 5 to 130 Hz, and pulse widths vary from 50 to 450 ms. The intensity of stimulation is compared with the motor threshold, with a starting value of 15–20 % of the energy needed to activate the motor components. A typical trial regimen may increase the intensity in 20 % increments up to a maximum level of stimulation that is 80 % of the motor threshold. Because MCS by definition does not elicit paresthesias of the kind commonly perceived in dorsal column or peripheral nerve stimulation, treatment stimulation benefit is tracked through a patient pain diary.

Once the trial is deemed successful, the patient is brought back to the operating room under general anesthesia to undergo generator placement. Most implanters prefer pocketing in the infraclavicular region, although multiple sites are acceptable. A pocket is fashioned for the pulse generator in the plane above the pectoralis fascia. A subcutaneous pouch is made at the area of the parietal boss to accommodate the extension connectors. A tunneling device is used to pass the extension cables in the subcutaneous plane between the parietal incision and the infraclavicular incision. The extension wires are brought through and the motor cortex stimulator leads are connected to the proximal ends of the extensions. Once the connections are secured and tested, both incisions are irrigated copiously and careful closure is performed (Figs. 33.8, 33.9, 33.10, 33.11, and 33.12).

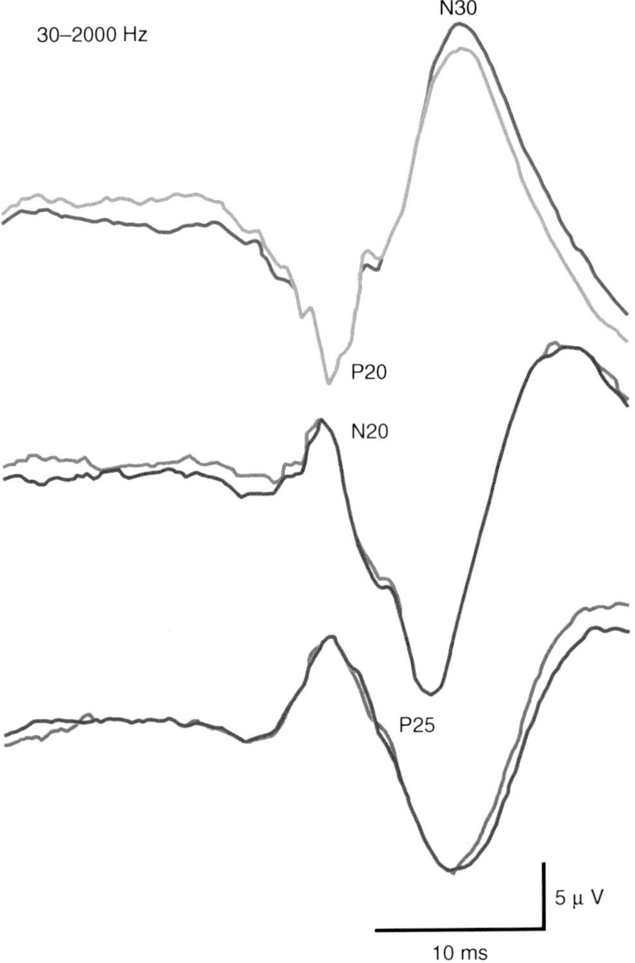

Fig. 33.1 SSEP waveforms show P20 and N20 components with phase reversal indicating an electrode overlying the central sulcus signifying the motor and sensory cortex

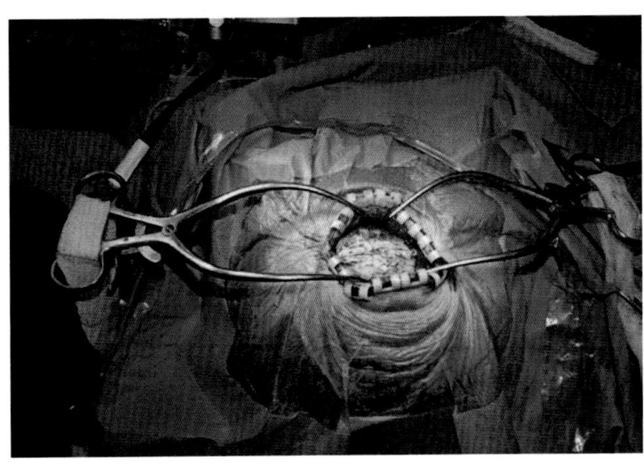

Fig. 33.3 Incision for exposure for craniotomy

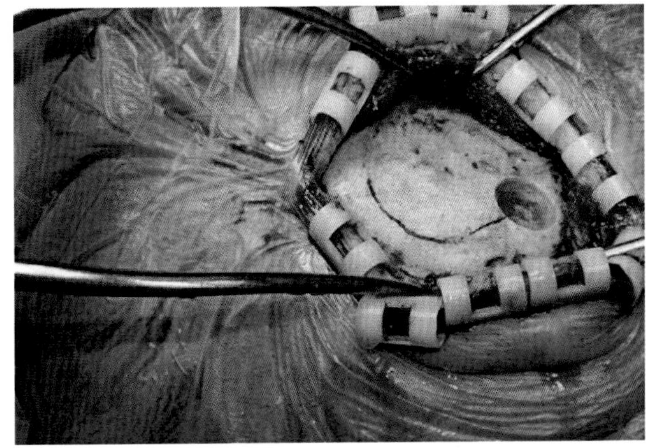

Fig. 33.4 Skull exposure with initiation of craniotomy

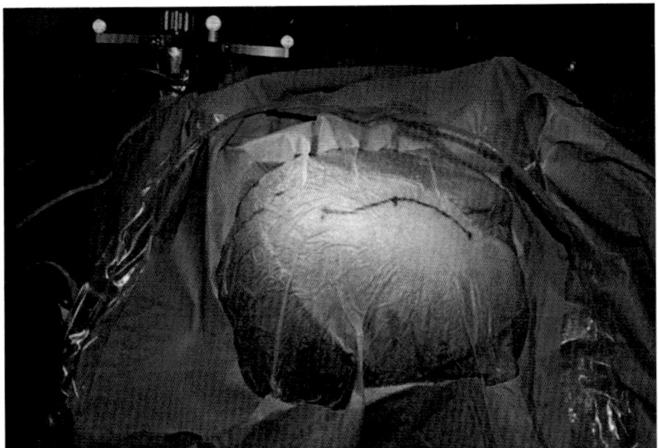

Fig. 33.2 Draping and planning the incision for the craniotomy approach

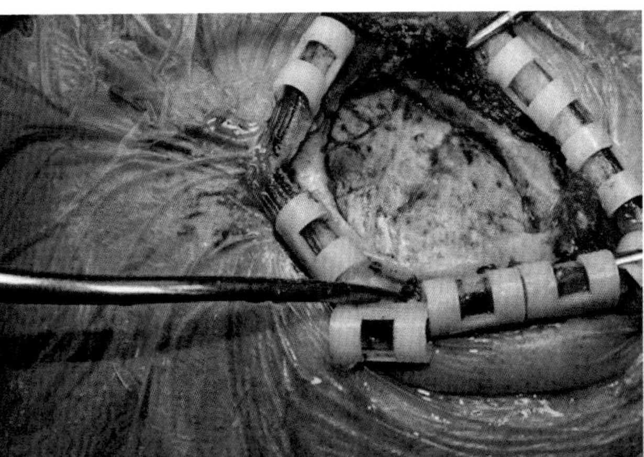

Fig. 33.5 Craniotomy with proper exposure over the central sulcus based on preoperative mapping

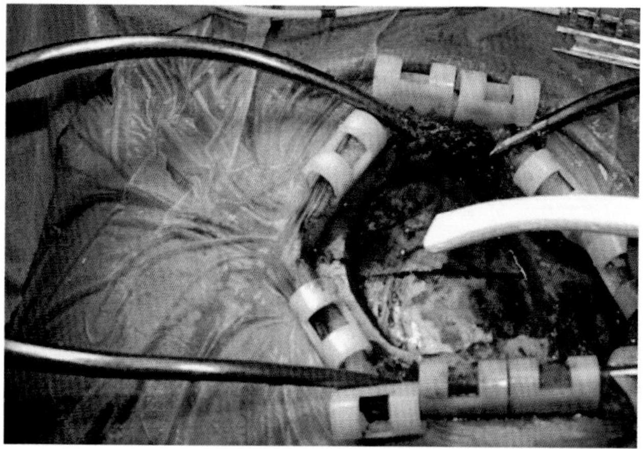

Fig. 33.6 Electrophysiological mapping for lead placement

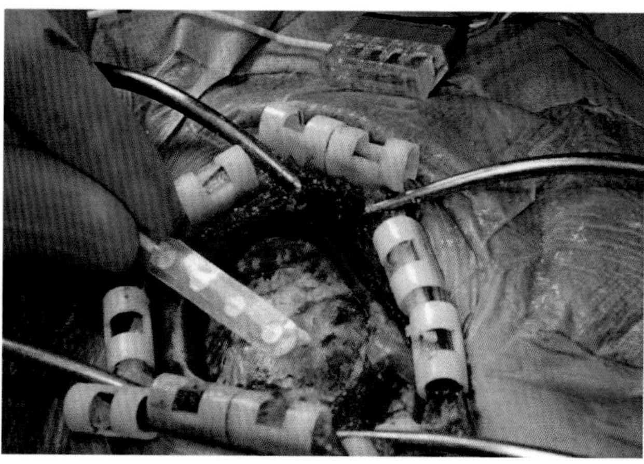

Fig. 33.7 Epidural exposure lead placement

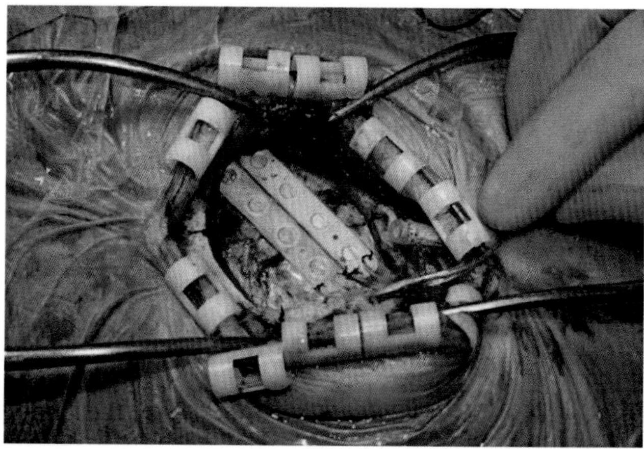

Fig. 33.8 Leads in proper position for MCS

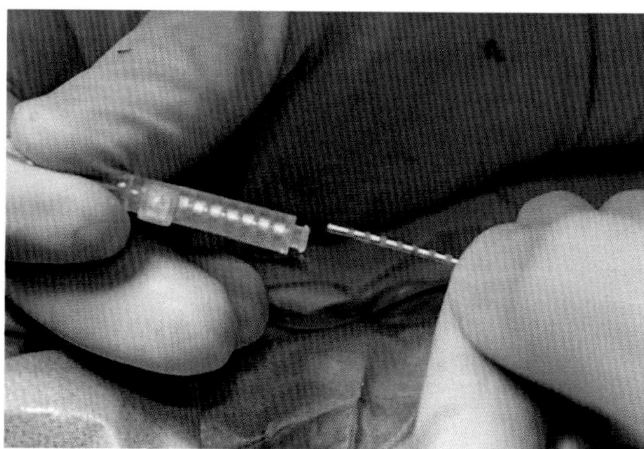

Fig. 33.9 Securing the connections

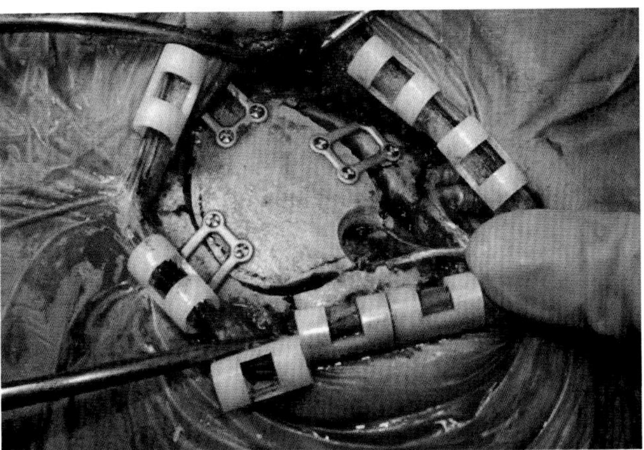

Fig. 33.10 Replacing the bone from the craniotomy prior to closure

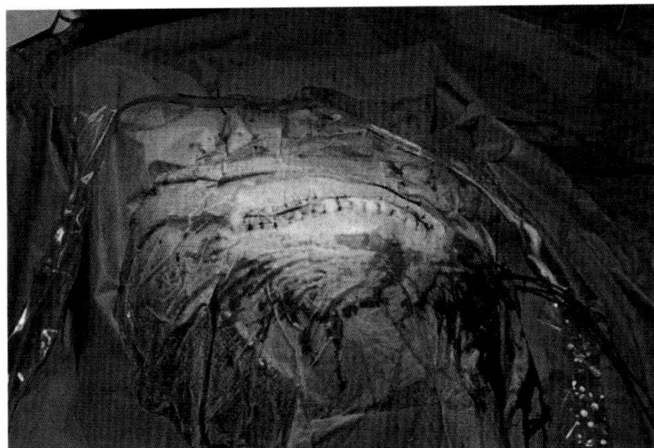

Fig. 33.11 Closure of the incision

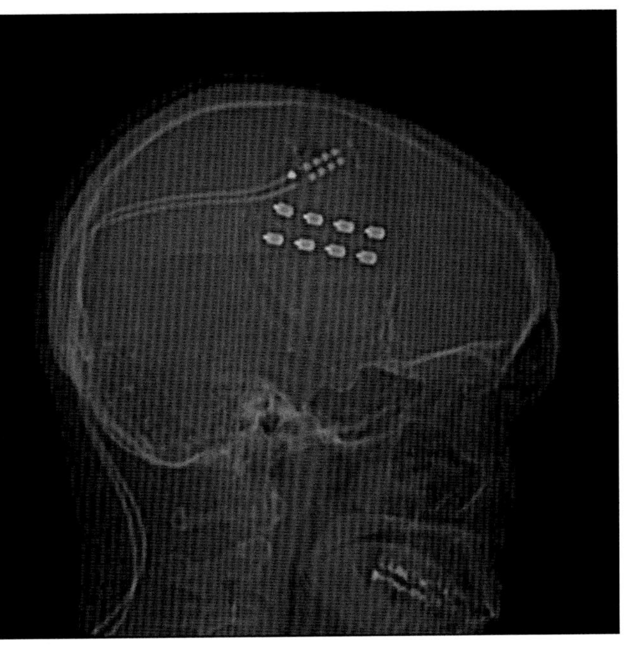

Fig. 33.12 Postoperative radiographs show two 1×4 leads centered over the face-motor area and the premotor and motor sulci based on intraoperative neurophysiological mapping

33.3 Risk Assessment

1. Despite the encouraging reports in the literature on the utility of MCS for refractory neuropathic pain, only a handful of centers perform the procedure, and many clinicians are not aware of it as a therapeutic option. MCS requires a relatively involved trial process in order to determine its benefit for an individual patient. Furthermore, the effect of MCS can wane over time, requiring cycling or reprogramming.
2. One of the most serious events that can occur during placement of MCS is intracranial bleeding (epidural or subdural). These complications can lead to severe neurological dysfunction and even death.
3. Infection risks are very serious when implanting MCS leads. Infection may result in meningitis, osteomyelitis, sepsis, and death.
4. Reported neurological deficits have included stroke, hemiparesis, confusion, abnormal involuntary movements, and development of motor loss in one or more limbs.
5. The most commonly reported complication is seizure. This event can occur in the intraoperative setting or immediate postoperative period. Recording the motor threshold is important to avoid this in the postoperative setting. There is a risk of seizures during stimulator programming, although the development of epilepsy has not been reported.

33.4 Risk Avoidance

1. Prior to surgery, the physician should complete a thorough physical examination with an eye to identifying any infection or lesions that might heighten perioperative infection risk. Surgery should be delayed if there is any doubt about the safety of moving forward.
2. Prior to surgery, the physician should review the patient's medications and ensure that all medical conditions are under adequate control prior to moving forward. Drugs that affect bleeding should be discussed with the proper medical specialist and discontinued when safe and advisable.
3. Close attention is paid to coagulation status and meticulous hemostasis at the time of surgery.
4. Preoperative, intraoperative, and postoperative antibiotics are recommended. Appropriate use of perioperative antibiotics and antibiotic-containing irrigation during surgery aid in minimizing infection risk. Some clinicians may opt to continue antibiotics during the trial period when the extensions are externalized, although there is no agreement in the clinical literature on this practice.
5. It is critical to have the patient keep a good diary of the pain level and patterns prior to the implant and during the course of the trial. Because the patient cannot feel a sensory change during the trial, the ability to keep proper records is critical in determining the success of the trial.
6. Pain relief is most commonly achieved at amplitudes of 6 V or less, with mean amplitudes of 5 V or less in most studies. Amplitudes above 6 V are more likely to be associated with seizures during programming.
7. When tunneling the permanent system, the clinician must be careful to avoid blood vessels along the path of the procedure. The carotid and jugular vessels are of particular concern.
8. The position of the generator pocket should be carefully planned to allow patient comfort and to avoid tissue irritation or skin erosion.

33.5 Conclusions

MCS stimulation is an important component of the pain treatment continuum. It is a technologically advanced procedure that requires skill and advanced training. With additional study it will likely become a more widespread tool in the treatment of difficult pain syndromes.

References

1. Tsubokawa T, Katayama Y, Yamamoto T, Hirayama T, Koyama S. Treatment of thalamic pain by chronic motor cortex stimulation. Pacing Clin Electrophysiol. 1991;14(1):131–4.
2. Rasche D, Rupppoit M, Stippich C, Unterberg A, Tronnier V. Motor cortex stimulation for the long-term relief of chronic neuropathic pain: a 10 year experience. Pain. 2006;121:43–52.

Suggested Reading

Henderson J, Lad S. Motor cortex stimulation and neuropathic facial pain. Neurosurg Focus. 2006;21, E6.

Levy R, Ruland S, Weinand M, Lowry D, Dafer R, Bakay R. Cortical stimulation for the rehabilitation of patients with hemiparetic stroke: a multicenter feasibility study of safety and efficacy. J Neurosurg. 2008;108:707–14.

Osenbach R. Motor cortex stimulation for intractable pain. Neurosurg Focus. 2006;21, E7.

34 Stimulation of the Peripheral Nervous System: Occipital Techniques for the Treatment of Occipital Neuritis and Transformed Migraine

Nameer R. Haider and Timothy R. Deer

34.1 Introduction

Pain in the occiput that radiates cephalad or laterally is often secondary to abnormalities of the divisions of the occipital nerve. The occipital nerve is involved in pain syndromes originating from nerve trauma, myofascial spasm causing compression, cervicogenic disease, cervical spondylosis, posterior fossa surgery, and transformed migraine. Inflammation of the C2 nerve root will also cause severe symptoms in this region, consistent with cervical radiculitis. The transformed migraine begins with pain in the occipital nerve distribution and then evolves into a full migraine headache. Neurostimulation has also been employed in the treatment of chronic tension-type headache, hemicrania continua, short-lasting unilateral neuralgiform headaches, and cluster headaches. Treatment of these headache conditions may include direct stimulation of the greater and lesser occipital, supraorbital and supratrochlear, auriculotemporal, and infraorbital nerves. More recently, 360° cranial stimulation has been described as well. This is a concept of stimulating nerve structures in the posterior and anterior extracranial regions simultaneously.

The treatments of headache pain syndromes include oral medications, physical therapy, nerve blocks, and radiofrequency ablation. In the past, occipital neurectomy, which involved the destruction of the nerve, was performed by neurosurgery, but this fell out of favor because of deafferentation syndrome and the potential worsening of the pain syndrome. Cryotherapy and pulsed radiofrequency appear to have some efficacy but unfortunately are short lived in duration and require the patient to undergo multiple procedures over time. Surgical decompression of the occipital nerves has also been described but has not been seen acceptable success. Stimulation of the nerves has evolved over the past decade and has become a standard treatment of chronic headache pain that does not respond to conservative measures.

N.R. Haider, MD (✉)
Minimally Invasive Pain Institute, Washington, DC, USA
e-mail: drhaider@killpain.com

T.R. Deer, MD (✉)
The Center for Pain Relief, 400 Court Street, Suite 100, Charleston, WV 25301, USA
e-mail: DocTDeer@aol.com

T.R. Deer, J.E. Pope (eds.), *Atlas of Implantable Therapies for Pain Management*, DOI 10.1007/978-1-4939-2110-2_34

34.2 Technical Overview

Prior to considering the technical aspects of implantation of extracranial leads, the clinician must confirm the diagnosis of corresponding neuralgia. The clinician should have a clear mental picture of the neuroanatomy including the branches of the respective nerves (Figs. 34.1, 34.2, and 34.3).

The diagnostic workup for peripheral cranial neuralgia includes a history of pain originating or ending in the nerve area and a physical examination that includes tenderness over the respective nerve and nerve root distribution. Some implanters have recommended confirmation of the neuropathic pain generator by a good temporary response to injection of local anesthetic that provides relief for the duration of the medication used, but there has been no prospective confirmation that this is predictable of a good outcome.

Once the patient is felt to be an appropriate candidate for stimulation, the anatomy is reexamined and the skin is evaluated for lesions, texture, and bony prominences. The peripheral nerves branch into multiple fibers and the coverage of the appropriate pain pattern should be considered when planning the types and number of leads and electrodes needed. The respective cranial region is shaved to remove hair, which can be a nidus for infection. The trial leads are often placed via a single needle stick on the affected side(s), and the permanent leads are most commonly placed via a midline incision for occipital neural stimulation, parietal/temporal incision for a auriculotemporal nerve stimulation, and incision just behind the hairline for supraorbital/supratrochlear stimulation. Infraorbital stimulation requires needle entry over the maxillary region (Fig. 34.2).

By using a widely spaced octipolar lead array, the area of stimulation increases, covering the multiple branches of the nerve. With temporary leads, once the implant is placed by fluoroscopy, the leads are secured to the skin by a suture or tape. In permanent occipital nerve implants, the surgical process begins by making an incision at the midline just below or above the occipital prominence. Tissue separation can be achieved with the blunt use of a surgical scissor to minimize trauma. Once the fascia is visualized, a cautery tool is used to achieve hemostasis. In some younger and healthier patients blunt dissection will not be possible and sharp dissection is needed. This can lead to increased bleeding, and the implanter must focus on hemostasis. Once hemostasis is acceptable, a needle is placed in the desired path of the planned lead placement. Local anesthetic should be placed only at the needle entry location. If local anesthetic is placed in the path of the needle, it will be difficult to confirm stimulation on the operating room table. Use of epinephrine in local anesthetic may reduce bleeding. Fluoroscopy is important to guide and confirm the needle path, but ultrasound is an acceptable alternative for guidance. In many cases, the needle must be slightly bent to achieve the desired depth and course of the lead implant. Needles with a plastic stylet are often easier to use because the metal stylet may be difficult to remove once the needle is bent. The depth of the needle should be just below the dermis in the subcutaneous tissue. The needle bevel should be directed downward to avoid placing the tip of the lead too superficially. Once the stylet is removed, the lead is placed to the tip of the needle using fluoroscopy to confirm placement. The needle is then pulled distally while the lead is held in position using radiograph confirmation, while the tissue is stabilized by holding pressure above the lead.

Once the lead is in the desired location, a handheld programmer is used to activate the leads and achieve stimulation. In many cases an array with multiple cathodes is successful, which will help spread the current. When two leads are placed it is not uncommon to use one lead with primarily anodes and the other with primarily cathodes to create a cross-talk to cover a wider neuropathic pain profile.

For permanent implants, when the patient's stimulation is acceptable, the leads are anchored to the fascia with nonabsorbable suture. At each incisional site, a coil is then made as a form of strain relief and the leads are tunneled to the pocket. Pocketing options include the anterior chest wall in the subclavicular region, posterior axillary region, buttock, and flank. If pockets are made in more distal locations, it may be necessary to add lead extensions to reach the pocket (Figs. 34.3 and 34.4).

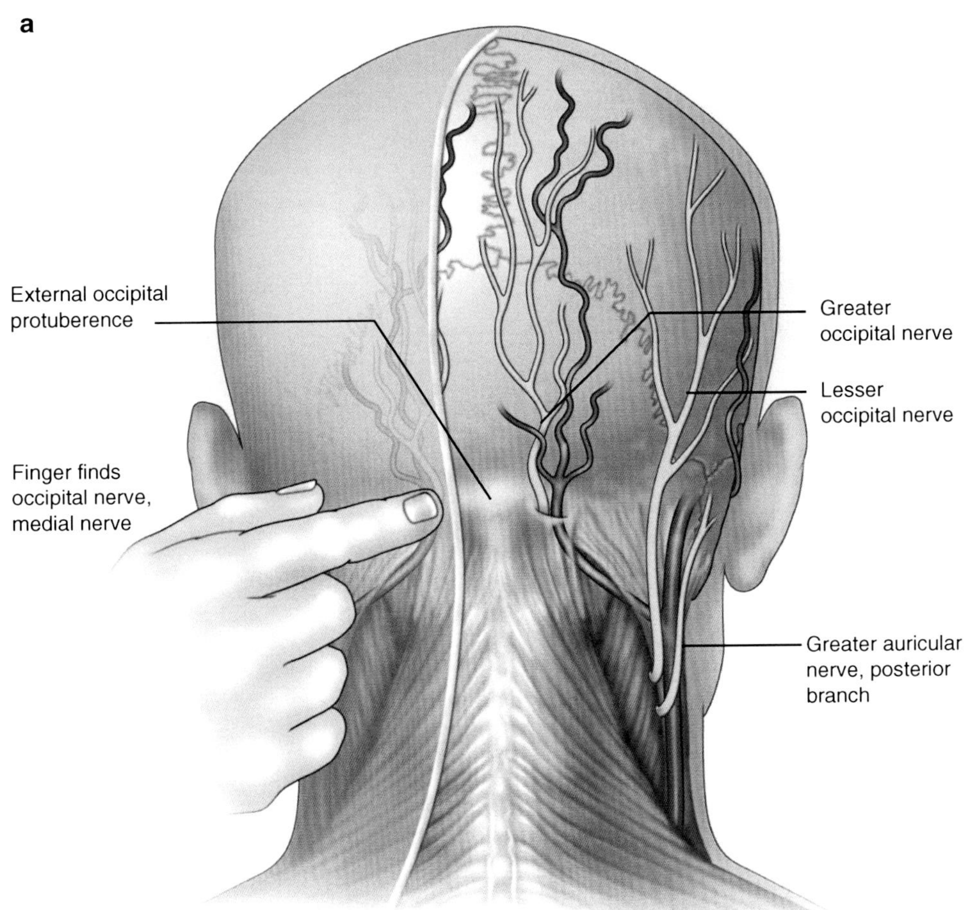

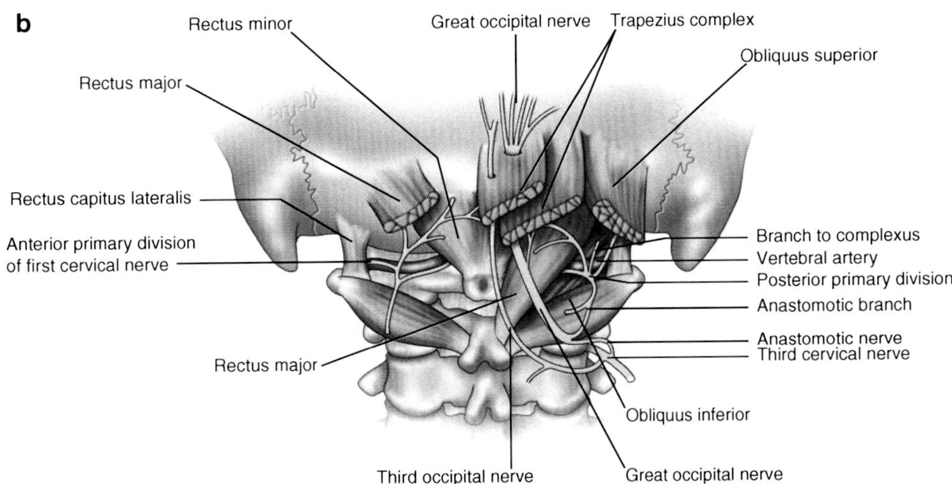

Fig. 34.1 (**a**, **b**) Neuroanatomy of the branches of the occipital nerve

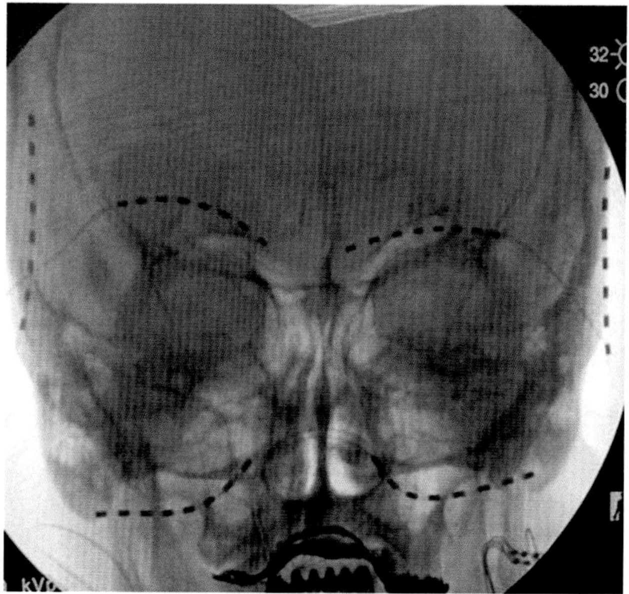

Fig. 34.2 Supraorbital, infraorbital, and auriculotemporal nerve stimulation

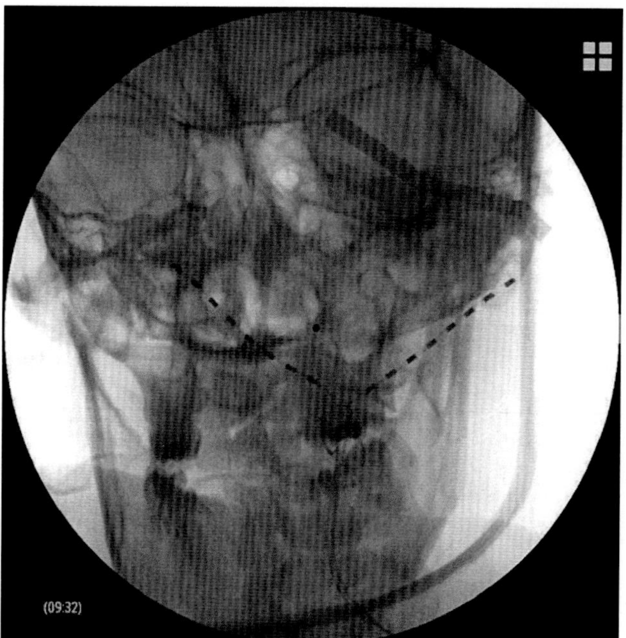

Fig. 34.3 Occipital nerve stimulation, AP view

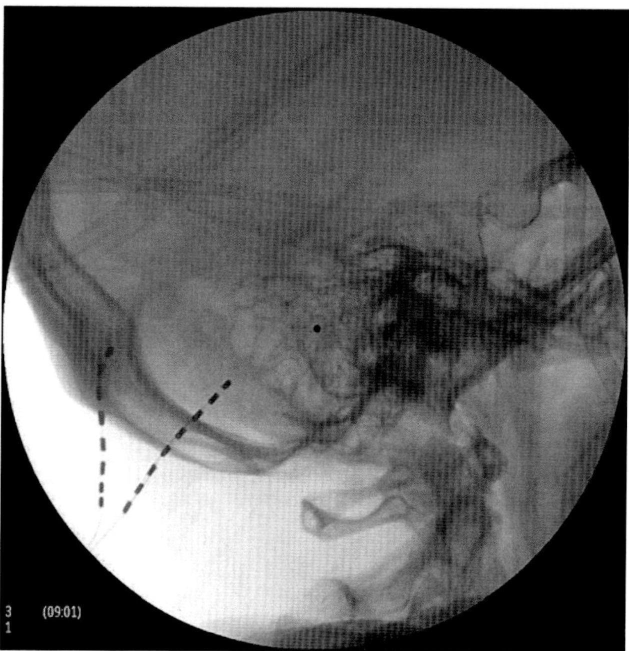

Fig. 34.4 Occipital nerve stimulation, lateral view

34.2.1 Method for Occipital Stimulation

The targets for the leads vary based on physician preference and can range from a lateral C1 approach to a perpendicular greater occipital nerve approach. The most common area for placement for the leads is at an angle from the midline to the lateral edge of the occipital bone, in order to capture fibers of both the greater and the lesser occipital nerves (Fig. 34.5). This placement allows for proper stimulation even in the event of mild-to-moderate migration.

34.2.2 Method for Supraorbital/ Supratrochlear Stimulation

The insertion site for the lead is just posterior to the anterior hairline of the temporal region, advancing a bent/curved needle with a plastic stylet over the supraorbital margin placing electrode contacts adjacent to supraorbital and supratrochlear nerves. Care must be taken not to perforate the skin and to keep the needle in the proper trajectory avoiding inferior placement of lead over orbit (Fig. 34.6).

34.2.3 Method for Auriculotemporal Stimulation

The insertional lead is performed posterior and superior to the ear, advancing the lead anteriorly over the auriculotemporal nerve (Fig. 34.7).

34.2.4 Method for Infraorbital Stimulation

The insertion of lead is performed using a bent/curved needle with a plastic stylet from the maxillary region immediately inferior to the orbit with electrode contacts overlying the nerve. If a wide-spaced eight-contact lead array is used, simultaneous stimulation of the infratrochlear, infraorbital, zygomaticofacial, lacrimal, and infraocular nerves may be achieved for treatment of cluster headache (Figs. 34.8 and 34.9).

34.2.5 Method for Halo 360° Cranial Stimulation

The targets for the leads using this technique include bilateral simulation of supraorbital, supratrochlear, zygomaticotemporal, auriculotemporal, greater occipital, and lesser occipital nerves. There is also stimulation noted of the terminal branches of bilateral zygomaticofacial, greater auricular, third occipital nerves and C2–3 nerve roots. This method requires use of a 32-contact internal pulse generator system and four leads each with eight electrode contacts, with wide 6-mm spacing between the adjacent electrode contacts. Bilateral leads are placed superior to the ear, advancing a needle with a bent/curved stylet anteriorly with the electrode contacts overlying bilateral supraorbital, supratrochlear, zygomaticotemporal and auriculotemporal nerves. Bilateral leads are simultaneously placed posteriorly overlying greater/lesser occipital, greater auricular, and branches of the third occipital nerves, as well as ascending branches of the posterior rami of C2 and C3 nerve roots. This method is promising, but the cost-to-benefit ratio is yet to be established considering the increased amount of hardware needed. Further evaluation may determine this to be an excellent method of treatment (Fig. 34.10).

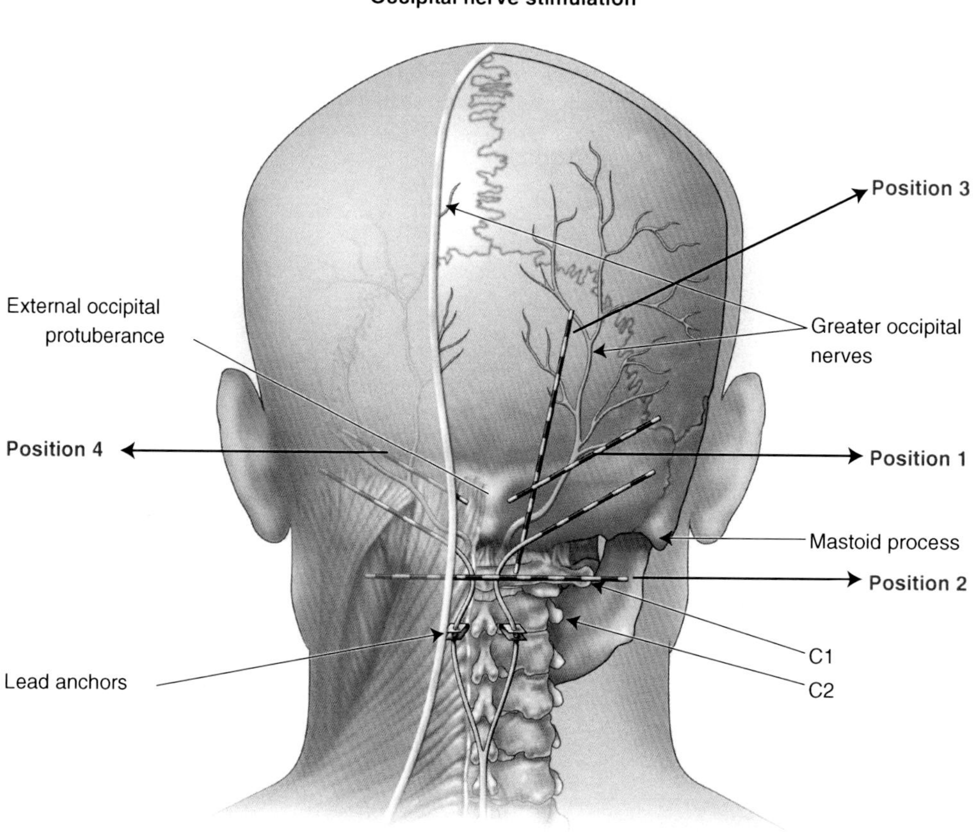

Fig. 34.5 Variability of lead orientation for occipital nerve stimulation

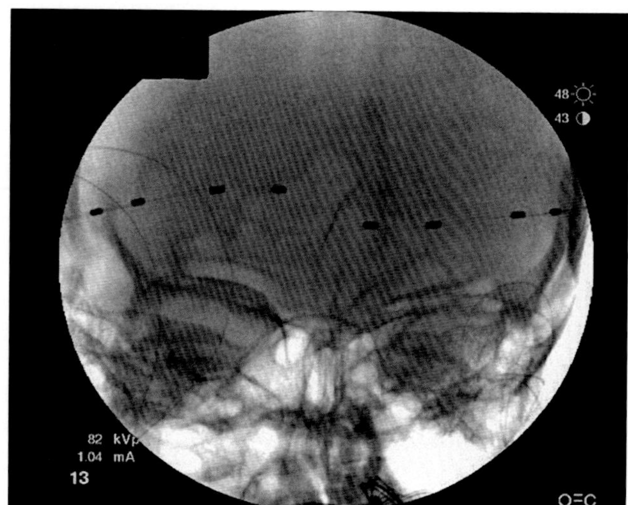

Fig. 34.6 Supraorbital stimulation

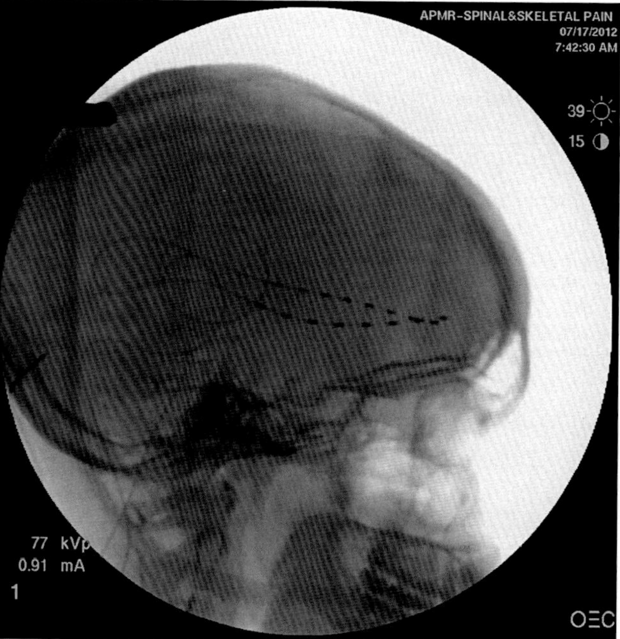

Fig. 34.7 Auriculotemporal stimulation, lateral view

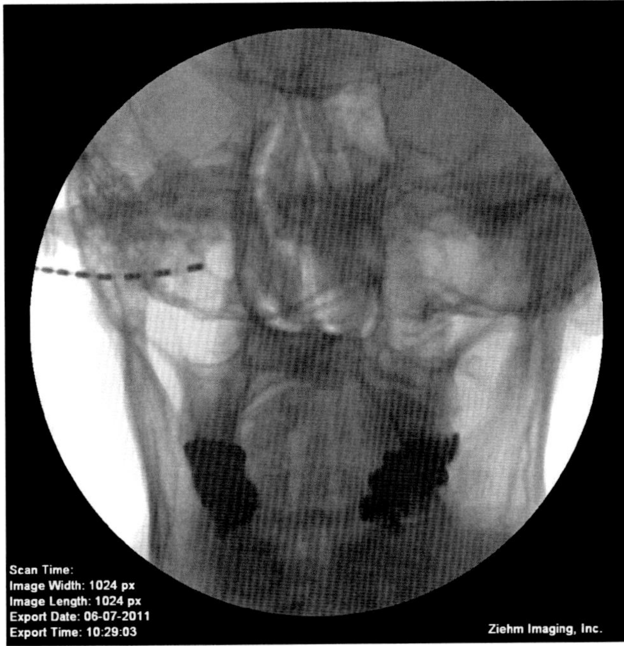

Fig. 34.8 Infraorbital nerve stimulation AP view

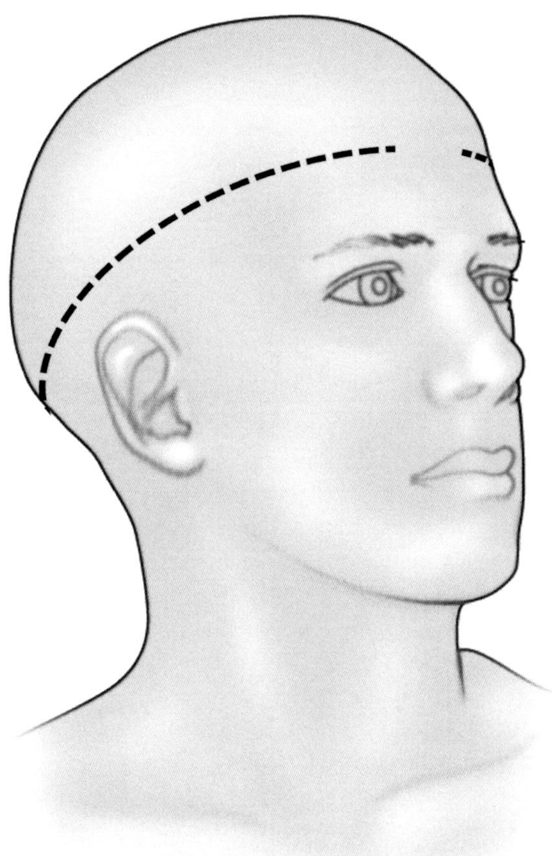

Fig. 34.10 Stimulation oblique view of Halo technique

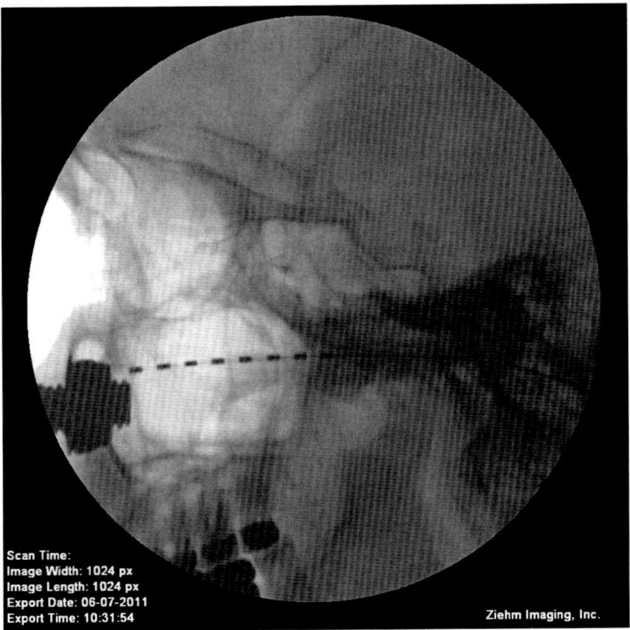

Fig. 34.9 Infraorbital stimulation lateral view

34.3 Risk Assessment

1. The depth of the leads and generator should be carefully considered. The ideal lead placement is in the tissue just below the dermis. If the lead is over a pressure point, the depth should be slightly increased. The generator depth should be 1.5 to 3.0 cm.
2. The tissue of the planned surgery should be evaluated for lesions or infection. If an area of irritation exists, surgery should be delayed.
3. The lead may be prone to erosion through the skin. Diabetic patients and those with a history of skin disorders should be approached carefully.
4. The patient's postoperative movement is a fine balance. If the patient is allowed to have unrestricted movement, it may cause lead migration, but if too-restricted, fibrosis can occur, which may cause restricted movement of the neck and pain with palpation over the wiring.
5. Injection and surgical manipulation of the occipital or temporal region could lead to extensive bleeding of the occipital or temporal arteries, respectively, or to arterial clotting. Either process could lead to tissue sloughing or a need to reoperate on the patient.
6. Proper surgical planning would include assessment of patient positioning and surgical planning for tunneling because a stab incision may need to be made between the internal pulse generator and the cranial leads in order to tunnel the leads from skull to the internal pulse generator pocket.

34.4 Risk Avoidance

1. Prior to surgery, the physician should review the patient's tissue for infection or lesions in the surgical area. The surgery should be delayed if there is any doubt about the safety of moving forward.
2. Prior to surgery, the physician should review the patient's medications and ensure that all medical conditions are under adequate control prior to moving forward. Drugs that affect bleeding should be discussed with the proper medical specialist and discontinued when safe and advisable.
3. Preoperative and intraoperative antibiotics are recommended. It is advisable to vigorously irrigate the wound prior to closure.
4. Preparing and draping of the occipital region can be difficult because of the need to operate in the region of the patient's head where there is also a need for airway access. This issue is very important when tunneling the leads. In positioning the patient, the pocket location is important. The options for pocketing can be the chest wall, which requires a lateral decubitus position, or the back or buttock, which can be done in the prone position.
5. It is critical to adequately measure the lead length and try to match it to the insertion and pocket location. There should be adequate length to allow for a stress-relief loop at both the lead anchoring site and the generator location. This will reduce the risk of both migration and fibrosis.
6. The tissue in the area of the occipital and temporal regions should be handled gently. It is important to separate the tissue with care and to minimize bleeding. The tissue should close evenly and without stress to maximize tissue circulation.
7. Postimplant, the patient's movement should be restricted for the first 6 weeks. At the end of 6 weeks, the patient may benefit from musculoskeletal treatment by a certified physical therapist.

Conclusions

Peripheral cranial stimulation is becoming a common procedure to treat chronic headaches. It is an alternative to more destructive procedures and to high-dose oral medications that may cause systemic side effects and complications as well as rebound headaches and addictive disorders. Peripheral extracranial nerve stimulation is a valuable low-risk procedure that will continue to improve as lead technology and programming are enhanced by future research and development.

Suggested Reading

Dodick DW, Silberstein SD, Reed KL, Deer TR, Slavin KV, Huh B, et al. Safety and efficacy of peripheral nerve stimulation of the occipital nerves for the management of chronic migraine: Long-term results from a randomized, multicenter, double-blinded, controlled study. Cephalalgia. 2014. pii: 0333102414543331. [Epub ahead of print].

Pope JE. Complications of cranial nerve stimulation. Reducing risks and complications of interventional pain procedures, Interventional and neuromodulatory techniques for pain management series, vol. 5. 1st ed. Philadelphia: Elsevier Saunders; 2012.

Pope JE, Deer TR, Grigsby EJ, Kim PS. Stimulation of the peripheral nerve and field. Comprehensive treatment of chronic pain by medical, interventional and integrative approaches. American Academy of Pain Medicine. New York: Springer; 2013.

Vaisman J, Markley H, Ordia J, Deer T. Supraorbital and supratrochlear stimulation for trigeminal autonomic cephalalgias. Curr Pain Headache Rep. 2014;18(4):409.

Part IV

Drug Delivery

35 History of Intrathecal Drug Delivery

Timothy R. Deer

Intrathecal infusions of analgesics have been utilized increasingly since the late 1980s for the treatment of persistent pain. Early credit goes to Leonard Corning, who administered neuraxial local anesthetic in 1885. Corning's work led to an interest in using this method to treat pain during surgery, with chronic pain being of little interest in the initial development of these methods. Morphine may have been administered spinally as early as 1901. The use of opioids in the spine then underwent a long void in advancement. A breakthrough came in 1971 with the discovery of specific opioid receptors in the spinal cord. Yaksh and Rudy demonstrated the efficacy of analgesia from intrathecal opioids in animal models in 1976, and Wang and colleagues reported the treatment of cancer pain with morphine in 1979. With the development of implantable, programmable, continuous drug delivery systems in the 1980s, the use of intraspinal opioids became part of the modern treatment algorithm. The availability of these devices led to interest in using pumps to treat cancer pain, noncancer pain, and intractable spasticity.

T.R. Deer, MD
The Center for Pain Relief, 400 Court Street, Suite 100,
Charleston, WV 25301, USA
e-mail: DocTDeer@aol.com

T.R. Deer, J.E. Pope (eds.), *Atlas of Implantable Therapies for Pain Management*, DOI 10.1007/978-1-4939-2110-2_35

35.1 Development of Delivery Systems

Although many clinicians recognized the value of spinal anesthetics in early studies, the short duration of action led to a search for methods of lengthening the period of effectiveness. Continuous catheter access was first proposed in 1935 by Dr. Grafton Love, a neurosurgeon at the Mayo Clinic. Dr. Love had an extensive background in the treatment of hydrocephalus with the use of continuously draining ureteral catheters placed in lateral ventricles. His treatment of meningitis patients prompted him to attempt the same technique by introducing an intrathecal catheter into the lumbar space.

The first clinical application of continuous spinal anesthesia was described in a 1940 report by Dr. William Leonard, a Philadelphia surgeon, who administered procaine to approximately 200 patients. Dr. Leonard utilized a control syringe attached to a malleable needle, which had been placed presurgically in the lumbar spine. This method was quickly adopted by other physicians in the field, who used it primarily in patients who were felt to be at high risk for the use of systemic approaches to anesthesia.

The next major advancement was in the form of a flexible epidural or intrathecal catheter. Dr. Samuel Manalan, an obstetrician from Indianapolis, Indiana, is credited with first administering caudal anesthesia, using an antiquated nylon catheter. This catheter was placed into the sacral canal through a 14-gauge needle and was left in place for varying periods, in some cases for as much as 18 h. Though the catheters were left indwelling, they were not used continuously; the method of anesthesia was based on a strategy of intermittent bolus injections.

The development of continuous intrathecal and lumbar catheter techniques was further advanced in 1944 by Edward Tuohy's introduction of a new catheter into the spinal interspace for the purpose of repeated delivery of the surgical anesthetic procaine. The Tuohy needle and catheter was the first of its kind because of its ability to direct its course to a predictable location in the spine. The technique was later enhanced by the development of a needle with a side exit deployment access area, designed by Hubor.

The Medtronic Synchromed II employs a rotor driven mechanism for drug delivery. This system has been recently plagued by inaccuracy and a higher chance of motor failure when off-label therapies are delivered. In 2012, Medasys received U.S. Food and Drug Administration approval for the Prometra pump, which uses a valve-gated dose-regulation system. Studies suggest that the Prometra pump has an accuracy of 97.1 %, improved from the delivery provided by the Synchromed II peristaltic system. Further, unpublished data suggest that the delivery kinetics of the Prometra system may innately further reduce the incidence of granuloma.

The final major advancement in the development of the delivery technique was the permanent implantation of the intrathecal and epidural catheter in combination with internal or external ports, reservoirs, and programmable pumps for the continuous injection or infusion of a wide variety of therapeutic agents. These catheters were implanted in the spine, and the drug was infused by accessing the port, which in most cases was implanted in the subcutaneous tissue. The first human clinical implant of a programmable intrathecal pump occurred in 1982, with widespread release of the system in the United States in 1991 by Medtronic Neurological, Minneapolis, Minnesota. The approved drug at that time was preservative-free morphine sulfate. Over the past two decades, the pump and catheter have remained similar in appearance and function.

Table 35.1 summarizes the significant events in the development of intrathecal drug delivery.

Table 35.1 Important milestones in intrathecal drug delivery

Year	Milestone
1885	Leonard Corning administers neuraxial local anesthetic
1901	Intraspinal morphine use is first reported
1935	Dr. Grafton Love first proposes continuous catheter access
1940	The first practical application of continuous spinal anesthesia is described by Dr. William Leonard, a Philadelphia surgeon, who administered procaine to approximately 200 patients
1944	Edward Tuohy introduces a catheter into the spinal interspace for the purpose of repeated delivery of the surgical anesthetic procaine
1976	Yaksh and Rudy demonstrate the efficacy of analgesia from intrathecal opioids in animal models
1979	Wang and colleagues report the treatment of cancer pain with morphine
1982	Medtronic Neurological (Minneapolis, Minnesota) reports the first clinical implant of a programmable intrathecal pump
1991	Medtronic Neurological (Minneapolis, Minnesota) releases a programmable intrathecal pump in the United States
2012	Medasys receives US Food and Drug Administration (FDA) approval for an implantable pump

35.2 Outlook for Future Developments

This decade will most likely see major changes in pump therapy for chronic diseases. Delivery tools continue to evolve, with several companies working on new technologies that may impact the size of the programmable pump, internal mechanisms, accuracy, safety, and catheter materials used to deliver the drug. The other area of interest in the intrathecal space is the development of new drugs that could be delivered to treat specific ailments. These drug developments have been slow to progress, but many clinicians remain hopeful that eventually we will be able to treat many new patients for diseases causing pain and other areas of human affliction.

Suggested Reading

Deer T, Winkelmüller W, Erdine S, Bedder M, Burchiel K. Intrathecal therapy for cancer and nonmalignant pain: patient selection and patient management. Neuromodulation. 1999;2:55–66.

Krames ES. A history of intraspinal analgesia: a small and personal journey. Neuromodulation. 2012;15(3):172–93.

Medasys Inc. announces FDA approval for implantable programmable drug pump. 2012. http://www.flowonix.com/press_releases/FDA_Clearance-Prometra.pdf. Accessed September 7, 2014.

Rauck R, Deer T, Rosen S, Padda G, Barsa J, Dunbar E, Dwarakanath G. Accuracy and efficacy of intrathecal administration of morphine sulfate for treatment of intractable pain using the Prometra® Programmable Pump. Neuromodulation. 2010;13:102–8.

Selection and Indications for Intrathecal Pump Placement

36

Timothy R. Deer and Jason E. Pope

The placement of an intrathecal catheter, tunneling of the catheter, pocketing for pump placement, and connection of the system is a complex process of interventions requiring great technical skill, but it can be argued that the selection of the patient who will receive the pump is of even greater importance. A device placed for the wrong indication in the wrong patient may provide disappointing results. Selection considers patient characteristics; indications consider the disease state being treated. This chapter focuses on proper patient selection for implantation of intrathecal drug infusion systems.

36.1 Factors to Determine Proper Selection for Pump Implantation

Intrathecal pumps are approved by the US Food and Drug Administration (FDA) for chronic use in patients with moderate to severe pain from cancer or noncancer causes. The implantation of a pump should be seen as part of a treatment continuum based on very specific selection criteria. The implanting physician often has a long-term relationship with the patient, but in some cases, the physician may be seen in consultation to determine whether pump implantation is appropriate. In both situations, a list of criteria similar to those shown on Table 36.1 is helpful when considering implantation. The patient does not have to meet every criterion for implantation, but these criteria should be considered.

Importantly, the intrathecal pump functions as a platform to deliver medication into the intrathecal space in an effort to treat pain or spasticity. (For the purposes of this chapter, we are focusing on patient selection for pain management.) Therefore, it does not define the medication selected, but simply provides a method of delivering it more sustainably. This paradigm—separating pump from medicine—is advantageous to note. Further, patient selection is also centered on a careful, algorithmic approach to intrathecal therapy, taking into account the type and location of the pain (Fig. 36.1). Although historically intrathecal therapy has been positioned as salvage therapy after trials of stimulation therapies, recently intrathecal therapy has been entering into the algorithm concurrent with other neuromodulation strategies.

T.R. Deer, MD (✉)
The Center for Pain Relief, 400 Court Street, Suite 100, Charleston, WV 25301, USA
e-mail: DocTDeer@aol.com

J.E. Pope
Summit Pain Alliance,
392 Tesconi Court, Santa Rosa, CA 95401, USA
e-mail: popeje@me.com

T.R. Deer, J.E. Pope (eds.), *Atlas of Implantable Therapies for Pain Management*, DOI 10.1007/978-1-4939-2110-2_36

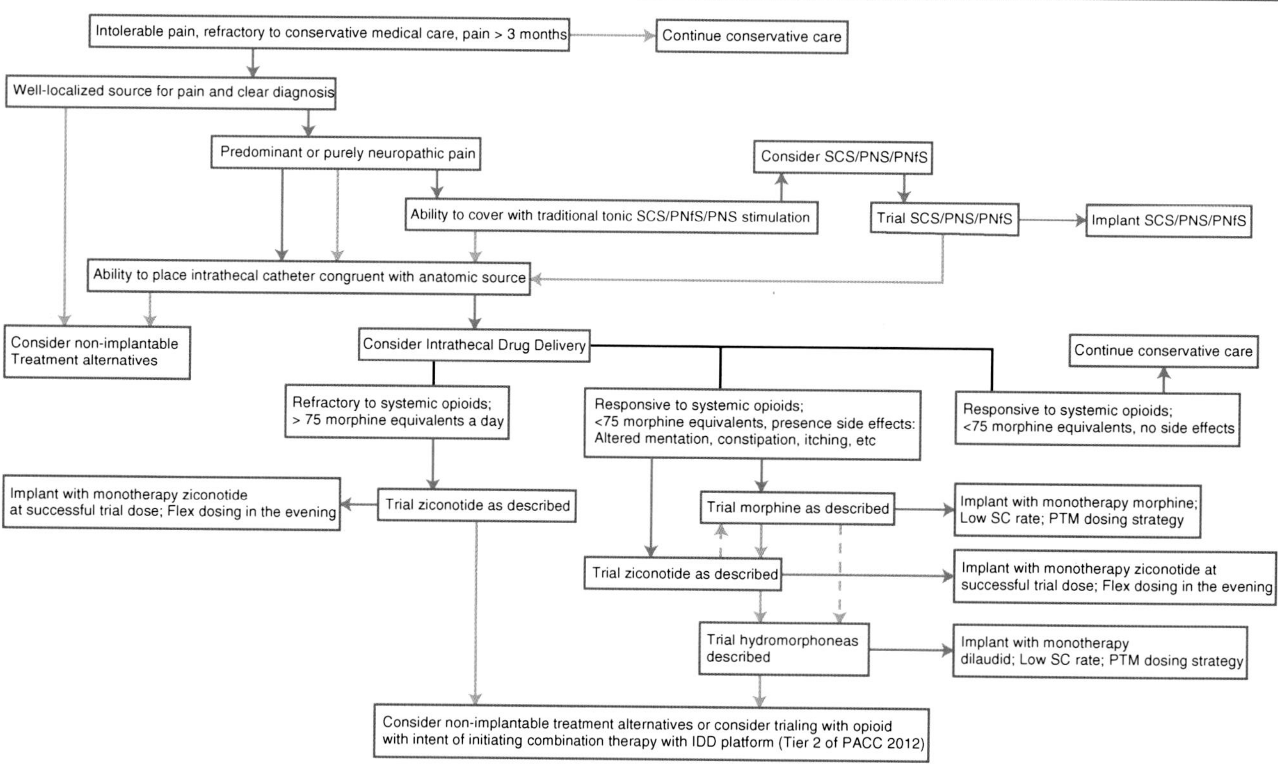

Fig. 36.1 Algorithmic approach to advanced pain care therapies. *Green arrows* indicate affirmative position; *orange arrows* indicate deaffirmative position; *hashed arrows* indicate physician preference

Table 36.1 Selection criteria for intrathecal pumps

More conservative treatment options have failed, or other options are unacceptable or not indicated.
A trial of neuraxial medications provides acceptable pain relief, tolerable side effects, and functional improvement, when indicated.
Oral or transdermal medications produce unacceptable side effects or an unacceptable level of relief.
The patient's spinal anatomy will allow for the placement of a spinal catheter.
The patient is medically stable, with no untreated bleeding disorders.
The patient is medically stable, with no untreated infectious processes.
The patient has no skin disorders that would preclude the implantation of a foreign body.
The patient is mentally stable, with no untreated severe depression or anxiety disorders.
No significant personality disorder, such as borderline or antisocial personality disorder, has been diagnosed in the patient.
The region of pain can be covered by the anatomic congruent placement of an intrathecal catheter.

36.2 Factors to Determine Proper Indications for Pump Implantation

Intrathecal pumps are indicated for chronic use in patients with moderate to severe pain of cancer and noncancer origin. The indications for these devices vary based on the disease process and the effect of the disease on the source of pain generation. Some of the more common indications are listed in Table 36.2.

Table 36.2 Selection criteria for intrathecal pumps

Cancer indications
Primary tumors causing pain from tissue invasion
Metastatic lesions causing pain from tissue invasion
Neuropathy from chemotherapy treatments
Nerve irritation or injury from radiation
Noncancer indications
Failed back surgery syndrome
Spinal canal stenosis
Foraminal stenosis
Compression fracture
Spondylolisthesis
Peripheral neuropathy
Truncal pain
Complex regional pain syndrome
Severe osteoarthritis
Rheumatoid arthritis
Connective tissue disorders

Conclusions

The decision to place an intrathecal device should not be entered into hastily. The physician and the patient should discuss the details of pump placement, risks of the procedure, and alternatives. Patients should have an acceptable indication for device placement and should meet acceptable selection criteria. If a patient's indication is uncommon or not all selection criteria are met, the situation should be considered on an individual basis.

Suggested Reading

Deer T, Winkelmüller W, Erdine S, Bedder M, Burchiel K. Intrathecal therapy for cancer and nonmalignant pain: patient selection and patient management. Neuromodulation. 1999;2:55–66.

Deer T, Krames E, Hassenbusch S, Burton A, Caraway D, Dupen S, et al. Polyanalgesic consensus conference 2007: recommendations for the management of pain by intrathecal (intraspinal) drug delivery: report of an interdisciplinary expert panel. Neuromodulation. 2007;10:300–28.

Deer TR, Prager J, Levy R, Burton A, Buchser E, Caraway D, et al. Polyanalgesic Consensus Conference – 2012: recommendations on trialing for intrathecal (intraspinal) drug delivery: report of an interdisciplinary expert panel. Neuromodulation. 2012;15:420–35.

Hassenbusch SJ, Portenoy RK, Cousins M, Buchser E, Deer TR, Du Pen SL, et al. Polyanalgesic Consensus Conference 2003: an update on the management of pain by intraspinal drug delivery–report of an expert panel. J Pain Symptom Manage. 2004;27:540–63.

Hayek SM, Deer TR, Pope JE, Panchal SJ, Patel VB. Intrathecal therapy for cancer and noncancer pain. Pain Physician. 2011;14:219–48.

Krames ES. Intraspinal opioid therapy for chronic nonmalignant pain: current practice and clinical guidelines. J Pain Symptom Manage. 1996;11:333–52.

Pope JE, Deer TR. Ziconotide: a clinical update and pharmacologic review. Expert Opin Pharmacother. 2013;14:957–66.

Smith TJ, Staats PS, Deer T, Stearns LJ, Rauck RL, et al.; Implantable Drug Delivery Systems Study Group. Randomized clinical trial of an implantable drug delivery system compared with comprehensive medical management for refractory cancer pain: impact on pain, drug-related toxicity, and survival. J Clin Oncol. 2002;20:4040–9

37 Placement of Intrathecal Needle and Catheter for Chronic Infusion

Timothy R. Deer, Michael H. Verdolin, and Jason E. Pope

37.1 Introduction

The procedure discussed in this chapter is an end point of a long process. The process includes initial patient evaluation, decision to treat an identified pain problem, creation of a pain algorithm, and eventually the decision to place an intrathecal pump. Once that decision is made, the patient is evaluated for psychological appropriateness and absence of absolute contraindications. Once these hurdles have been passed, the patient is scheduled for a trial injection or infusion. The success of the trial leads to a permanent implant.

The needle and catheter placement for chronic intrathecal infusion therapy seems trivial to many, as placement of needles and catheters occur regularly during preoperative care for short-term therapy. The authors would suggest respect for the procedure to improve the sustainability of long-term care and reduce device-related complications. This chapter focuses on the critical aspects of needle and catheter placement and discusses the pearls of placement. The catheter is the most common cause of system failure in the long-term delivery of intrathecal medications, and although, we cannot eliminate problems, we can reduce some of these issues with careful technique and vigilance.

T.R. Deer, MD (✉)
The Center for Pain Relief, 400 Court Street, Suite 100, Charleston, WV 25301, USA
e-mail: DocTDeer@aol.com

M.H. Verdolin
Verdolin Pain Specialists, Chula Vista, CA, USA
e-mail: mverdolin@att.net

J.E. Pope
Summit Pain Alliance,
392 Tesconi Court, Santa Rosa, CA 95401, USA
e-mail: popeje@me.com

T.R. Deer, J.E. Pope (eds.), *Atlas of Implantable Therapies for Pain Management*, DOI 10.1007/978-1-4939-2110-2_37

37.2 Technical Overview

The patient is positioned to establish the best possible path to successfully place the needle and catheter. The most common position is the lateral decubitus with flexion of the hips and cervical spine (Fig. 37.1). This position is based on the plan to place a pump in the abdominal wall. Prior to going to the operating room, the patient should be adequately evaluated for the placement of the pump. Table 37.1 illustrates issues to address prior to making initial incisions.

In some cases the preoperative evaluation will suggest that there is not an appropriate area to place a pump in the abdominal wall. Reasons may include lack of body fat, previous surgeries, or skin infection or poor quality of skin texture.

An alternative position is prone placement of the pump, which obviates the need for lateral decubitus position. In the lateral decubitus position, the patient should be aligned with both shoulders at equal tilt to avoid torsion of the trunk. The patient is prepared widely to encompass both the planned area of invasion and the surrounding tissues. Fluoroscopic imagery is used to assess the bony anatomy and to determine the level in which the needle will be placed. Once the clinician is pleased with the positioning, preparing, draping, and x-ray imaging, the procedure is initiated. In some cases the position is less than optimal because of the patient's pain being too great to be placed in the lateral decubitus position or because of body habitus and spinal abnormalities. In these cases the position can be modified to the prone orientation, realizing that, if the plan is to place the pocket into the abdominal wall, repositioning will be required. However, if there is adequate body mass to support the pump in the posterior flank or above the hip, then pump placement in the buttock or hip area may be considered, thus avoiding the need to reposition the patient during the procedure. It is important to realize that the prone position buttock placement of the pump should be used with pumps of a volume of 20 mL or less, given their inherent bulk when compared with neurostimulator implanted pulse generators. In addition, the pump should be placed at least 10 cm above the iliac crest to avoid uncomfortable pressure on the bony surface when the patient is sitting or lying down.

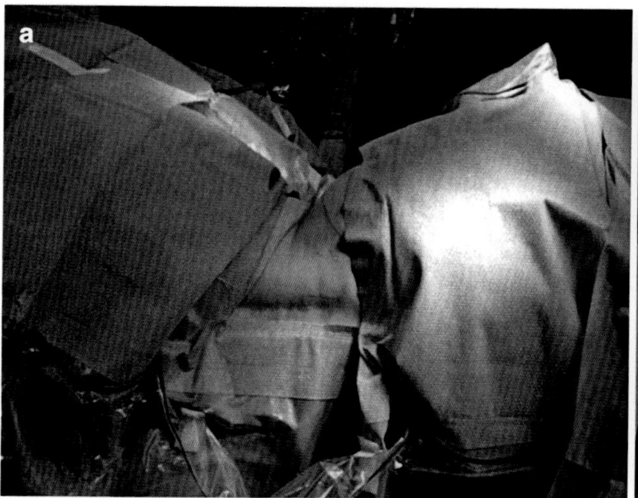

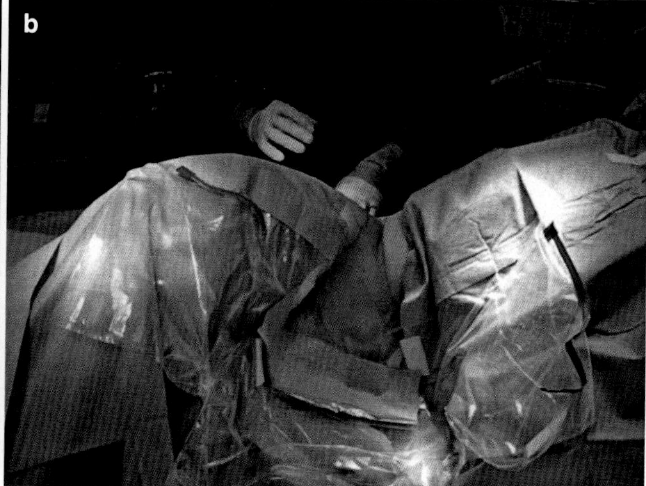

Fig. 37.1 Lateral decubitus positioning of patient (posterior view (**a**) and anterior view (**b**))

Table 37.1 Considerations prior to procedure

Issue to address	Method of investigation
Spinal anatomy for needle placement	Visual inspection of the spine
Spinal anatomy for needle placement	Plain films of the lumbar spine
Ability to thread catheter	Review previous procedures
Ability to thread catheter	MRI or CT if history of complex anatomical anatomy
Level of needle placement	Plain films of the lumbar spine and inspection of skin
Course of tunneling	Visual inspection of the patient's body
Pocket placement	Drawing of planned pocketing including palpation of rib and anterior iliac spine

37.2.1 Needle Placement

After satisfactory positioning, preparing, and draping, the fluoroscopic image is visualized to place local anesthetic one to two vertebral bodies below the planned site of entry. A paramedian approach is recommended to allow the catheter to avoid the constant wear and tear of the spinous processes (Fig. 37.2). The needle is positioned to walk off the lamina and enter the intrathecal space at an ideal angle of 30° to 45° (Fig. 37.3). In some cases the angle can be must be increased to 60° because of anatomical variation, but angles that exceed this mark may lead to excessive pressure on the catheter and subsequent catheter failure (Fig. 37.4). Another approach to imaging needle guidance includes the use of the contralateral oblique view (CLO). In the CLO view the image intensifier is inserted obliquely up to 45° away from the clinician (Fig. 37.5). The needle, in many cases, can be seen piercing the ligamentum flavum to enter the epidural space and then into the intrathecal space (Fig. 37.6).

Once the needle is positioned into the intrathecal space, the implanter should remove the stylet and visualize unobstructed flow of cerebrospinal fluid (CSF). In some settings physicians have attributed lack of flow to scarring or narrowing in the canal. No documented publication shows that a successful placement can be achieved with poor or no flow. In the setting of poor flow, the implanter should be suspicious of epidural or other placement outside of the CSF. The authors would recommend repositioning the catheter until flow is satisfactory. Once good flow of CSF is confirmed, the implanter can move forward with catheter placement.

Modern intrathecal catheters have improved steering ability and are more radiopaque. Ideally the catheter is placed in the posterior intrathecal space. The low angle of needle placement is important in this process. The level of tip placement varies on physician preference, but recent science suggests placement of the tip closest to the spinal cord level matching the dermatomal level of pain provides for improved chance of a satisfactory outcome. Some clinicians prefer to place the catheter below the conus to reduce the complication severity of a granuloma, but this has not been proven to be accurate. The improved position may be less helpful in pain relief and necessitate increased drug dosing, which may negate the benefit of placing the catheter below the conus.

A myelogram with compatible contrast may be performed for confirmation of intrathecal placement at the target level (Fig. 37.7). The decision process for level placement is outlined in Table 37.2. Once the catheter is ideally placed, a cutdown is made to the ligament and fascia, at which time the fatty tissue is debrided and a pursestring suture is placed along with an anchoring suture. The pursestring suture should be placed while the needle remains in place and secured prior to needle removal. The same suture may also be used to secure the anchor, but this is a decision based on physician preference. A newer anchor (Injex; Medtronic; Minneapolis, MN) has been released by one manufacturer that securely attaches to the catheter once deployed over a Teflon guide. This tightly gripping anchor eliminates the need to place an additional suture around the anchor wings of a butterfly anchor. Additional anchors are available from competitive manufacturers that also claim improved catheter stability. No comparative studies exist.

Once the catheter is anchored, a strain-relief loop is created and the catheter is then ready to tunnel to the desired pocket location for connection to the pump. A final film is taken to document the catheter course once it is attached to the intact system. It is imperative to verify free-flowing CSF from the proximal (pump) end of the catheter at all stages. Prior to wound closure vigorous irrigation is recommended. Figure 37.8 demonstrates slow curves paraspinally to the catheter prior to connection to the implantable device.

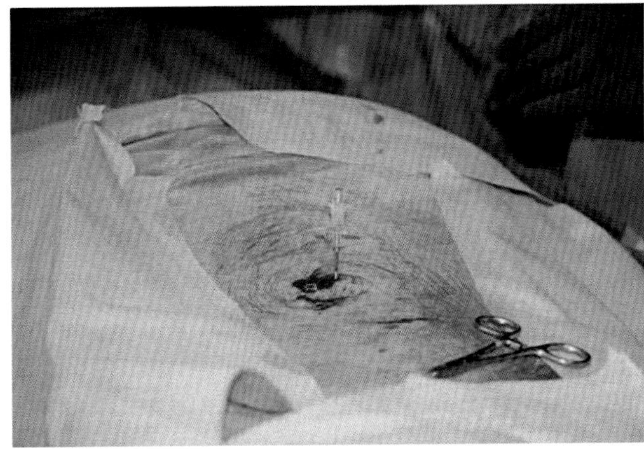

Fig. 37.2 Paramedian approach to needle placement

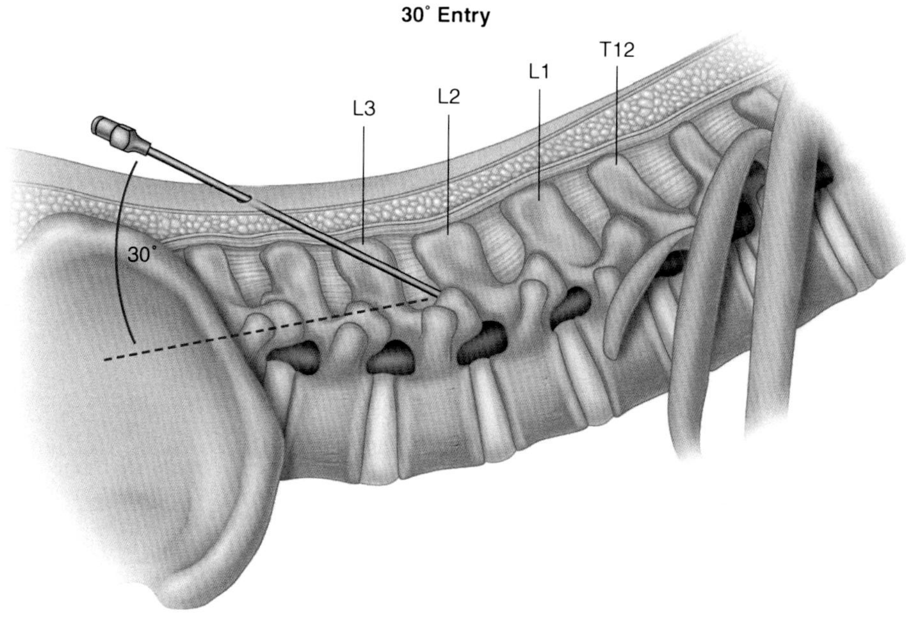

Fig. 37.3 Proper needle angle placement at 30°

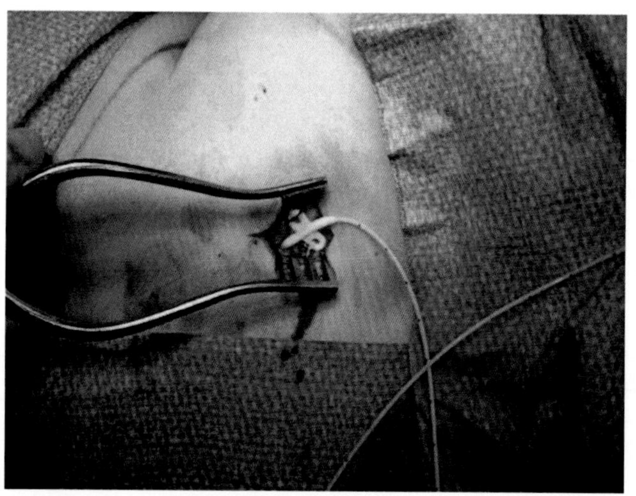

Fig. 37.4 Placement of anchor before catheter tunneling

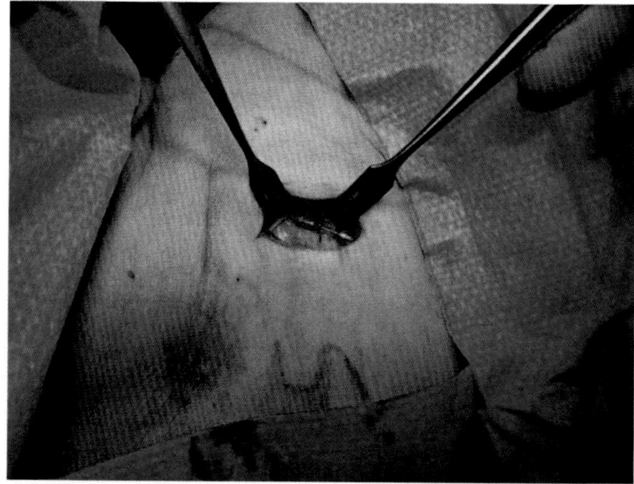

Fig. 37.5 Placement of anchors and stress relief loop, 2 catheter technique

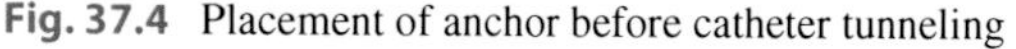

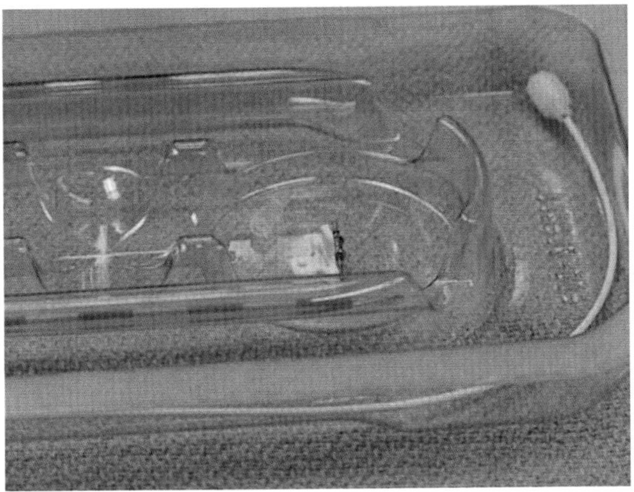

Fig. 37.6 Example of an intrathecal catheter with stylet, needle, anchor, and titanium connector

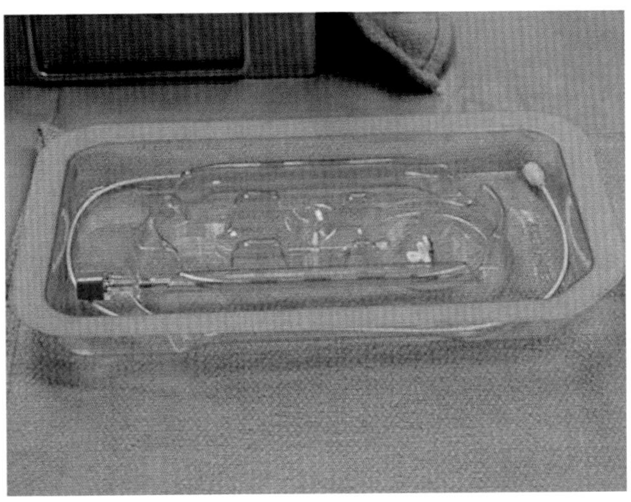

Fig. 37.7 Intrathecal catheter with needle and accessories

Table 37.2 Catheter location considerations[a]

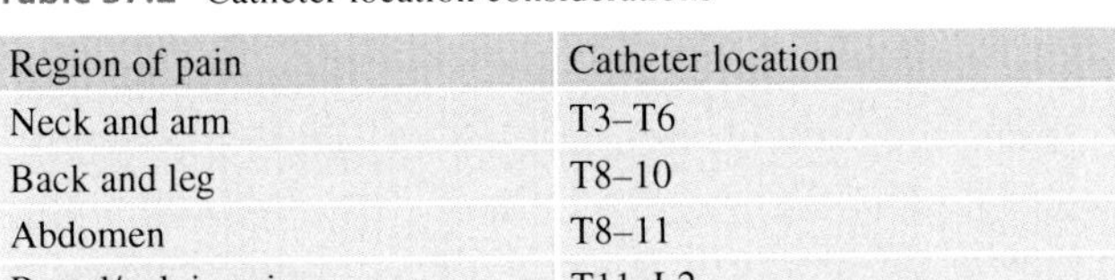

Region of pain	Catheter location
Neck and arm	T3–T6
Back and leg	T8–10
Abdomen	T8–11
Rectal/pelvic pain	T11–L2

[a]Physiochemical properties of the intrathecal medication chosen may either increase or limit spread. Increasing spread from hydrophilicity; increasing baricity above that of the cerebral spinal fluid may result in less cephalad migration

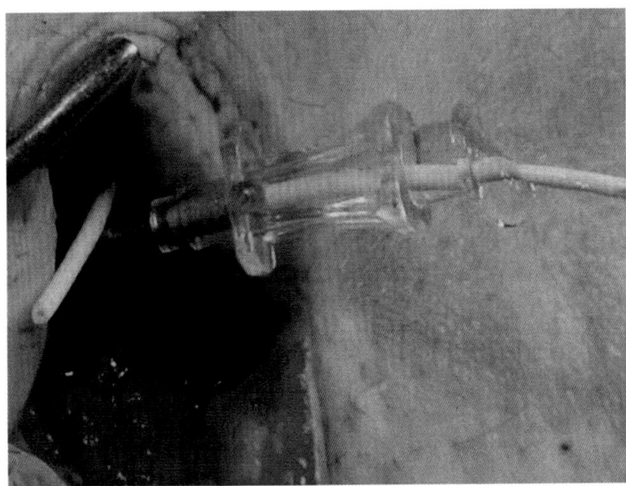

Fig. 37.8 Continuous CSF flow should be seen from the distal end of the catheter prior to connecting the system to the intrathecal device

37.3 Risk Assessment

The most significant risk of catheter placement is injury to the spinal cord or nerve roots. The injuries can range from nerve inflammation to serious cord injury resulting in paraplegia. The catheter angle required to achieve intrathecal placement may be very steep in complex anatomical cases. In severe and complex cases, this angle can approach 90°, which may make the entry easier, but can be difficult for threading the catheter. In these cases if the patient is under heavy sedation, this can be an additional risk considering the nerve roots in the region. This angle may allow easy entry into the space and subsequently may increase the torque on the catheter. This steep angle may increase the risk of tissue injury, lead to increased difficulty passing the catheter, and increase catheter movement or failure over time. Multiple entries into the intrathecal space may lead to a significant loss of CSF and also lead to CSF leak.

Ventral placement of the catheter is sometimes the only option when placement is performed. This may lead to significant risk of motor compromise should an inflammatory mass or granuloma develop. Catheter damage including tearing, fracture, or accidental removal may occur during needle or stylet removal. The implanter should not withdraw the catheter through the needle if the desired catheter course is not initially achieved.

The pursestring catheter may lead to catheter occlusion or obstructed flow. The anchor and anchoring suture may lead to catheter kinking or obstruction. The catheter wall may be insulted with a needle when suturing the anchor or during tissue closure.

37.4 Risk Avoidance

Risk avoidance is a key part of the practice of interventional pain. In order to improve compliance, the physician must have an ongoing commitment to improving patient care. A compliant patient is also critical, because an excellent physician can have a bad outcome with a noncompliant patient.

37.4.1 Nerve Injury

To avoid nerve or spinal cord injury, the physician can take several precautions. Attention should be paid to proper and aligned positioning to optimize the ability to place the needle easily. The fluoroscopic image should be modified by changing the beam to correct for patient rotation, spinal kyphosis, scoliosis, or abnormal body habitus. This will allow needle placement in a gun barrel approach. When possible, a laser-guided imaging technique can be helpful. The CLO fluoroscopic view may obviate some of these concerns, particularly if the chosen pump position is placement above the buttock, allowing use of the prone position throughout the procedure.

37.4.2 Anesthesia

The choice of anesthesia technique is based on surgeon and anesthesiologist preference; however, the use of monitored sedation with direct patient communication can provide an early warning for the implanter of impending nerve injury or spinal cord damage. An alternative would be a wakeup test in patients undergoing general anesthesia, but in some settings general anesthesia is needed for the entire procedure because of patient disease state, body habitus, pain level, or anxiety level.

37.4.3 Needle Entry

The entry of the needle below the level of the conus will also reduce the risk of cord injury, although the cord can still be invaded with forceful catheter advancement. The angle of entry for the needle can be optimized by proper positioning, paramedian approach, careful anatomical observation, and in some cases by making a cutdown to improve the ability to drop the hub of the needle and therefore lowering the angle. A cutdown approach is very helpful in obese patients. In patients with a large body habitus, the use of a longer (6 in.) needle may also be of value. Proper needle angle, use of bevel position, positioning, and attention to CSF flow will reduce the need to make multiple entries into the intrathecal space. Using a shallow angle and a paramedian approach leads to easier catheter placement and tends to encourage lead placement to the posterior intrathecal space.

37.4.4 Catheter Placement, Needle Removal, Purse-String Placement, and Anchoring

Careful attention should be given to resistance to withdrawing the needle or stylet. When significant resistance occurs, the implanter should remove the entire system and reinitiate the procedure. Pulling the needle out against significant resistance can lead to catheter damage or fracture and should be avoided. It is important to secure the purse-string around the needle and tie the suture prior to removing the needle. Tying the suture after removing the needle can lead to occlusion of the catheter and failure of the system.

The anchor should be carefully placed against the fascia to ensure that the catheter does not have the tendency to occlude or kink. The catheter should have a smooth course through the anchor and into a strain-relief loop prior to being tunneled to the pocket.

37.4.5 Wound Closure

When closing the tissues and skin of the area of the catheter, careful attention must be paid to avoid hitting the catheter with the needle. This can lead to fluid leak and failure of the system. Avoidance methods include careful vigilance to the catheter and the use of blunt instruments to retract the catheter to avoid injury to the device (Fig. 37.9).

Injecting flowable hemostatic solutions into the wound after deep closure may also promote hemostasis improve healing.

Prone positioning and posterior pump placement should be selected only in those patients with adequate tissue to support the pump. Erosion can be minimized by only using pumps of 20 mL or smaller.

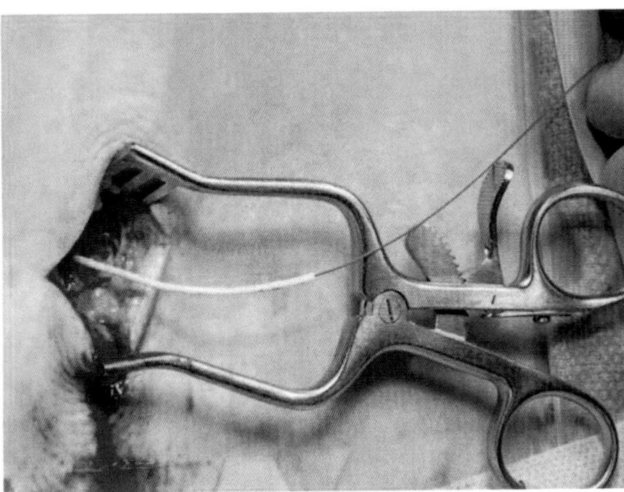

Fig. 37.9 Stylet removal from the catheter. CSF flow should be observed after stylet removal

37.4.6 Infection

Irrigation of the wound is very important in the time before closing. High-volume irrigation and preoperative intravenous antibiotics are very important to reduce the risk of infection.

Conclusions

Intrathecal pump placement is a complex procedure that requires significant training and clinical execution. The needle placement and catheter placement allows for the overall success of the therapy. Each step of this process must be carefully planned and performed. Clinical experience is very important in continuingly improving techniques with these methods.

37.5 Supplemental Images

See Figs. 37.10, 37.11, and 37.12.

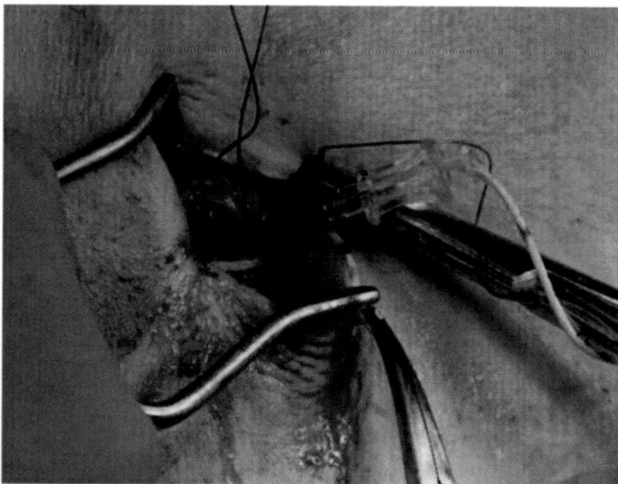

Fig. 37.10 Fascia should be exposed prior to placing the purse-string suture around the needle at the ligament entry. A purse-string suture may promote fibrosis around the catheter and reduce CSF leaks and hygroma formation

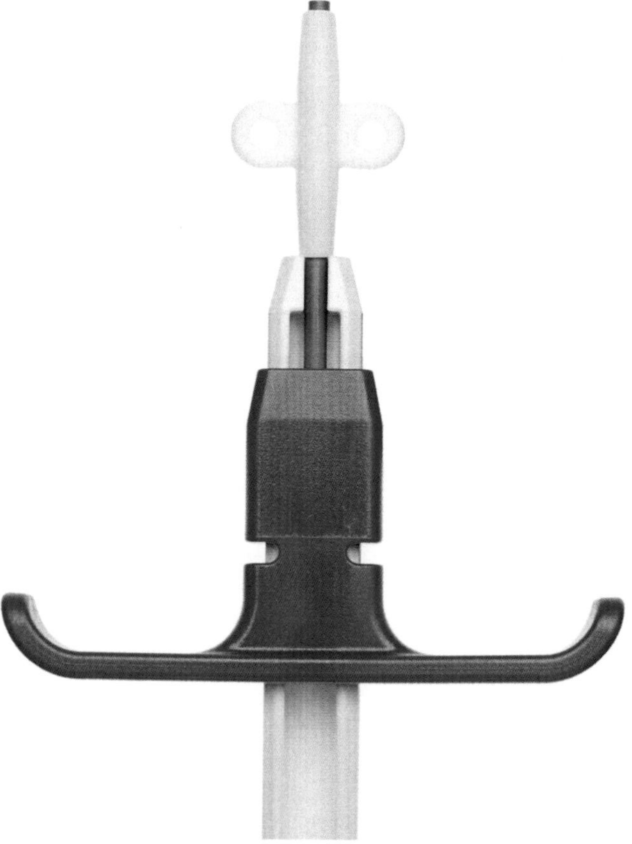

Fig. 37.11 Injex deployment system for anchor with Teflon guide and wing-type anchor with wings. The Ethibond 2-0 suture is anchored to the fascia first and then the distal ends are passed through the eyelets of the wings and tied down prior to deployment of the anchor that firmly and permanently grips the catheter (Reprinted with the permission of Medtronic, Inc.)

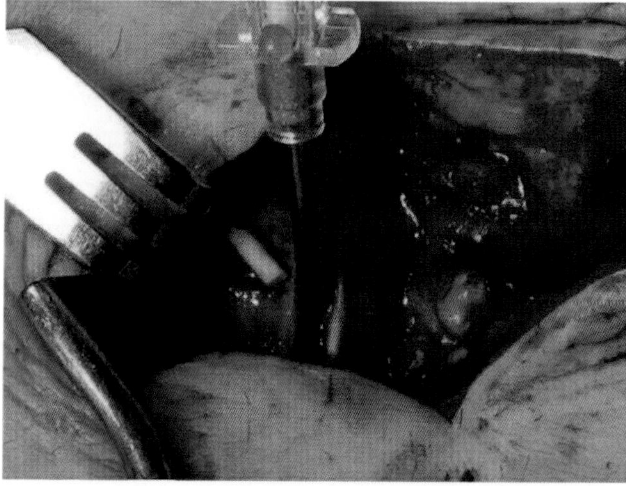

Fig. 37.12 Alternatively after using the newer Injex anchoring system, flowable hemostat may be injected into the wound after deep closure to promote hemostasis, sealing of the tissues, and rapid healing

Suggested Reading

Deer T, Krames E, Hassenbusch S, et al. Polyanalgesic consensus conference 2007: recommendations for the management of pain by intrathecal (intraspinal) drug delivery: report of an interdisciplinary expert panel. Neuromodulation. 2007;10:300–28.

Furman M, Jasper N, Hwei L. Fluoroscopic contralateral oblique view in interlaminar interventions: a technical note. Pain Med. 2012;13:1389–96.

Pope JE, Deer TR. Guide to implantable devices for intrathecal therapy. Pract Pain Manage. 2013. http://www.practicalpainmanagement.com/treatments/interventional/pumps/guide-implantable-devices-intrathecal-therapy.

Pope JE, Deer TR. Chapter 88: Intrathecal drug delivery: an overview of modern concepts in advanced pain care. McGraw-Hill's principles and practice in pain medicine, vol. 3. New York: McGraw-Hill; (in press).

Radhakrishnan L, Duarte R, Mutagi H, Kapur S. Complications of intrathecal drug delivery system implantation for chronic pain: a retrospective review of 62 patients over 16 years: 638. Reg Anesth Pain Med. 2008;33, e201.

Smith T, Staats P, Deer T, et al. Implantable Drug Delivery Systems Study Group. Randomized clinical trial of an implantable drug delivery system compared with comprehensive medical management for refractory cancer pain: impact on pain, drug-related toxicity, and survival. J Clin Oncol. 2002;20:4040–9.

38 Securing and Anchoring Permanent Intrathecal Catheters

Timothy R. Deer, Michael H. Verdolin, and Jason E. Pope

38.1 Introduction

Catheter migration is an important problem when considering complications of intrathecal drug infusion systems. Catheter migration can result in loss of efficacy, drug-withdrawal, and the need for surgical revision. The methods of securing the catheter vary owing to physician preference.

38.2 Anchoring Overview

The first steps of ensuring a stable catheter is to place the needle in the spine at an appropriate low angle and to obtain a good course of the catheter in the cerebrospinal fluid (CSF). Once the catheter is in a good position with low torque, the implanter should place a purse-string suture. Many implanters do not understand the purpose of the purse-string suture. The intent is to use this purse-string suture around the needle to improve tissue tension and fibrosis around the catheter entry site. The purse-string suture does not anchor the catheter but is meant to stabilize the tissue around the entry point. Once the purse-string suture is in place, the implanter must anchor the catheter. A variety of Silastic anchors to secure the catheter to the ligament or fascia are available for physician selection.

Classic Silastic anchors are in the shape of an elbow, tube, or butterfly. A newly developed anchor (Injex; Medtronic; Minneapolis, MN) and a reinforced catheter system (Ascenda; Medtronic; Minneapolis, MN) may allow for the deployment of a constricting anchor over the catheter that obviates the need for further suturing beyond the winged ends and allows for rapid securing with reduced migration risk. The clinical advantage of this anchor has not been studied in a comparative fashion, and longitudinal follow up is needed.

This chapter examines both the options of securing the catheter and the associated problems with catheter movement.

T.R. Deer, MD (✉)
The Center for Pain Relief, 400 Court Street, Suite 100, Charleston, WV 25301, USA
e-mail: DocTDeer@aol.com

M.H. Verdolin
Verdolin Pain Specialists, 891 Kuhn Drive, Chula Vista, CA 91914, USA
e-mail: mverdolin@att.net

J.E. Pope
Summit Pain Alliance, 392 Tesconi Court, Santa Rosa, CA 95401, USA
e-mail: popeje@me.com

T.R. Deer, J.E. Pope (eds.), *Atlas of Implantable Therapies for Pain Management*, DOI 10.1007/978-1-4939-2110-2_38

38.3 Technical Overview

The process of securing and anchoring the catheter involves several steps that help ensure a good outcome (Table 38.1).

Once the needle and catheter are in good position, the physician must debride all fatty tissue from the area surrounding the needle, exposing the fascia and ligament. At this point the physician should place a purse-string suture around the needle. The goals of a purse-string suture are to secure the tissue that surrounds the catheter to reduce the short-term risk of CSF leak around the catheter and to reduce the risks of catheter migration in the long term by allowing the tissue to fibrose around the catheter. The purse-string is placed by using a nonabsorbable suture such as Ethibond or silk around the catheter while it is still in the needle. The suture is placed in the fascia and ligament in a purse-string orientation with at least four entries and exists is a circular pattern encompassing the needle. The suture is then tied while the needle is in place. This allows for a tight occlusion of the tissue without worry of damaging the catheter, which can result in catheter fracture or occlusion (Table 38.1).

Many anchor choices exist for physician preference in securing the catheter. Anchors are shaped in an elbow orientation, tubular form, bumpy tubular form, or butterfly shape.

Alternatives to these anchors exist with the introduction of a form-fitting bi-wing anchor on a Teflon-coated deployment device that tracks the catheter into the tissue deep to the incision.

Injection of a flowable hemostatic foam may be helpful in tissue healing and CSF leakage. The use of Gelfoam may also be helpful in reducing the risk of chronic CSF leak (Fig. 38.1a, b).

Once the catheter is anchored, it is important to leave a strain-relief loop in the catheter before it is tunneled to the pocket. This will be critical in the first few weeks of tissue healing when the body movement may affect catheter security.

Table 38.1 Risks and action to ensure successful anchoring

Migration risk	Physician action
Fatty tissue at anchoring site	Debride fatty tissue around the needle entry site exposing fascia and ligament for proper anchoring
Anchoring to muscle	When using an exaggerated paramedian approach, the physician should dissect medially until approaching ligament or fascia, avoiding anchoring to muscle, which may lead to migration with contraction
Lead anchor gap	The anchor should be as close to the lead entry into the ligament or fascia as possible, avoiding room for migration distal to the anchor, with newer systems allowing for a distal tracking of the catheter to "plug" the gap
Suturing with silk	Avoid silk sutures when anchoring
Dependence on the anchor	The anchor should be seen as one component of securing the system. Total dependence on the anchor can lead to poor outcomes.
Hematoma below anchor	Hemostasis should be obtained prior to closing the wound. Bleeding can lead to catheter movement owing to hematoma compression placing pressure on the anchor.
Minimal migration changes	The catheter should be placed in an area of the spine that will not be affected by minimal migration movements. If the catheter tip is in the CSF, a good outcome may be preserved even in the presence of movement.

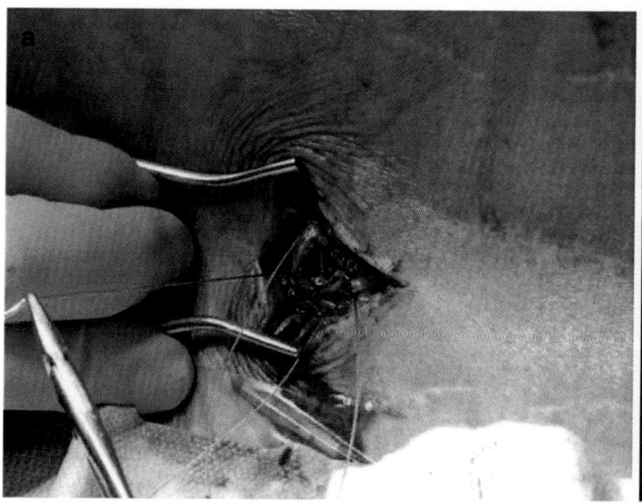

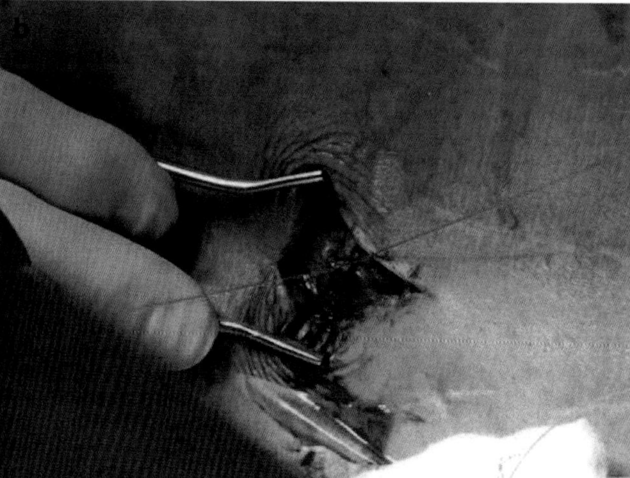

Fig. 38.1 (**a**) Purse-string suture. (**b**) "Butterfly" anchor on the catheter

38.3.1 Anchor Types

Anchoring can be performed with a variety of anchors depending on manufacturer, but there are only a few basic anchor types. These include a "butterfly" anchor, which secures the catheter by wrapping around the catheter. A suture is placed through a singular suture hole to lay the catheter and anchor down against the fascia. An advantage of this type of anchor is the ability to use the same suture used for the purse-string to also secure the catheter and anchor. To accomplish this task, the suture must exit the fascia caudad to the needle entry site (Fig. 38.2).

The "long tubular" anchor is placed over the catheter at the proximal tip and is slid downward to the spinal entry site to abut the fascia or ligament. This type of anchor may have one, two, or three suture holes, and it is important to ensure that sutures are placed that work well in concert so that there is no strain on the catheter materials that can lead to kinking or catheter trauma.

The "macaroni" anchor (Fig. 38.3) is a curved anchor with grooves in which the catheter rests. This anchor requires a stabilizing suture to hold down the anchor and an additional suture or two to hold the catheter in place in the anchor. The advantage of the macaroni anchor is that it directs the catheter in a subtle angle as it exits the anchor to avoid strain on the material. The disadvantage is the need to align the sutures in an exact location to reduce kinking. In some patients the ability to place the sutures in the exact location needed is difficult.

The new Injex anchor is a bi-wing type anchor on a deployment device shaped like a syringe. The catheter passes through a metal center and exits through the handle. The bi-wing has a distal flexible tip that follows the catheter deep to the incision site. The eyelets accommodate nonabsorbable suture (e.g., Ethibond), which is previously anchored to fascia. The suture is then tied to the bi-wing, and once in place, the plunger is depressed while stabilizing the anchor. The internal sleeve is Teflon-coated, allowing for the anchor to slide off the deployment device. As the inner metal cannula is removed during deployment, the internal diameter of the anchor shrinks to tightly and irrevocably grip the catheter without kinking or occluding it. A newly released intrathecal catheter (Ascenda) is also reinforced internally, reducing the risk of fracture or inadvertent tearing. The deployment device is then slid off the distal end of the catheter and disposed of, leaving the anchor in place adhered to the fascia, with the tip following and stabilizing the catheter deep to the incision, and gripping it permanently to prevent slip (Fig. 38.4). This method allows for a suture-less strategy to secure the anchor to the catheter and offers a simplified anchoring approach. The surgeon now only has to secure the anchor to the lumbodorsal fascia

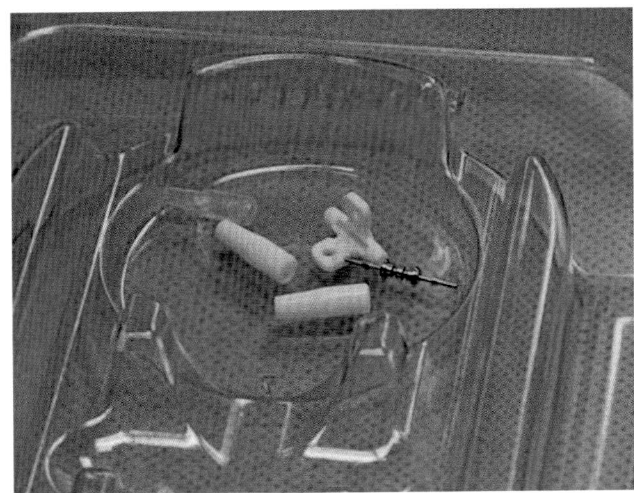

Fig. 38.2 Winged anchor with stainless steel pin and splicing catheter connectors.

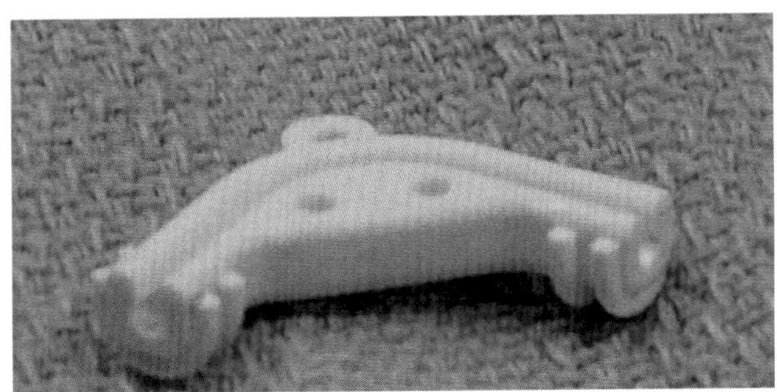

Fig. 38.3 Common "macaroni" anchor Injex bi-wing anchor ready for deployment after securing 2-0 Ethibond suture (already knotted to fascia). Injex bi-wing anchor in place with catheter ready for tunneling to pump pocket.

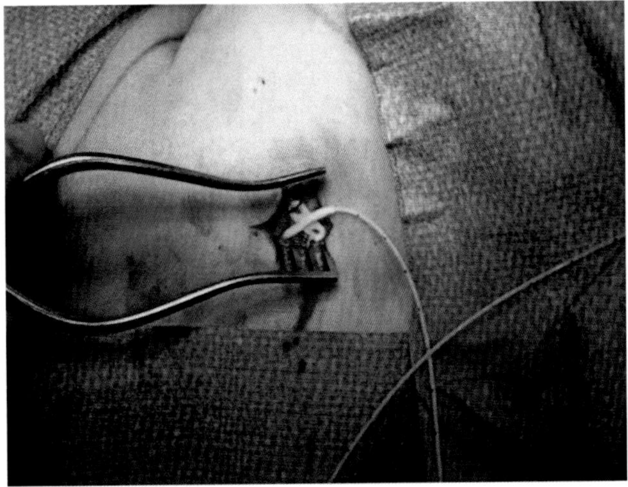

Fig. 38.4 Injex anchor is a bi-winged anchor that is a suture-less strategy that has simplified the anchoring procedure.

38.4 Suturing and Anchoring Materials

The suture used to anchor the catheter should be nonabsorbable and durable. In the past many texts and articles have recommended silk as a mainstay of anchoring. Over time the use of silk can lead to migration. This occurs because of silk degradation and eventually a high risk of suture breakdown. Ethibond and other similar sutures provide a sturdy nonabsorbable suture that will reduce the risk of long-term migration. The type of anchor the clinician chooses may be of minimal significance. Manufacturers often point out advantages to their anchoring systems and clinicians develop preferences based on individual experiences, but to date, no long-term studies have been performed comparing anchors from competing companies, or for anchors made from the same company.

38.4.1 The Deer-Stewart Anchoring Method

In our experience the commitment to excellence in anchoring is worth adding a few minutes to the surgical procedure. To adequately secure the catheter that has been placed percutaneously, it is important to space the sutures properly. This requires a purse-string that is initiated 0.5 cm distal to the needle entry into the ligament and fascia. The exit of the purse-string should be 0.1 cm from the entry point. The suture is then secured with a surgeon's knot and left uncut. The needle and stylet are then removed and an anchor is placed. The author prefers the butterfly anchor, which is placed over the catheter and advanced to the entry point to the ligament. The purse-string suture is then used to secure the anchor and catheter. This method avoids the need to place a suture while the vulnerable catheter material is exposed to the risk of puncture. Once the anchor is secured, a strain relief loop of 2–3 cm is placed in the incision prior to tunneling (Fig. 38.5a–h).

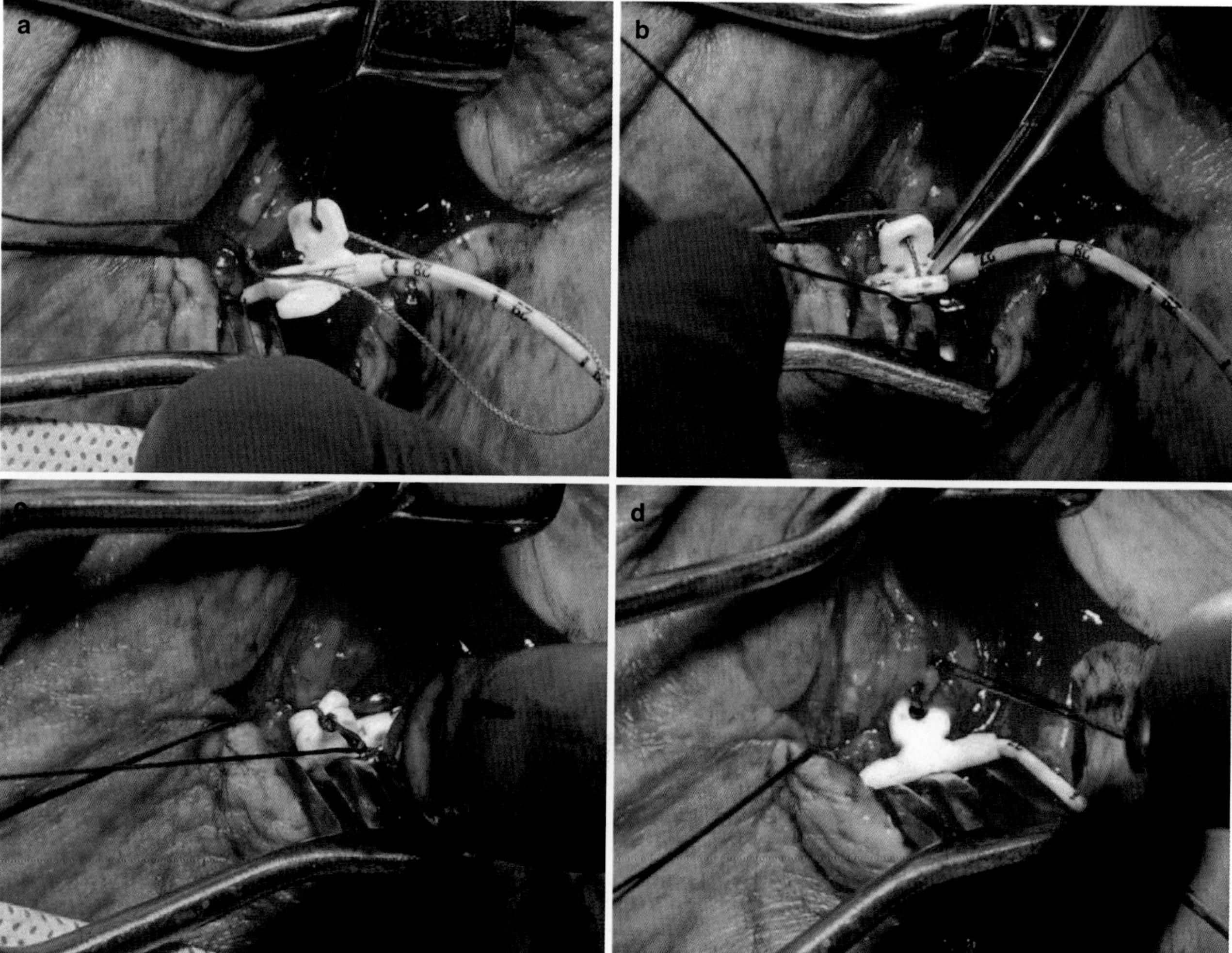

Fig. 38.5 (**a**–**h**) Deer-Stewart Method of securing the bi-winged anchor, employing purse string stitch.

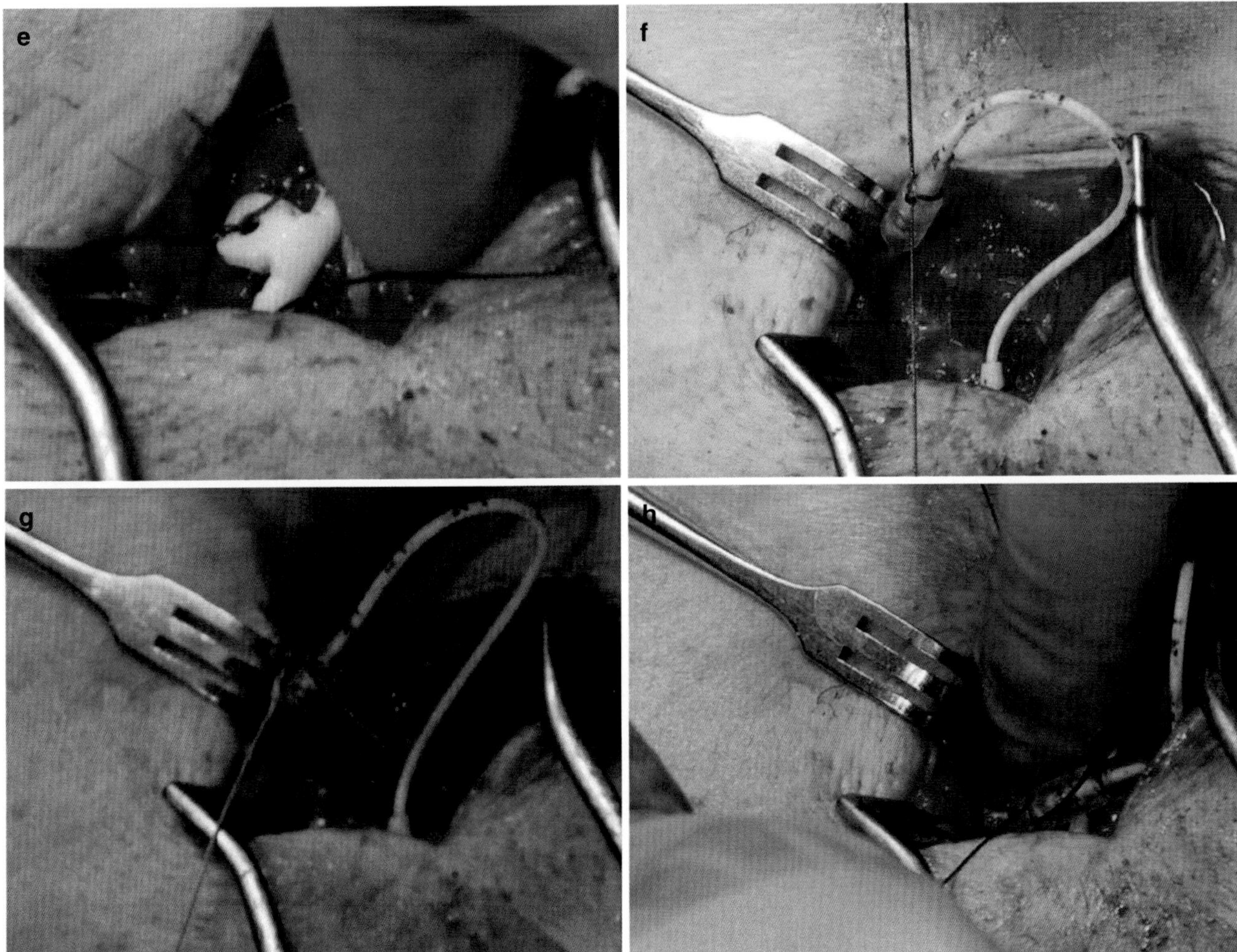

Fig. 38.5 (continued)

38.5 Risk Assessment

The incidence of migration for intrathecal catheters is low but can be problematic, leading to loss of efficacy, withdrawal, or mechanical failure of the device. In some cases the catheter can totally exit the spine and move into the abdominal pocket (Figs. 38.6 and 38.7).

Failure to create a proper purse-string suture can lead to CSF leak around the catheter and the development of a hygroma in the posterior incision or into the abdominal pocket (Fig. 38.8).

Failure to properly remove adipose tissue can lead to anchoring to a necrotic area of tissue that will lead to migration. When anchoring occurs to the muscle tissue, migration can occur as the patient undergoes normal movement requiring muscle contraction. Suture breakage can occur. This may lead to shifting of the catheter or anchor. The purse-string suture can lead to catheter occlusion. Kinking of the catheter can lead to fracture or kinking. This can occur at the spine exit point or the catheter entry or exit into the anchor. This can occur even with ideal needle entry, optimal catheter placement, and superb anchoring technique.

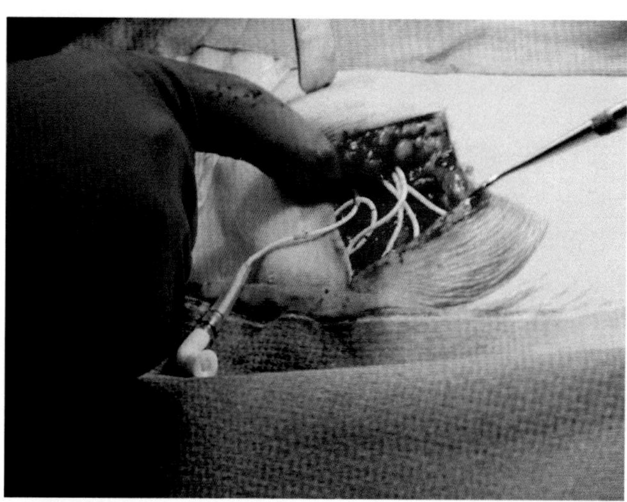

Fig. 38.6 Migration of the catheter into the pocket

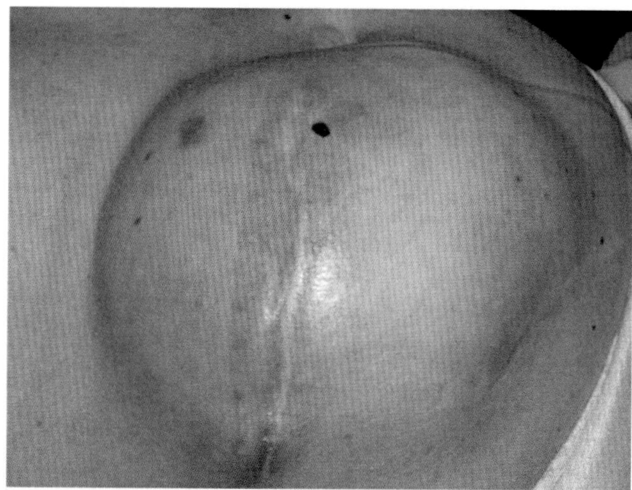

Fig. 38.8 Hygroma of pocket

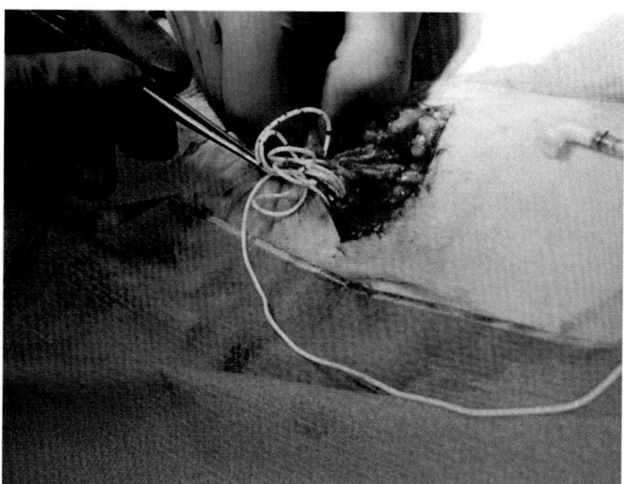

Fig. 38.7 Fibrosis of tissue around the catheter in the pocket that may have contributed to migration of the catheter into the pocket

38.6 Risk Avoidance

Migration can be reduced by using an angle of 45° or less for needle entry and by using a paramedian approach with needle placement. Anchoring should occur only after all fatty tissue has been debrided from the area surrounding the needle. The implanter should view a shiny fascial layer with the ligament and fascia in view prior to anchoring. When the paramedian approach is used in an extreme manner, the amount of fascia and ligament available for anchoring is unacceptable. This can lead to anchoring to muscle or adipose. The paramedian approach should be used in all cases of implantation; however, the needle entry point should remain in the area of the spine that allows for proper anchoring.

A proper purse-string should pull the tissue surrounding the needle entry site around the catheter to help with fibrosis to reduce the risk of CSF leak or hygroma.

Nonabsorbable suture should be used for anchoring. When possible, silk should be avoided because its long-term stability is worrisome. In thin patients it is important to use a double or triple layer closure to reduce the risk of discomfort at the anchor placement site. If an unacceptable tissue layer is present to cushion the anchor, the surgeon can make a pocket in the muscle adjacent to the anchor to place any excess catheter. Trimming the catheter in the pocket should be able to reduce this risk. The catheter should have a strain-relief loop at both the anchor site and the area beneath the pump.

Conclusions

An ideal outcome with an intrathecal drug infusion system requires several successful processes. Anchoring of the catheter is a very important component, particularly in regard to the long-term stability of the system. It is important to create a smooth transition for the catheter out of the spine, entering and exiting the anchor, and leaving the dorsal incision in the tunneling path. Attention to securing the catheter can improve outcomes and patient satisfaction and reduce the need for revisions.

Suggested Reading

Follett K, Burchiel K, Deer T, et al. Prevention of intrathecal drug delivery catheter-related complications. Neuromodulation. 2003;6:3–41.

McIntyre P, Deer T, Hayek S. Complications of spinal infusion therapies. Tech Reg Anesth Pain Manag. 2007;11:183–92.

Pope JE, Deer TR. Guide to implantable devices for intrathecal therapy. Pract Pain Manage. 2013. http://www.practicalpainmanagement.com/treatments/interventional/pumps/guide-implantable-devices-intrathecal-therapy.

Pope JE, Deer TR. Intrathecal drug delivery: an overview of modern concepts in advanced pain care. In: McGraw-Hill's principles and practice in pain medicine, vol 3. New York: McGraw-Hill (in press).

Tunneling Permanent Intrathecal Catheters

39

Timothy R. Deer, Michael H. Verdolin, and Jason E. Pope

39.1 Introduction

Once the intrathecal catheter is successfully placed in the spinal canal, the stylet and needle are removed, the purse-string suture is secured, and the anchor is successfully placed, the physician must pass the catheter from the dorsal incision at the spine to the pocket that has been created for the intrathecal pump. The process of tunneling can be viewed as a simple "passage" of the catheter, but the technique is important; if the tunneling is done improperly, the outcome can be poor. In most clinical settings, the pump pocket is in the abdominal wall, so tunneling is from the lumbar spine to the abdomen. Depending on the patient's body habitus, this course could be short or long. It may require a single pass or an intermediate incision at the mid flank.

Alternative pump locations in the lower back or buttock may allow shorter catheter "runs" with fewer complications, particularly in large patients or those with abdominal abnormalities or poor skin condition. The biggest issues with posterior pump placement is patient comfort and skin erosion. The implanter should consider a low-volume pump if a posterior approach is planned.

T.R. Deer, MD (✉)
The Center for Pain Relief, 400 Court Street, Suite 100, Charleston, WV 25301, USA
e-mail: DocTDeer@aol.com

M.H. Verdolin
Verdolin Pain Specialists, 891 Kuhn Drive, Chula Vista, CA 91914, USA
e-mail: mverdolin@att.net

J.E. Pope
Summit Pain Alliance, 392 Tesconi Court, Santa Rosa, CA 95401, USA
e-mail: popeje@me.com

T.R. Deer, J.E. Pope (eds.), *Atlas of Implantable Therapies for Pain Management*, DOI 10.1007/978-1-4939-2110-2_39

39.2 Technical Overview

Before going into the operating theater, it is important to evaluate the patient's body habitus and determine the ideal location for pocket placement. Once the pump pocket site has been located and the pocket has been made, the physician can determine the best path for tunneling the catheter. When making this determination, the physician should consider the patient's bony structure, including the rib margin and the bones of the sacrum. The pathway of tunneling should be finalized and a permanent marker should be used to mark the course for local anesthetic placement, as shown in Fig. 39.1. The ideal local anesthetic varies based on physician selection, with lidocaine and bupivacaine being the most common selections. When using lidocaine, the addition of a small amount of bicarbonate may lead to less pain on injection with a normal dilution ratio of 9:1 (lidocaine:bicarbonate). The addition of epinephrine may decrease bleeding at the time of tunneling. The local anesthetic placement should be accompanied by intermittent aspiration to avoid intravascular injection, with attention to depth in order to avoid puncture of inadvertent structures. Local anesthetic placement is depicted in Fig. 39.2. Alternatively, some physicians prefer to provide analgesia by giving a very small dose of intrathecal bupivacaine (2.5 mg or less) through the catheter before maturing the pump pocket and tunneling. This procedure should be coordinated with the anesthesiologist to ensure that the patient's blood pressure can support such a maneuver, and in any case the intrathecal anesthetic dose should be delivered at the level of the conus or below, to provide adequate analgesia in the desired dermatomes and avoid a "high spinal."

Once the patient has been properly anesthetized by using local anesthesia and intravenous sedation, or intrathecal analgesia, the physician is ready to tunnel. Conventional tunneling rods are of fairly large diameter and require passage over a distance that may lead to improper depth. This problem can be managed by bending the tunneling device to the contours of the body, or by making a two-pass tunneling approach. In this method, the physician makes an incision along the course of the tunneling path, tunnels to that incision, and then tunnels in a second step to complete the catheter pass. Figures 39.3 and 39.4 show the options for the one-pass and two-pass methods. Figure 39.5 demonstrates the placement of the catheter into the tunneling rod.

During the course of tunneling, the physician should use palpation to determine that the tunneling rod is staying at proper depth. Ideally, the tunneling rod should be palpable in the subcutaneous tissue, deep enough to avoid invading the dermis, but superficial enough to avoid penetrating unintended structures (Figs. 39.6 and 39.7).

The physician may tunnel from the spinal incision to the pocket or from the opposite direction. Regardless of the direction chosen, the physician must be aware of the risk of injuring the catheter as it enters the spinal structures, and should be vigilant in avoiding the catheter on either entry or exit of the tissues with the rigid tunneling device. Once tunneling is completed, the catheter should be prepared in the pocket for attachment to the pump with proper trimming and confirmation of proper cerebral spinal flow (Fig. 39.8). To help avoid catheter migration, a strain relief loop should be created in the spinal incision prior to wound closure.

Permanent location of the pump in a posterior location rather than in the abdomen has some advantages: The patient is in the prone position for the entire procedure, which greatly simplifies the implantation and increases the speed of placement. The tunneling distance is also significantly shortened, reducing the risk of accidental perforation of internal structures (*eg*, kidney, colon) or other tunneling misadventures, and decreasing postoperative pain and possible kinking or fracture over long distances. However, the patient must have adequate tissue mass posteriorly to support the pump. Pumps of greater than 20 mL volume may be too large to place posteriorly. Additionally, the pump should be placed at least 10 cm above the iliac crest to avoid placement in the buttock and development of discomfort from resting on the periosteum, leading to possible cluneal neuralgia.

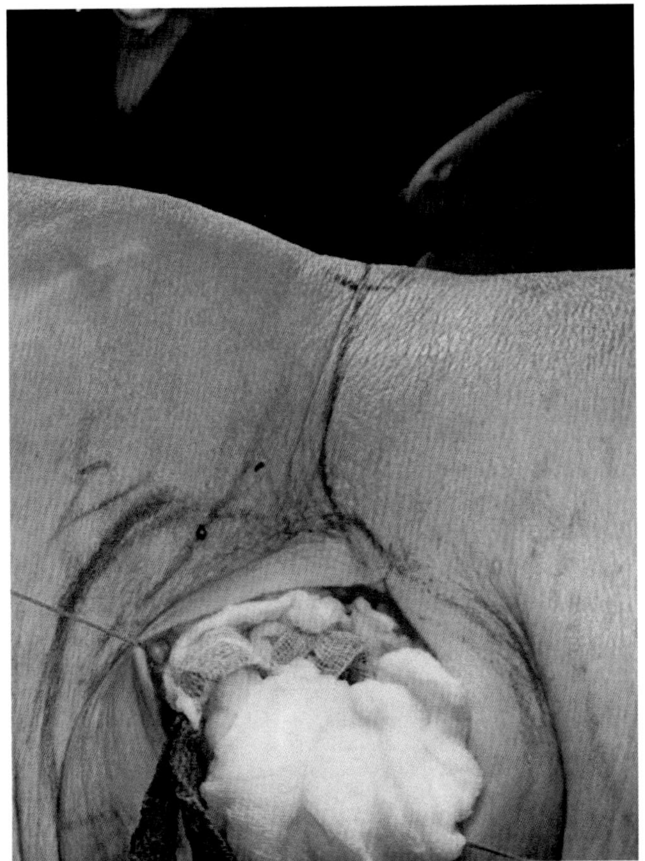

Fig. 39.1 Marking the skin for the tunneling course using the two-step technique

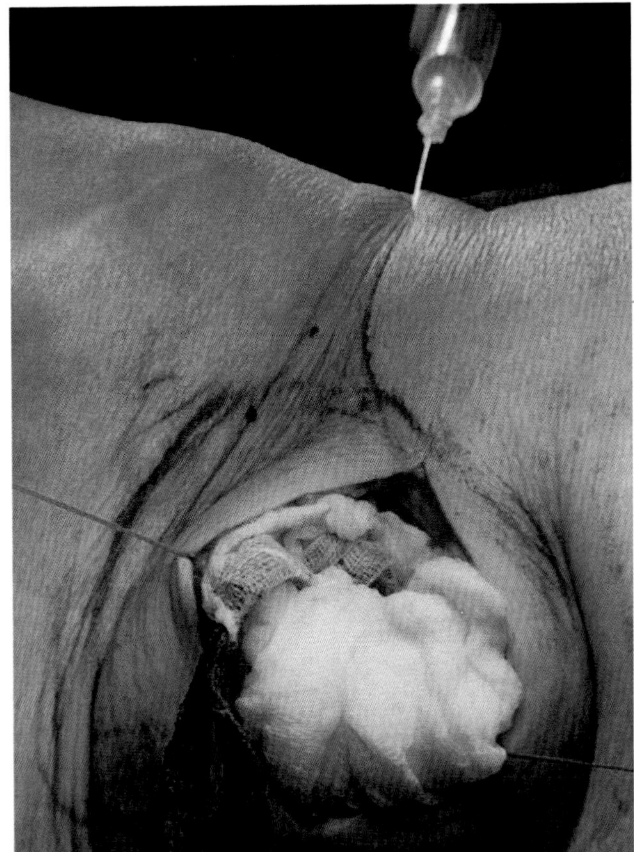

Fig. 39.2 Local anesthesia for tunneling

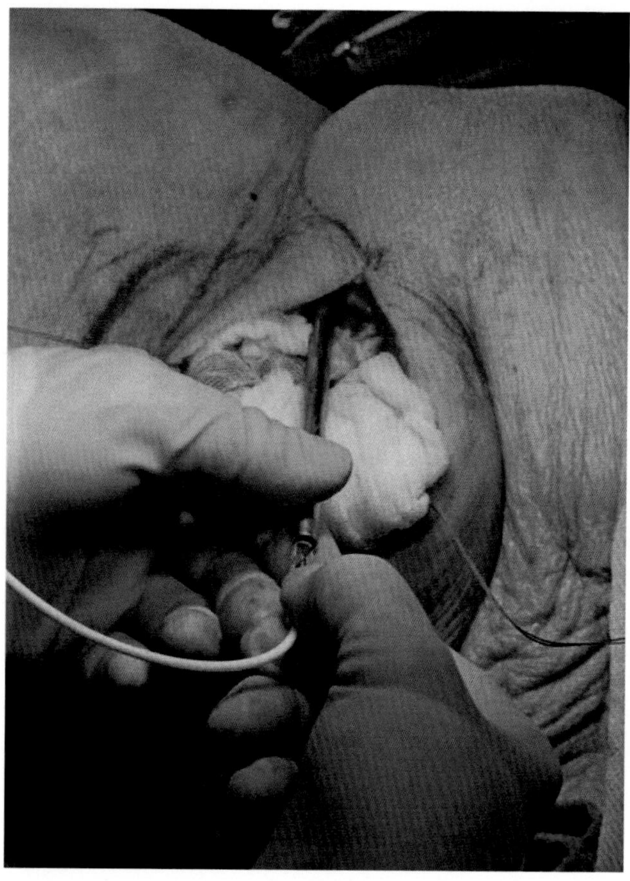

Fig. 39.3 Completion of step one with the tunneling rod in the spinal incision

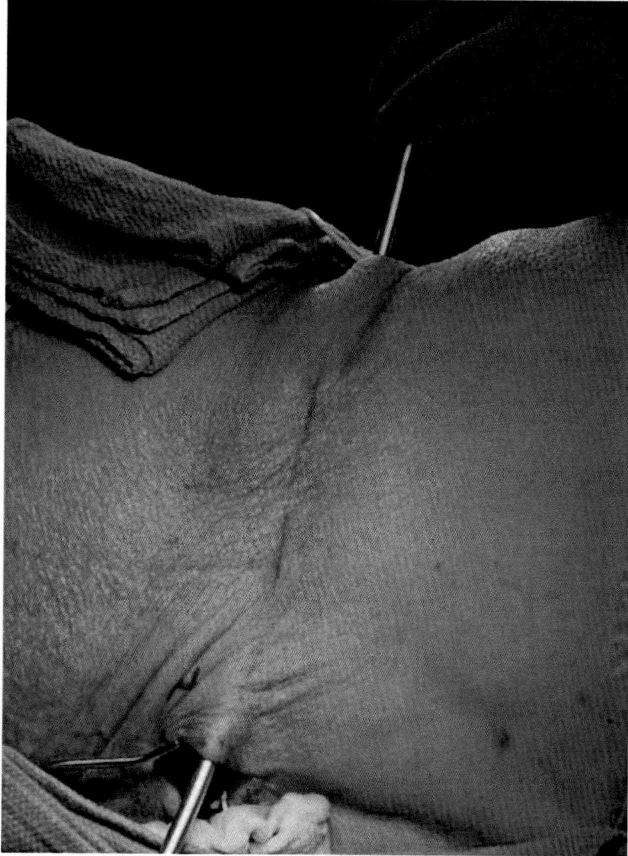

Fig. 39.4 Two-pass tunneling approach

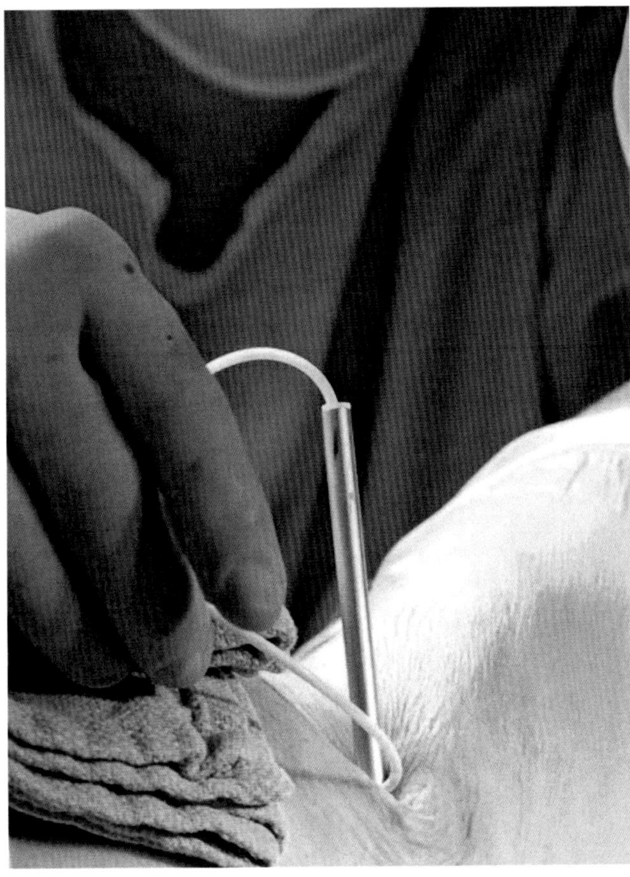

Fig. 39.5 Placement of the lead into the tunneling rod

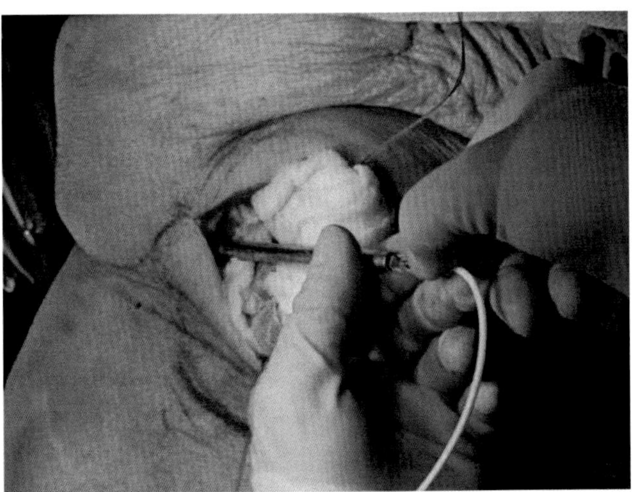

Fig. 39.6 The tunneling rod must stay in the proper tissue plane to ensure that the lead is not superficial, which can lead to erosion, or deep, which can result in patient injury

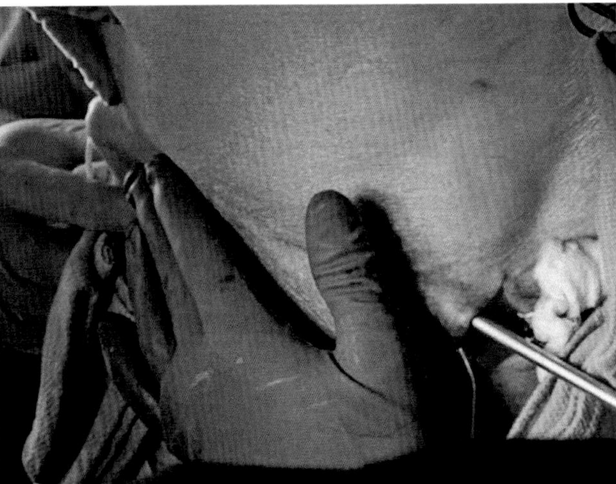

Fig. 39.7 The tunneling rod should be palpable as it is passed in the tissue to monitor depth

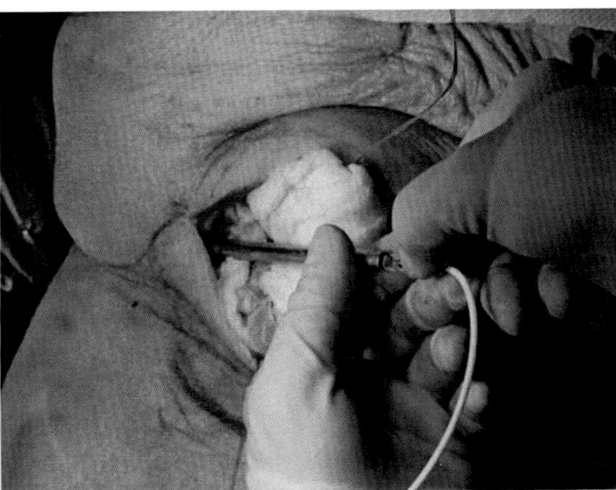

Fig. 39.8 The tunneling process is completed when the lead is secured to the IPG

39.3 Risk Assessment

Complications from the tunneling component of the procedure are rare in the overall consideration of pump morbidity. Table 39.1 reviews some of the more common problems seen in clinical settings:

- A hematoma can develop when the tunneling rod disrupts a vessel during passage.
- Tunneling too superficially can lead to discomfort and in some cases erosion through the tissue.
- Tunneling too deep can puncture the bowel, lung, or other vital structures.
- Infection can develop in the tract if the tunneling rod or catheter becomes contaminated.
- In obese patients, the ability to tunnel may be limited due to inadequate length of tunneling tools.
- In emaciated patients, tunneling may be difficult secondary to lack of subcutaneous fat.
- Posterior pump placement or placement in a location other than the abdomen is off- label and may be associated with compression over the iliac crest or erosion through the skin.

Table 39.1 Reducing risks of tunneling for intrathecal pumps

Tunneling risk	Physician action
Too deep: may puncture viscera	Enter tissue in the subcutaneous tissue and palpate the tunneling rod as it is advanced
Too shallow: may erode	Enter tissue in the subcutaneous tissue and palpate the tunneling rod as it is advanced
Large body habitus	Use a two-pass technique
High risk of infection	Use a one-pass technique
Hematoma along the tract	Check preoperative clotting factors, apply pressure if swelling develops, use surgical drainage if needed
Emaciated patients	Avoid tunneling in the dermis

39.4 Risk Avoidance

Even though complications of tunneling are rare, the clinician should take all possible steps to avoid risks to the patient:

- In patients with a high risk of bleeding, preoperative laboratory evaluation should be carefully reviewed with a focus on platelet function and clotting indices. If any sign of swelling develops in the tunneling course, pressure should be applied in the postoperative period with compression dressings and ice packs.
- When advancing the tunneling rod, the physician should palpate the tunneling rod, with a focus on avoiding the dermis. In severely protein-deficient patients, this may be difficult to accomplish, but it is critical to avoid erosion. Further, the physician should be aware of the location of the tip of the tunneling tool at all times.
- The clinician should be able to palpate the tunneling rod through its entire passage (Fig. 39.7). In this way, the doctor can avoid the risk of tunneling at depths that may lead to tissue damage.
- Tunneling may require the physician to be placed in physically uncomfortable positions to achieve the proper angle to place the rod, possibly getting outside of the sterile field and contaminating the tunneling tool or the catheter. This problem highlights the need for wide prepping and draping of patients receiving an intrathecal device. Vigorous irrigation of the tunneling tract with antibiotic solution may also be helpful.
- For obese patients, the tunneling distance required should be measured at the time of marking the course. This distance should be compared to the length of the tunneling tool. If the distance is longer than the available tunneling device, a two-step technique should be used. This alteration in technique will lead to a successful procedure and reduce the risk of improper depth of tunneling.
- If an alternative pump location outside of the abdomen is chosen, using a smaller volume pump may reduce the risk of erosion, and placement at least 10 cm above the iliac crest, off the midline, will reduce the chances of cluneal neuralgia from periosteal impingement. Additionally, patients must have adequate tissue mass to support the pump in the subcutaneous tissues. In some patients, the lack of body fat makes it necessary to create a pump pocket that is deep to the underlying muscular fascia.

Conclusions

The placement of a permanent intrathecal device requires attention to detail and vigilance at each step of the procedure. Much of the physician's attention is placed on the placement of the catheter and the creation of a pocket, but it is very important to adequately consider the tunneling element of the process, which has a profound impact on the achievement of a successful outcome.

Suggested Reading

Follett KA, Burchiel K, Deer T, Dupen S, Prager J, Turner MS, et al. Prevention of intrathecal drug delivery catheter-related complications. Neuromodulation. 2003;6:32–41.

McIntyre P, Deer T, Hayek S. Complications of spinal infusion therapies. Tech Reg Anesth Pain Manag. 2007;11:183–92.

Pope JE, Deer TR. Guide to implantable devices for intrathecal therapy. Pract Pain Manag. 2013. http://www.practicalpainmanagement.com/treatments/interventional/pumps/guide-implantable-devices-intrathecal-therapy. Accessed 15 Feb 2014.

Pope JE, Deer TR. Intrathecal drug delivery: an overview of modern concepts in advanced pain care. In: McGraw-Hill's principles and practice in pain medicine, vol. 3. New York: McGraw-Hill; 2015.

40 Pocketing for Intrathecal Drug Delivery Systems

Timothy R. Deer and C. Douglas Stewart

40.1 Introduction

Creating a pocket in the subcutaneous tissue is an important part of placing the permanent intrathecal drug delivery system (IDDS). For many with surgical experience the creation of the pocket seems trivial on the surface. The focus of much of the implantation of the intrathecal pump is on the proper delivery of the catheter to the spinal fluid and the subsequent anchoring and tunneling. Many critical aspects also exist for creating a pump pocket. These points are examined in this chapter.

T.R. Deer, MD (✉) • C.D. Stewart
The Center for Pain Relief, 400 Court Street, Suite 100,
Charleston, WV 25301, USA
e-mail: DocTDeer@aol.com; dstewart@centerforpainrelief.com

T.R. Deer, J.E. Pope (eds.), *Atlas of Implantable Therapies for Pain Management*, DOI 10.1007/978-1-4939-2110-2_40

40.2 Technical Overview

The incision of skin, separation of tissue planes, and hemostasis of the wound are factors we must focus on when creating a pump pocket. Several steps must be taken into consideration prior to doing the surgical components of the procedure. The physician should closely examine the patient's bony structure to evaluate the location of the most inferior rib margin and the anatomy of the anterior iliac spine. Attention should also be given to the patient's existing scars and skin lesions that may affect pocket creation.

Langer's lines, sometimes called cleavage lines, are topological lines drawn on a map of the human body (Fig. 40.1). They correspond to the natural orientation of collagen fibers in the dermis.

Knowing the direction of Langer's lines within a specific area of the skin is important for surgical operations, particularly cosmetic surgery. If a surgeon has a choice about where and in what direction to place an incision, he or she may choose to cut in the direction of Langer's lines. Incisions made parallel to Langer's lines may heal better and produce less scarring than those that cut across these lines. Conversely, incisions perpendicular to Langer's lines have a tendency to pucker and remain obvious, although sometimes this is unavoidable. The same could be said for taking care not to cut across old scar or hypertrophic scar. Almost assuredly the outcome will be poor.

Evaluation of local infection should be performed on the skin with the pocket location being altered based on any infectious-appearing areas. An evaluation of skin turgor and texture should be performed to determine whether the patient has acceptable nutrition to tolerate the placement of the device in the subcutaneous tissue or whether a need exists to place the device below the fascia. The patient should consider visiting with her or his primary care doctor to optimize comorbidities and nutritional status prior to surgery. Finally an evaluation should be done to determine whether the patient has skin viability to handle the procedure. This point may be important in patients on long-term high-dose steroids, with renal disease, or with chronic skin diseases.

Once the preoperative assessment is completed, the patient is taken to the operating theater and positioned. When positioning the patient, the placement of the pocket must be given consideration. The abdomen must be properly exposed and draping should allow for easy visual inspection of the surgical field, rib margin, pelvis, and umbilicus. This exposure will allow the physician to properly utilize the information obtained in the preoperative period. In some settings because of body habitus, previous surgeries, or skin issues, the pocket is placed in the lumbar region posteriorly. In these settings the patient can be positioned in the prone position.

Another area of concern is the need to maintain a sterile field on the abdomen while placing the catheter, using fluoroscopy, and anchoring the catheter. This often requires manipulating the fluoroscopy machine from an anteroposterior view to a lateral view with close contact above the abdomen. The author recommends using a three-quarter sheet over the abdomen until it is time to make the pocket. This will reduce the risk of secondary contamination (Fig. 40.2).

Once the patient has been properly prepared, the surgeon makes the skin incision to initiate pocket formation. Prior to incision the patient must be properly anesthetized with either local anesthesia, intravenous sedation, or both. The incision should be made with the skin retracted to a taut orientation. A #11 or #15 blade is the most commonly used instrument for incision. The incision can be made to the desired depth, which can be used as an entry point for pocket dissection, or the incision can be made just below the dermis and the depth can be achieved with cutting electrothermal dissection. The normal depth of the pocket ranges from 1 to 3 cm based on physician preference. The pocket can be made by sharp dissection with surgical scissors or by blunt dissection with the surgeon's hand or the blunt portion of an instrument. The method of pocket dissection chosen is based on physician preference and training. The pocket should be 110–120 % of the total volume of the pump. The physician may use the pump to measure the pocket size as dissection is carried out. If the pocket is too large, it may lead to pump movement and even result in the pump flipping. If the pocket is too small, it may lead to tissue pressure and possible discomfort or, in worse-case scenarios, tissue erosion with loss of the device. Unfortunately, even with careful attention to detail, the patient may develop some of these issues over time owing to the health of the adipose, fascia, and skin tissues.

Regardless of dissection technique, the tissue should be manipulated gently to avoid the later complication of seroma. If epinephrine is placed in the local anesthetic, it may retard some small vessel bleeding, but it can also cause a delay that can lead to bleeding after wound closure. The physician must be aware of this issue. Hemostasis can be achieved by electrocautery, suturing of the vessel, and applying pressure by packing the wound with antibiotic-soaked surgical tapes.

Once the pocket has been properly sized, the pump has been tested for proper fit, and the catheter has been tunneled to the pocket, the physician can connect the pump to the catheter and secure the connection to avoid disruption of the system. Prior to placing the pump into the pocket for the final time, the nonabsorbable suture is placed into the tissue. The suture can then be applied to suture loops on the pump, which will secure its position. The authors prefer suture loop pumps, but an alternative is to use a Dacron pouch, which allows suturing of the pouch to hold to the pump in place. The downside of the pouch is scarring over time that may make future revisions difficult. As the pump is placed in the pocket, the implanting doctor needs to pay attention to the location of the side port and pump catheter connector. The shape of this part of the pump can irritate the tissue and potentially cause pain. The patient's body habitus should be considered when placing the side port and the connector and the position should be noted in the operative note if it varies in individual patients.

Once the clinician is pleased with the pump pocket and device placement, the pocket must be closed. The pocket should be irrigated vigorously with antibiotic solution and then the tissue brought together with a two- to three-layer closure. The choice of suture is at the discretion of the implanter. The author prefers absorbable monofilament suture such as monocryl. Sterile surgical tapes can be applied on the skin surface or staples may be used in some cases. An abdominal binder can be helpful in reducing postoperative pain and may help in the reduction of pocket seroma or hematoma.

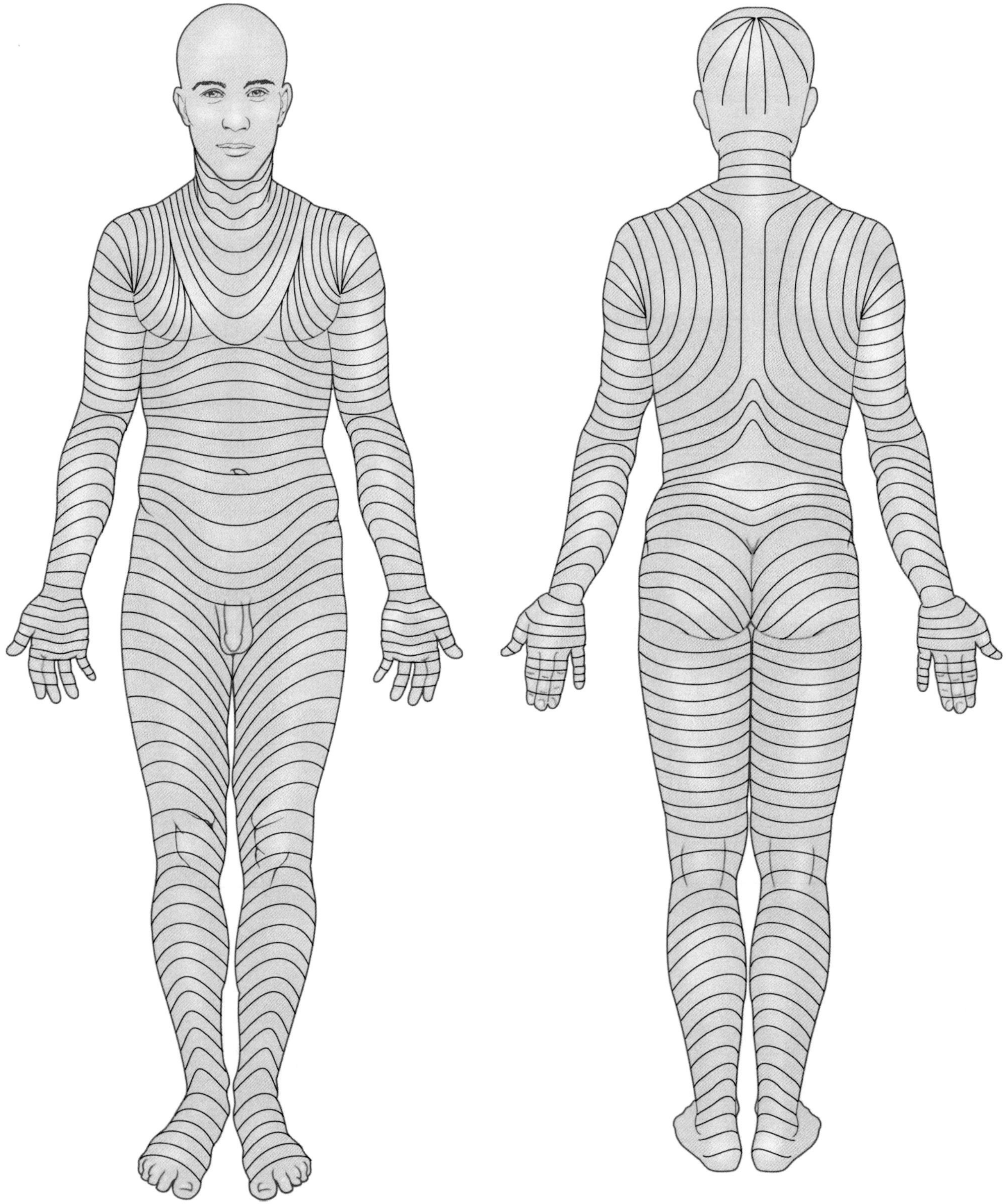

Fig. 40.1 Langer's lines

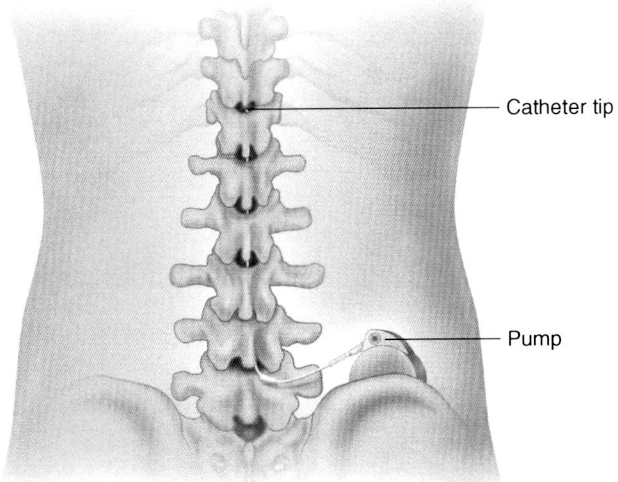

Fig. 40.2 Fluoroscopy unit with lateral view

40.3 Risk Assessment

1. The pocket may become infected. This can be superficial or involve the deeper tissues and the deviceBleeding within the pocket can cause a hematoma resulting in wound dehiscence and breakdown and ultimate loss of the device.
2. Seroma occurs when the tissue seeps serosanguineous fluid that results in pocket pressure and potential pain, wound dehiscence, and loss of the device.
3. A pocket that is too large can lead to pocket flipping, seroma formation, and eventual catheter complications.
4. A pocket that is too small may lead to pain, tissue necrosis, and erosion of the metal through the skin.
5. A pocket that is created close to the rib or anterior superior iliac spine can lead to discomfort when sitting, lying, or changing positions.

40.4 Risk Avoidance

1. Careful attention to detail is critical in preventing infection. This involves preoperative assessment, prophylactic antibiotics, proper preparing and draping, tissue irrigation, and attention to wound closure.
2. The avoidance of pocket bleeding can be achieved by attention to preoperative clotting indices, careful handling of the tissue during dissection, and hemostasis by electrocautery, suturing of vessels, and tissue pressure to clot small bleeding vessels that may not be initially obvious.
3. Seroma cannot always be avoided, but the likelihood of seroma can be reduced by paying careful attention to detail when dissecting the pocket. The tissue should be handled carefully, electrocautery should be used judiciously, and bleeding vessels should be controlled prior to wound closure. It is also important to size the pocket properly for the device. Tissue pressure in the postoperative period may be helpful in reducing seroma. This can be achieved by abdominal binders, elastic wraps, or pressure dressings.
4. Pocket sizing should be done carefully, checking the pocket with the actual device when the size of the pocket is felt to be adequate. In this method the pocket can slowly increase in size until it is 10–20 % bigger than the volume of the pump. In the future, sizing templates would be helpful in achieving proper size and depth of the pump.
5. The physician should ensure that there is 5 cm or more between the pump location and the bony landmarks of the ribs and the bones of the pelvis. This should allow for enough room when standing, sitting, and lying, avoiding bony irritation of the pump site. In cases of scoliosis, kyphosis, small stature, and other body habitus irregularities, the placement of the pump may be in contact with the bone even with the best effort to avoid such contact.

Conclusions

Successful pump placement requires attention to detail and execution of several critical steps. The placement of the pocket is more than simply making an incision and separating tissue. It involves the use of strategy, careful planning, and surgical skill to create a pocket that results in a good initial outcome and reduces the need for future revisions and reoperations. The other issue is patient satisfaction and comfort, which can be enhanced by following the edicts noted in this chapter.

40.5 Supplemental Images

See Figs. 40.3, 40.4, 40.5, 40.6, and 40.7.

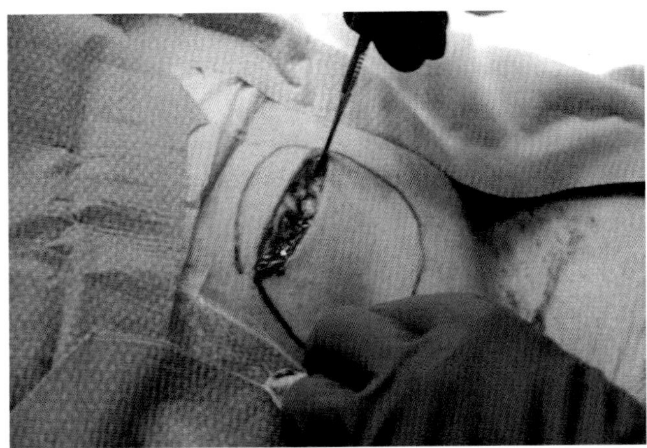

Fig. 40.3 Appropriate pocket incision length and location

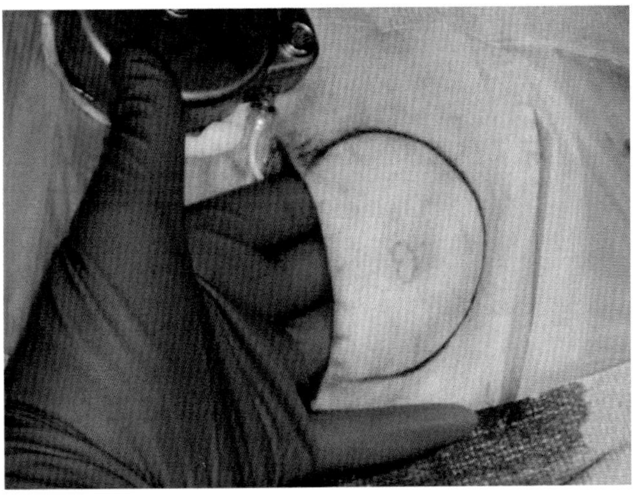

Fig. 40.4 The physician should evaluate pocket depth and size prior to pump implant

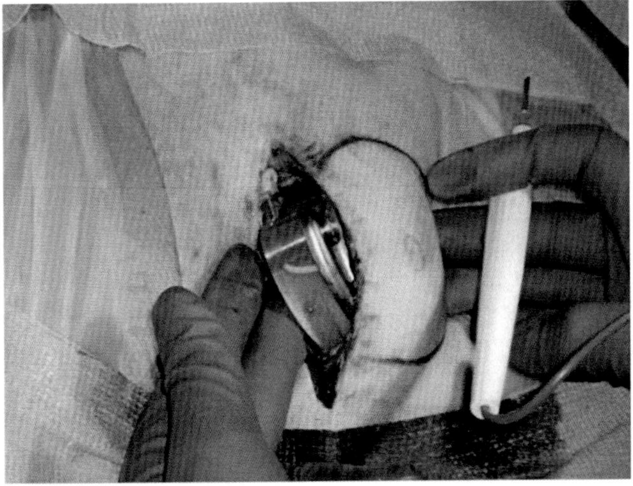

Fig. 40.5 Proper orientation of the pump in the pocket with the side port at the 1 o'clock orientation

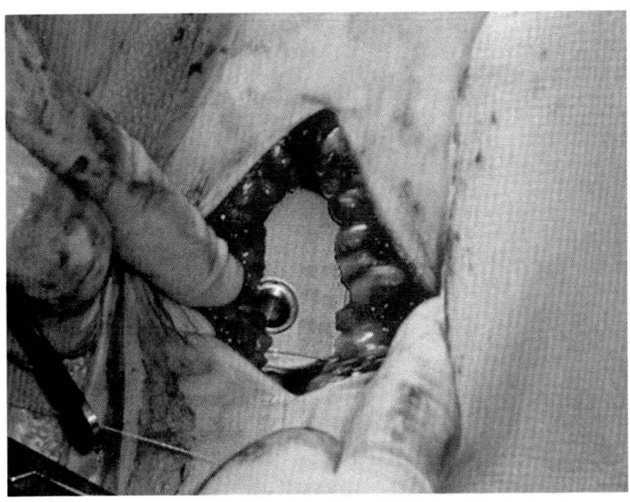

Fig. 40.6 The tissue must be loose enough to close without pressure on the tissue edges

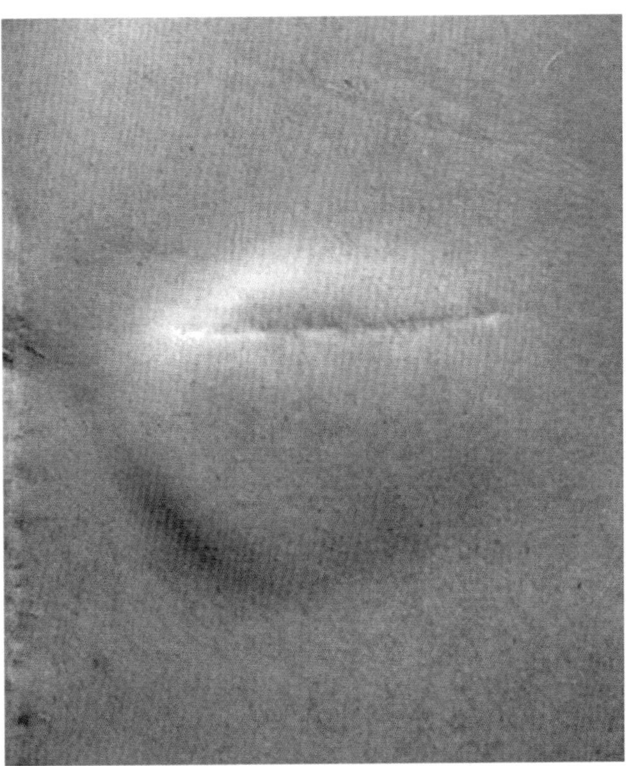

Fig. 40.7 Placement of the reservoir posteriorly in the flank

Suggested Reading

Belverud S, Mogilner A, Schulder M. Intrathecal pumps. Neurotherapeutics. 2008;5:114–22.

Corrado P, Alperson B, Wright M. Perceived success and failure of intrathecal infusion pump implantation in chronic pain patients. Neuromodulation. 2008;11:98–102.

Townsend CM, Beauchamp RD, Evers BM, Mattox L, editors. Sabiston textbook of surgery: the biological basis of modern surgical practice. 19th ed. Philadelphia: Elsevier Saunders; 2012.

Turner J, Sears J, Loeser D. Programmable intrathecal opioid delivery systems for chronic noncancer pain: a systemic review of effectiveness and complications. Clin J Pain. 2007;23:180–95.

41 Drug Selection for Intrathecal Drug Delivery

Karina Gritsenko, Veronica Carullo, Timothy R. Deer, and Jason E. Pope

The use of intrathecal agents to treat pain and other diseases, such as spasticity, is based on the principle that delivering drugs directly to the cerebral spinal fluid (CSF) bypasses the first-pass effect and results in increased potency and reduced systemic side-effects as compared to other routes of delivery such as the oral or transdermal approach. This may improve efficacy and sustainability, as compared to epidural, intravenous, oral, or transdermal preparations.

Importantly, the intrathecal drug delivery system itself functions as a platform to deliver medications into the intrathecal space; it does not assign the medication chosen for delivery. The selection of the proper drug to use in an individual patient is complicated by the disease state, previous failures of systemic medications, patient characteristics, and the location and pathology of the chronic pain state. Further, the traditional approach of regarding the intrathecal drug delivery system as salvage therapy is outdated; advancements are improving outcomes and influencing drug choice and dosing strategies. This chapter examines the options for drug delivery in the intrathecal space. These principles can be applied when managing a trial to see whether someone is a candidate for an implant or in the setting of managing a permanent implant.

K. Gritsenko
Montefiore Medical Center, Albert Einstein College of Medicine, 3400 Bainbridge Avenue, MMC-MAP, Room LL400, Bronx, NY 10467, USA
e-mail: karina.gritsenko@gmail.com

V. Carullo
Pediatric Pain Management Service, Montefiore Medical Center, Albert Einstein College of Medicine, Bronx, NY, USA
e-mail: vcarullo@montefiore.org

T.R. Deer, MD (✉)
The Center for Pain Relief, 400 Court Street, Suite 100, Charleston, WV 25301, USA
e-mail: DocTDeer@aol.com

J.E. Pope
Summit Pain Alliance, 392 Tesconi Court, Santa Rosa, CA 95401, USA
e-mail: popeje@me.com

T.R. Deer, J.E. Pope (eds.), *Atlas of Implantable Therapies for Pain Management*, DOI 10.1007/978-1-4939-2110-2_41

41.1 Technical Overview

In the United States, the Food and Drug Administration (FDA) has approved three drugs for chronic, continuous intrathecal use. These agents are morphine and ziconotide for the treatment of pain, and baclofen for the treatment of spasticity. It has become common practice in the United States, and throughout the world, to use other agents in patients who have unacceptable relief or adverse effects from the use of these three standard substances. This strategy is termed off-label use. (Monotherapy with the aforementioned agents is on-label.) The authors do not recommend or endorse the off-label use of medications, and the decision to use drugs in an off-label fashion is a case-to-case decision made by the managing physician. If the treating physician decides to employ off-label medications or off-label combination therapy, several safety factors should be considered:

- Animal and human safety data support the use of the agent.
- Other clinicians in the field use the drug in a similar fashion.
- Studies or consensus guidelines in the literature support the off-label use of the medications.

As a guide to clinical practice and an effort to improve patient safety, algorithms have been created by well-published experts on the proper selection and dosing of both on-label and off-label medications based on patient response. These algorithmic selections are based on animal safety data, human safety data, clinical efficacy publications, and clinical experience. These consensus algorithms shape current practices on drug selection and continue to evolve, with new studies and clinical experience.

The most recent peer-reviewed consensus guideline statement for intrathecal therapy was the Polyanalgesic Consensus Conference (PACC) of 2012. This is the fourth such effort to standardize and provide an evidence-based foundation for the implementation and management of intrathecal therapy. The first, by Portenoy and Hassenbusch in 2000, recommended morphine as the only first-line agent for the treatment of pain, with an algorithm for alternatives if morphine failed or had unacceptable side effects. The second line of therapy based on established criteria included hydromorphone as an alternative opioid, or the addition of a nonopioid adjuvant such as bupivacaine or clonidine to morphine in neuropathic states. In a 2003 update, use of hydromorphone was advanced to a first-line agent equal to morphine. The reasoning included equivalent efficacy data, equivalent or superior safety data, and the possibility of reduced risk of intrathecal granuloma with hydromorphone. In 2007, the advancement in the field warranted yet another update to this living document. This consensus of experts determined that first-line therapies should include morphine, hydromorphone, and ziconotide. Other significant changes included adding fentanyl as a solo agent as a second-line option, and adding combination therapies including opioids with bupivacaine or clonidine, but also with ziconotide.

The latest iteration of the PACC guidelines was in 2012, and included updates to the existing algorithm. Importantly, the pain was divided into neuropathic or nociceptive pain, which may influence the medication employed. Other notable differences included increasing the maximum dose of hydromorphone to 10 mg per day, compared with the 2007 recommendation of 4 mg per day (Tables 41.1, 41.2, and 41.3). The algorithms described, and line of therapy, are outlined in Tables 41.4 and 41.5.

In selecting the proper drug for each patient, the physician should attempt to determine the type of pain. Other important features in selecting an intrathecal medicine includes the region of pain and the ability to place a catheter congruently. Each medicine has different physicochemical properties that influence medication spread. Dose titration and vigilance will improve the efficacy of the therapy The occurrence of adverse effects also may have a profound effect on the need for adjustments to infusion combinations.

Drug algorithm selection is not only used during continuous, chronic intrathecal infusion, but also is used by many physicians during patient screening. When the patient fails to respond to an opioid alone during the trial, many physicians will change to ziconotide or add an adjuvant such as bupivacaine or clonidine.

Table 41.1 Polyanalgesic Consensus Conference 2012 recommendations for starting doses of intrathecal agents

Agent	Starting dose
Morphine	0.1–0.5 mg/day
Hydromorphone	0.02–0.5 mg/day
Fentanyl	25–75 μg/day
Bupivacaine	1–4 mg/day
Clonidine	40–100 μg/day
Ziconotide	0.5–2.4 μg/day

From Deer et al. (2012) with permission

Table 41.2 Polyanalgesic Consensus Conference 2012 recommendations for maximum concentration of intrathecal agents

Agent	Maximum concentration
Morphine	20 mg/mL
Hydromorphone	15 mg/mL
Fentanyl	10,000 μg/mL
Bupivacaine	30 mg/mL
Clonidine	1000 μg/mL
Ziconotide	100 μg/mL

From Deer et al. (2012) with permission

Table 41.3 Polyanalgesic Consensus Conference 2012 recommendations for maximum dose of intrathecal agents

Agent	Maximum dose
Morphine	15 mg/day
Hydromorphone	10 mg/day
Fentanyl	None
Bupivacaine	10 mg/day
Clonidine	600 μg/day
Ziconotide	19.2 μg/day

From Deer et al. (2012) with permission

Table 41.4 Polyanalgesic Consensus Conference 2012 recommendations for neuropathic pain

Line 1	Morphine	Ziconotide		Morphine + bupivacaine
Line 2	Hydromorphone	Hydromorphone + bupivacaine *or* Hydromorphone + clonidine		Morphine + clonidine
Line 3	Clonidine	Ziconotide + opioid	Fentanyl	Fentanyl + bupivacaine *or* Fentanyl + clonidine
Line 4	Opioid + clonidine + bupivacaine		Bupivacaine + clonidine	
Line 5	Baclofen			

From Deer et al. (2012) with permission
Line 1: Morphine and ziconotide are approved by the US Food and Drug Administration for IT therapy and are recommended as first-line therapy for neuropathic pain. The combination of morphine and bupivacaine is recommended for neuropathic pain on the basis of clinical use and apparent safety. **Line 2**: Hydromorphone, alone or in combination with bupivacaine or clonidine, is recommended. Alternatively, the combination of morphine and clonidine may be used. **Line 3**: Third-line recommendations for neuropathic pain include clonidine, ziconotide plus an opioid, and fentanyl alone or in combination with bupivacaine or clonidine. **Line 4**: The combination of bupivacaine and clonidine (with or without an opioid drug) is recommended. **Line 5**: Baclofen is recommended on the basis of safety, although reports of efficacy are limited

Table 41.5 Polyanalgesic Consensus Conference 2012 recommendations for nociceptive pain

Line 1	Morphine	Hydromorphone	Ziconotide	Fentanyl
Line 2	Morphine + bupivacaine	Ziconotide + opioid	Hydromorphone + bupivacaine	Fentanyl + bupivacaine
Line 3	Opioid (morphine, hydromorphone, or fentanyl) + clonidine			Sufentanil
Line 4	Opioid + clonidine + bupivacaine		Sufentanil + bupivacaine or clonidine	
Line 5	Sufentanil + bupivacaine + clonidine			

From Deer et al. (2012) with permission
Line 1: Morphine and ziconotide are approved by the US Food and Drug Administration for IT therapy and are recommended as first-line therapy for nociceptive pain. Hydromorphone is recommended on the basis of widespread clinical use and apparent safety. Fentanyl has been upgraded to first-line use by the consensus conference. **Line 2**: Bupivacaine in combination with morphine, hydromorphone, or fentanyl is recommended. Alternatively, the combination of ziconotide and an opioid drug can be employed. **Line 3**: Recommendations include clonidine plus an opioid (i.e., morphine, hydromorphone, or fentanyl) or sufentanil monotherapy. **Line 4**: The triple combination of an opioid, clonidine, and bupivacaine is recommended. An alternate recommendation is sufentanil in combination with either bupivacaine or clonidine. **Line 5**: The triple combination of sufentanil, bupivacaine, and clonidine is suggested

41.2 End of Life

The 2012 PACC group realized that the use of intrathecal agents in the terminally ill patient may differ from their use in someone who is a candidate for long-term therapy. Higher concentrations of agents, and the use of agents that are not normally recommended (such as tetracaine, ropivacaine, and meperidine), may be appropriate for the terminally ill patient. A frank discussion of risks and benefits should occur with the health care team, the patient, and the patient's significant others. As the medications are to be used off-label, the treating physician should weigh the risks and the benefits of the therapy.

41.3 Future Research and Development

The future use of intrathecal drug delivery devices may include new drugs, new delivery strategies, new dosing paradigms, and software innovations. Practitioners should be mindful of the limitations of the currently available devices. Unfortunately, there is not a robust advent of new intrathecal agents, but hardware and software innovations soon to be on the horizon may continue to advance the pain-care algorithm.

41.4 Risk Assessment

- Intrathecal opioids may cause tolerance, and the drug effect may be lost over time. Selecting patients with lower systemic opioids for intrathecal drug delivery may mitigate tolerance. Some authors contend that combination therapy may offset the speed of dose escalation with monotherapy.
- Intrathecal opioids may affect the hormonal axis, causing changes in antidiuretic hormone and testosterone. A common complication is peripheral edema, which may occur early in the course of therapy and may be difficult to control during ongoing opioid therapy.
- Intrathecal opioids have been associated with inflammatory masses, also called granulomas, which can result in failure of the system and may lead to neurologic symptoms.
- Intrathecal clonidine has been seen to have an impact on blood pressure and may cause sedation. Withdrawal can be fatal because of rebound hypertension.
- Intrathecal bupivacaine may cause numbness, edema, urinary retention, and change in proprioception.
- Intrathecal ziconotide may cause drowsiness, dizziness, and hallucinations. It is contraindicated in patients with psychosis.
- Currently available intrathecal delivery platforms have limitations that can affect patient care. These include MRI incompatibility, the fear of overdose, unexpected overinfusion, and the lack of an extremely low minimal rate while the Personal Therapy Manager (PTM; Medtronic, Minneapolis, MN) is employed.

41.5 Risk Avoidance

- Some practitioners believe that tolerance can be avoided or slowed either by increasing dosages at prolonged intervals of several months or by adding synergistic drugs to lessen the need for opioids.
- Patients with long-term opioid therapy may require hormone replacement and testing. This is a problem not only with the intrathecal use of opioids, but also with other routes of opioid administration and with chronic pain in general. The most commonly replaced drug is testosterone, but other hormones also may be affected. The development of pedal edema may be directly related to intrathecal opioid and can be treated with mild antidiuretics, compression stockings, and leg elevation. If the problem is not resolved, the patient may benefit from drug substitution. The primary care doctor should also evaluate the patient to rule out other causes of fluid retention.
- The formation of intrathecal inflammatory masses has been shown to be directly related to high concentrations and dosage of opioids and may represent a pharmacokinetic failure. The PACC in 2012 set recommended concentrations for drug infusion (*see* Table 41.2). Warning signs of inflammatory masses include loss of analgesic effect or changes in proprioception, sensation, or motor function. The masses can be diagnosed by MRI or CT myelography.
- Intrathecal clonidine is well tolerated by most patients, with no change in blood pressure or consciousness. The dose should be initiated at low levels such as 10–30 μg/day, and interval changes should be small. The risk of complications is greater when the catheter is in the high thoracic or cervical region.
- Intrathecal bupivacaine has been shown to improve efficacy and reduce the need for opioids for equianalgesic effect. To reduce the risk of complications and side effects, the dose should be initiated at a low level of 1–3 mg per day, with any change being made at very small intervals.

- The use of ziconotide has gained momentum, as it is a first-line therapy for both nociceptive and neuropathic pain. Further, as a nonopioid, it is not associated with cardiopulmonary depression with overdose, and no fatal events have been reported. It also appears to be nongranulomagenic. The dosing strategy of "starting low and titrating slow" improves patient tolerability.
- The reader is directed to the device manufacturer for current information on the limitations of the available intrathecal platforms. It is of paramount importance to understand the different risks and limitations of each device before beginning therapy.

Conclusions

Intrathecal drug delivery offers a different, complementary neuromodulation pathway for patients when conservative medical care has failed. Treating intrathecal therapy as a salvage therapy is an antiquated and misguided attitude. Improving efficacy and mitigation of therapy-related complications centers on improved patient selection, trialing, and drug selection. Success commonly can be achieved with monotherapy. When considering drugs that are not approved for first-line use, the physician should take a scientific approach centered on patient safety; choosing agents on the basis of physician preference, anecdotal reports, or off-label marketing is not acceptable. Algorithmic thought, vigilance, and an attention to both a good outcome and safety must be the overriding hierarchy of intrathecal therapies.

Suggested Reading

Bennett G, Burchiel K, Buchser E, Classen A, Deer T, Du Pen S, et al. Clinical guidelines for intraspinal infusion: report of an expert panel. Polyanalgesic Consensus Conference 2000. J Pain Symptom Manage. 2000;20:S37–43.

Deer TR, Prager J, Levy R, Rathmell J, Buchser E, Burton A, et al. Polyanalgesic Consensus Conference 2012: recommendations for the management of pain by intrathecal (intraspinal) drug delivery: report of an interdisciplinary expert panel. Neuromodulation. 2012;15:436–64; discussion 464–6.

Hassenbusch SJ, Portenoy RK, Cousins M, Buchser E, Deer TR, Du Pen SL, et al. Polyanalgesic Consensus Conference 2003: an update on the management of pain by intraspinal drug delivery —report of an expert panel. J Pain Symptom Manage. 2004;27:540–63.

Hayek SM, Deer TR, Pope JE, Panchal SJ, Patel VB. Intrathecal therapy for cancer and noncancer pain. Pain Physician. 2011;14: 219–48.

Pope JE, Deer TR. Ziconotide: a clinical update and pharmacologic review. Expert Opin Pharmacother. 2013;14:957–66.

Smith TJ, Staats PS, Deer T, Stearns LJ, Rauck RL, Boortz-Marx RL, et al. Randomized clinical trial of an implantable drug delivery system compared with comprehensive medical management for refractory cancer pain: impact on pain, drug-related toxicity, and survival. J Clin Oncol. 2002;20:4040–9.

Intrathecal Pump Refills

42

Karina Gritsenko, Veronica Carullo, and Timothy R. Deer

42.1 Introduction

It is extremely important to ensure an appropriate level of understanding and training regarding the initial placement of intrathecal catheters and intrathecal pumps; the maintenance of these devices, however, specifically the refill process, is equally important. In a perfect setting, the pump is placed without incident, the patient does well on a continuing basis, and the pump is refilled at regular intervals. Many implanting doctors spend little or no time in training to learn the refill technique. Although this procedure seems limited in technical difficulty, and lacking in excitement, it is very important for the continued desired outcome of acceptable pain relief and absence of complications, which may be serious if this relatively simple task is not done properly. Vigilance is an essential part of this simple but also essential part of intrathecal drug delivery and care. In settings where a team approach is implemented, the administrative person in charge of nurse education must be committed to proper training of nurses and physician extenders performing this procedure.

K. Gritsenko
Montefiore Medical Center, Albert Einstein College of Medicine, 3400 Bainbridge Avenue, MMC-MAP, Room LL400, Bronx, NY 10467, USA
e-mail: karina.gritsenko@gmail.com

V. Carullo
Pediatric Pain Management Service, Montefiore Medical Center, Albert Einstein College of Medicine, Bronx, NY, USA
e-mail: vcarullo@montefiore.org

T.R. Deer, MD (✉)
The Center for Pain Relief, 400 Court Street, Suite 100, Charleston, WV 25301, USA
e-mail: DocTDeer@aol.com

42.2 Technical Overview: How to Conduct a Refill

Once the patient has been implanted with the intrathecal pump, telemetry is performed to establish an initial starting dose and alarm date. The patients initially are seen frequently in the physician's office to monitor for postoperative infection, assess their analgesic response to the intrathecal drug therapy or side effects that may occur with dose changes, and identify the need for dosage adjustments. Most office evaluations of the intrathecal device system include interrogation of the patient's pump to assess medication settings and reservoir volumes, establishment of the alarm date, and scheduling of an office infusion center or home refill service appointment at least 1 week before the alarm date to ensure the pump will be refilled before the depletion of medication from the pump reservoir.

Before refilling the pump, the patient is assessed by the physician or team member with regard to pain relief, neurological function, and any potential complications. The prescribed drug is reviewed to confirm proper concentration, volume, and dosing. The procedure is explained to the patient and informed consent documents are completed. The patient is placed on the examination table in the supine position and the baseline pump telemetry assessment is performed based on manufacturer's recommendations. The pump telemetry informs the physician of the patient's demographic information and the pump and catheter specifications including model number, serial number, and catheter length. Pump telemetry also informs the physician of the medication settings of the pump including drug concentration and dosage, pump reservoir volume, and alarm date. All of these components are critical in order to establish the pre-procedure volume baseline so that a comparison can be conducted following pump refill. Understanding of this data is essential to avoid any untoward sequelae related to improper administration of the medication or improper programming, especially in the setting of any planned medication changes, where precision is of utmost importance. In settings where

T.R. Deer, J.E. Pope (eds.), *Atlas of Implantable Therapies for Pain Management*, DOI 10.1007/978-1-4939-2110-2_42

the refill is performed by an infusion center or home refill service it is still important that the patient be evaluated by the physician at some interval to examine them and note the stability of neurological function.

Available programmable pumps have information on the calculated volume of the pump, but actual volumes are not determined by the reading of the device. In pumps that are constant flow and "nonprogrammable," the volume is based on timing and the number of days between refill events. These pumps cannot be interrogated by telemetry, and give no computerized information to the managing physician. The number of nonprogrammable pumps in the United States is limited and physicians who are not familiar with the devices should consult with the manufacturer's insert and technical support before moving forward. Programmable pumps are the most common type of implant in both the United States and in most international settings where pump therapies are offered. Most commonly, a Medtronic (Minneapolis, MN) device has been used.

Recently, a new programmable pump system, the Prometra Programmable Infusion Pump system (Flowonix; Mt. Olive, NJ), approved in 2012, has been studied and has become a presence in the market. This system works via an electrically programmed valve-gated system which is non-peristaltic and will mitigate the need for complex gears and rotors. In theory, the newer technology is unique in that the care team is able to access the actual volume in the computer without aspirating the pump. Based on an industry-sponsored multicenter study, there is additional literature supporting a lesser likelihood of pump pocket subcutaneous refills due to a larger refill septum and higher reservoir pressures in the system itself so any additional medication would be returned into the medication syringe. As this is a relatively newly approved device, complications of these new pump mechanisms are not currently known and will need to be continue to be assessed.

In terms of the pump refill process itself, sterile kits are available. The pump refill kit should include sterile drape, a pump template; proper non-coring Huber needles for intrathecal pump port access; syringes; micropore filters to reduce the risk of introduction of contaminants; and tubing with proper stopcocks that allow change in flow direction, stoppage of flow, and evaluation of pump pressure. The prepping process should be performed with a solution that is proper for local pathogens and should be done widely outside the area of planned pump refill. The prep should be initiated at the center of the pump site and then moved outward in a circular motion until the entire pump area is cleansed. This process should be repeated on at least three occasions. Once the pump is properly prepped, the field should be covered with a fenestrated drape. Each kit contains a sterile, plastic template that can be placed onto the skin for guidance and mimicking of the shape of the pump and the location of the central port. The central port of the pump is accessed by using a template and inserting the non-coring Huber needle of the appropriate gauge perfectly parallel with the center port in the pump. The pump lumen is secured when the physician or nurse feels the needle contact a metal surface, after passing through a rubbery port structure. At times, fluoroscopic imaging or ultrasound imaging has been used in order to locate the port to minimize complication risk, especially in patients with an atypical body habitus or high bmi numbers. The medication remaining in the pump is withdrawn and measured, comparing the actual volume with the programmer reservoir volume found upon the initial pump telemetry. After rechecking and verifying the new medication concentration with the concentration noted on the initial telemetry, the new medication is injected into the pump, aspirating every 5 mL to verify continued needle placement in the pump. With the Prometra device, it is suggested that an additional safety measure is present due to the higher reservoir pressures in the system itself so any additional medication would be returned into the medication syringe as an additional safety measure if there is a change in the pressure during injection. Once all of the medication is injected into the pump, the needle is withdrawn from the pump and a bandage is applied to the puncture site. The pump programmer is then used to verify the drug concentration, make dosage adjustments, and reset the reservoir volume to reflect the amount of medication placed in the pump. The new alarm date is noted and the patient is given an appointment for at least 1 week before the alarm date. All tracings should be confirmed by at least two members of the clinical team. The physician should always be the person to determine the settings of dosing after the refill, even in settings in which the physician does not actively participate in the procedure.

42.3 Risk Assessment

1. The greatest risk to the patient during the refill process is placing the wrong drug or concentration into the device or subcutaneously outside of the device. This can lead to death or serious injury or, in contrast, to opioid withdrawal if the medication is not injected into the planned location or if there is a syringe swap or medication error.
2. Infection is a risk of pump refill. This can lead to localized infection, as well as meningitis, abscess, or death.
3. The patient can develop sensitivity to the prepping solution leading to a rash over the refill site.
4. The catheter can be damaged with the placement of the needle for pump refill.
5. Pump programming is an essential part of every refill. Improper programming can lead to overdose, under dose, withdrawal, serious neurological injury, or death.
6. Overfilling of the pump can lead to damage to the bellows and pump failure.
7. Inadvertent placement of the drug into the subcutaneous area can lead to abnormal reactions to the drug in the immediate period after pump refill.
8. Pocket refills continue to be a concern, but with the assistance of available technologies, including more commonly accessible fluoroscopy or portable ultrasound devices and the advent of improving pump refill system devices, the hope is to mitigate complications related to pump refill errors, especially in the obese population.

42.4 Risk Avoidance

1. Prior to refilling the pump, the physician and nurse should review the prescribed drug, concentration, and dose and double check it against the drug delivered by the pharmacy provider.
2. Careful attention to sterile technique, use of micro-pore filters, and sterile handling of the drug solutions are critical in reducing infection. Any redness or swelling of the pump pocket should lead to close observation, and may necessitate incision and drainage of the pump.
3. The patient's skin should be evaluated prior to each refill. If a rash develops, the cleaning solution should be changed, and if necessary, a dermatologist should be consulted.
4. The catheter should be placed below the pump at the time of implant. If the catheter moves to an area in front of the device, it may be injured. This is why it is critical to aspirate after every 5 mL is injected.
5. All programming should be prescribed by the physician and confirmed by at least two members of the clinical team including the physician.
6. The pump volume to be replaced should be reviewed at the time of each refill. The volume should never be exceeded. Excessive filling of the pump could lead to injury of the internal pump mechanics, and failure of the device.
7. It is important to place the needle through the rubber port and then to feel it stop at the metal back portion of the lumen. Once it is in proper position, the existing drug should be aspirated and compared to the calculated volume. If the volumes are within 25 %, it considered reasonable for refill. In cases where the aspirated volume is more than 25 % of the expected volume, the physician should do additional workup on the integrity of the pump. Once the refill process is started, the drug should be aspirated at 5 mL intervals.
8. If there is any difficulty in finding the port itself, use adjuvant devices such as ultrasound or fluoroscopy to locate the device and prevent any untoward events.

Conclusions

The procedure of refilling a pump appears simplistic to the casual observer. The serious nature of this process may be undervalued by many practices and physicians. The pump refill process is very important and should be taken very seriously with attention given to pre-refill preparation, vigilance during refill, and follow-up afterward to access any potential complications.

42.5 Supplemental Images

See Figs. 42.1, 42.2, 42.3, 42.4, 42.5, 42.6, 42.7, 42.8, 42.9, 42.10, 42.11, and 42.12.

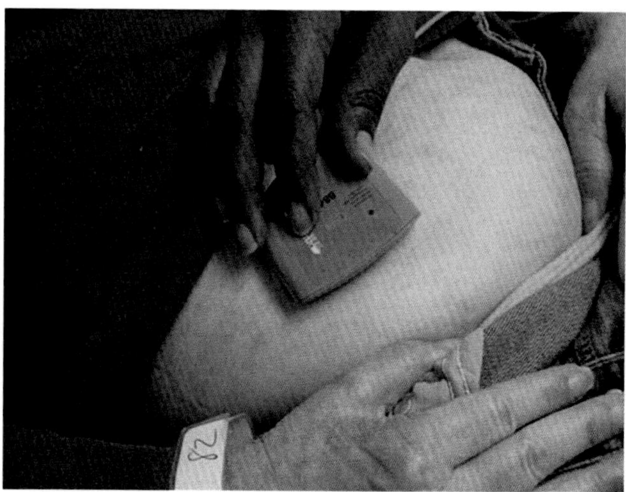

Fig. 42.1 Computer telemetry to access the status of the pump before pump refill

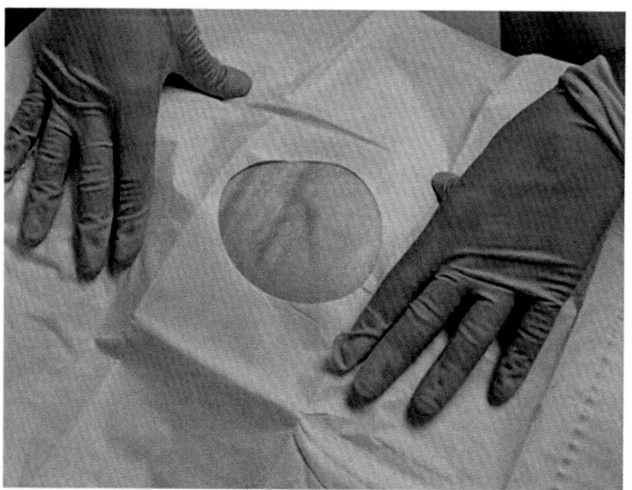

Fig. 42.2 After carefully prepping the abdomen on multiple occasions, sterile drapes are placed

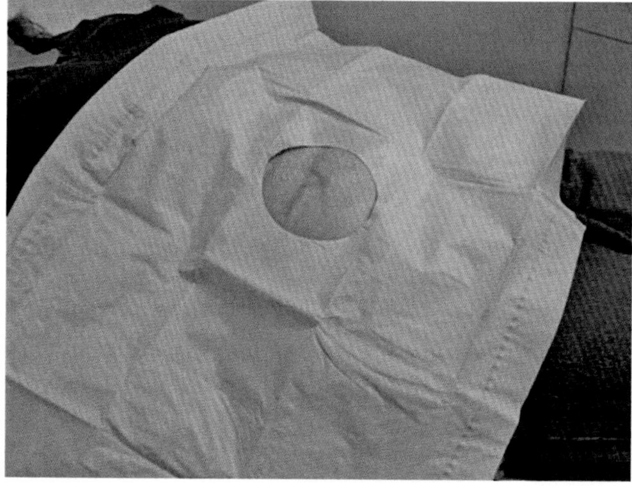

Fig. 42.3 The patient should be assessed to orientation of the pump, and as to evidence of any skin abnormalities

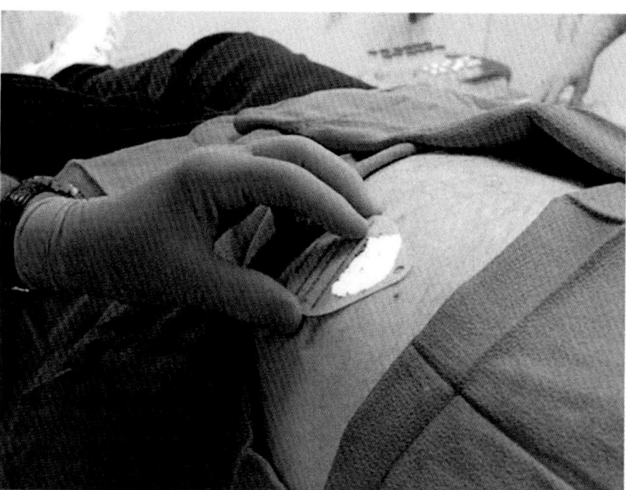

Fig. 42.4 In some cases, laser-guided fluoroscopy can be used to refill the pump. This may be very helpful in the obese patient or in a patient with an abnormal abdominal wall secondary to scar or poor tissue integrity

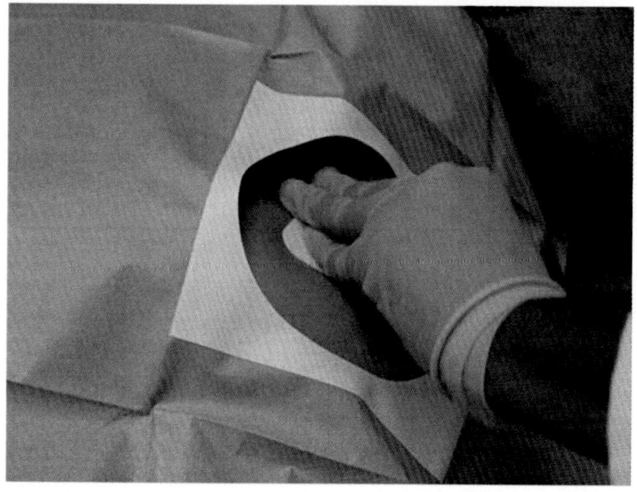

Fig. 42.5 Sterile dressings are placed once the pump is refilled

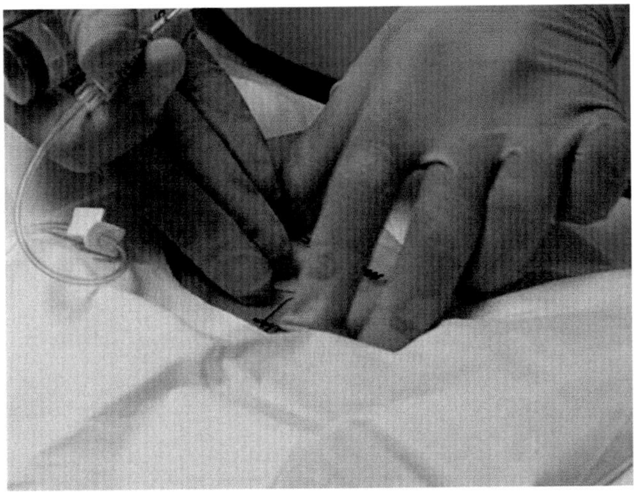

Fig. 42.6 A template can be used to help identify the port of the intrathecal pump

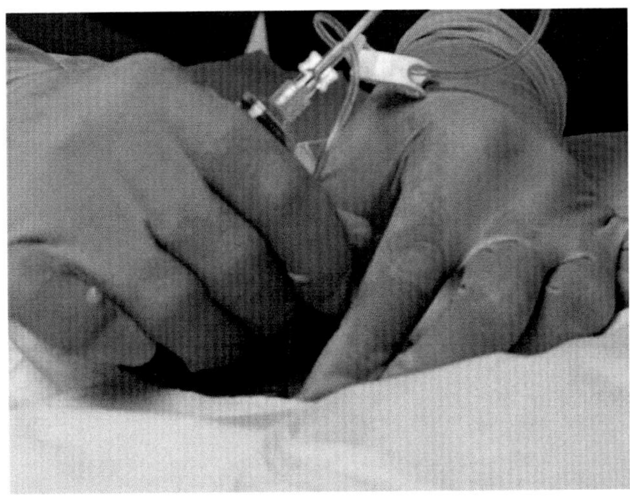

Fig. 42.8 The needle should be secured in the pump lumen and secured based on landmarks and successful aspiration throughout the aspiration and injection of any medication

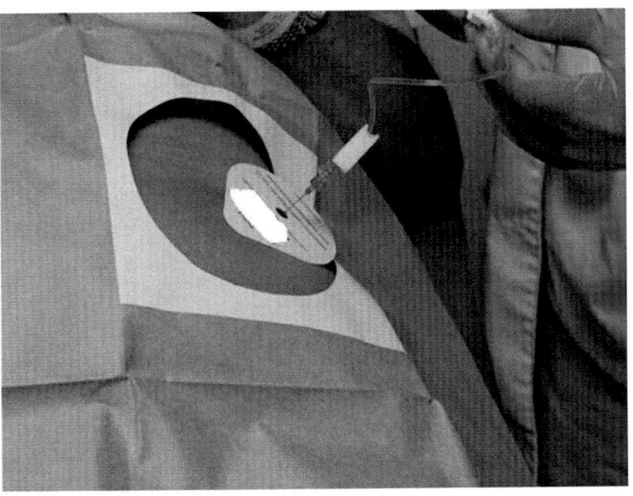

Fig. 42.7 After securing the needle in the lumen, the pump should be aspirated and compared to the expected volume. One should hold the needle in place

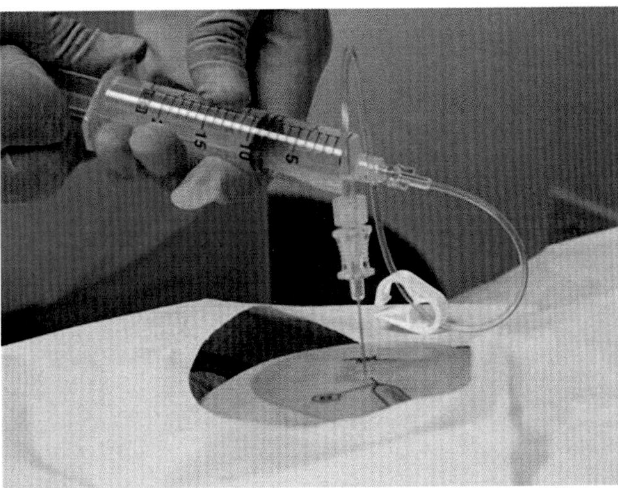

Fig. 42.9 The infusate should be delivered in small increments with frequent aspiration to assure that the needle does not slip outside of the lumen

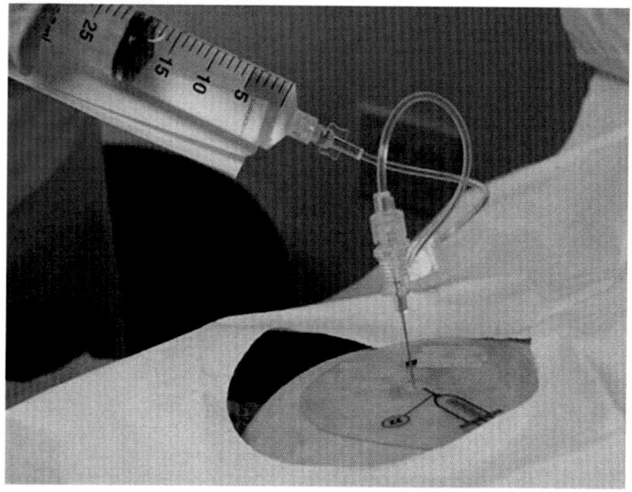

Fig. 42.10 An example of pump refill using sterile morphine with intermittent aspiration and filling

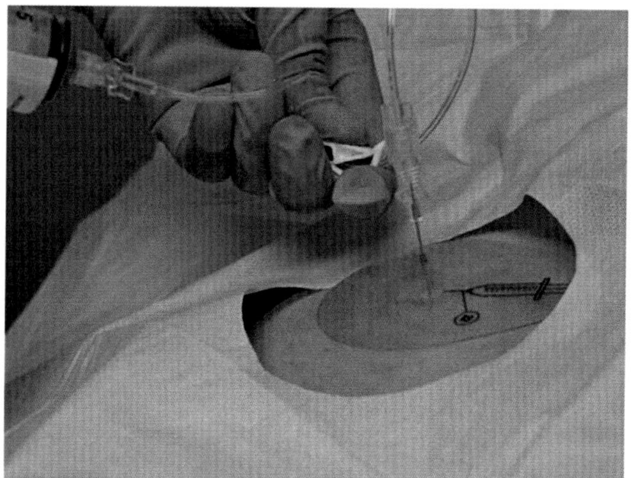

Fig. 42.11 The tubing should be clamped off prior to removing the needle to avoid drug leaking into the surrounding tissue

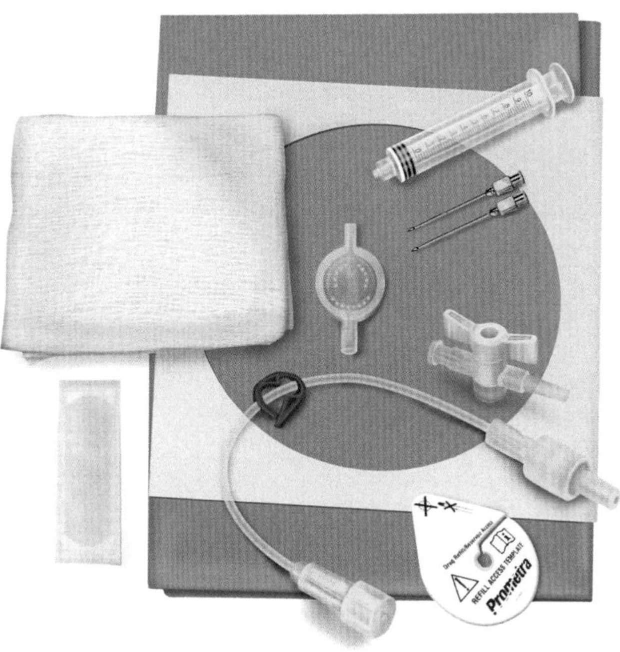

Fig. 42.12 A sample pump refill kit for the Prometra pump, including syringe with cap, stopcock, extension tubing with clamp, fenestrated drape, fenestrated sterile drape, filter, non-coring needs, refill template

Suggested Reading

Codman 3000. Updated 2003. Available at http://www.codmanpumps.com/PDFs/Chemo03.pdf.

Gofeld M, McQueen CK. Ultrasound guided intrathecal pump access and prevention of pocket fill. Pain Med. 2011;12:607–11.

Medtronic SynchroMed II Infusion System: Programming Reference Guide. Available at https://professional.medtronic.com/wcm/groups/mdtcom_sg/@mdt/@neuro/documents/documents/pump-nvsn-quik-gd.pdf.

Prometra 3rd Generation Implantable Device: North American Neuromodulation Society (NANS) 2013 presentation. Prometra product information. Available at: http://www.fda.gov/MedicalDevices/ProductsandMedicalProcedures/DeviceApprovalsandClearances/Recently-ApprovedDevices/ucm293502.htm.

Shankar H. Ultrasound guided localization of difficult to access refill port of the intrathecal pump reservoir. Neuromodulation. 2009;12:215–8.

43 Complications of Intrathecal Drug Delivery

Karina Gritsenko, Veronica Carullo, and Timothy R. Deer

43.1 Introduction

Intrathecal pumps are an option that allows patients who suffer from moderate-to-severe pain to have an improvement in quality of life, reduction in pain, improvement in systemic side effects, and change in function. They also are an option for patients who are at the end of life to improve alertness, reduce fatigue and nausea, and improve survival in the cancer population. This has been noted to be both clinically beneficial and cost effective, especially in those patients who are expected to survive longer than 6 months [1]. Unfortunately, despite the many positive attributes of these devices, they are not without risks. The complications can be classified as surgical, device related, or drug related. This chapter focuses on the complications of intrathecal drug delivery and options to assess and reduce risks (Fig. 43.1).

The reported incidence of adverse events range from 3 to 24 %, most of which are minor and related to the drug infused. The risks of serious events such as neural injury appear to be markedly less than 1 %. The majority of device complications occurs with the pump at the time of implant and maintenance of the therapy, including refills and programming.

K. Gritsenko
Montefiore Medical Center, Albert Einstein College of Medicine, 3400 Bainbridge Avenue, MMC-MAP, Room LL400, Bronx, NY 10467, USA
e-mail: karina.gritsenko@gmail.com

V. Carullo
Pediatric Pain Management Service, Montefiore Medical Center, Albert Einstein College of Medicine, Bronx, NY, USA
e-mail: vcarullo@montefiore.org

T.R. Deer, MD (✉)
The Center for Pain Relief, 400 Court Street, Suite 100, Charleston, WV 25301, USA
e-mail: DocTDeer@aol.com

T.R. Deer, J.E. Pope (eds.), *Atlas of Implantable Therapies for Pain Management*, DOI 10.1007/978-1-4939-2110-2_43

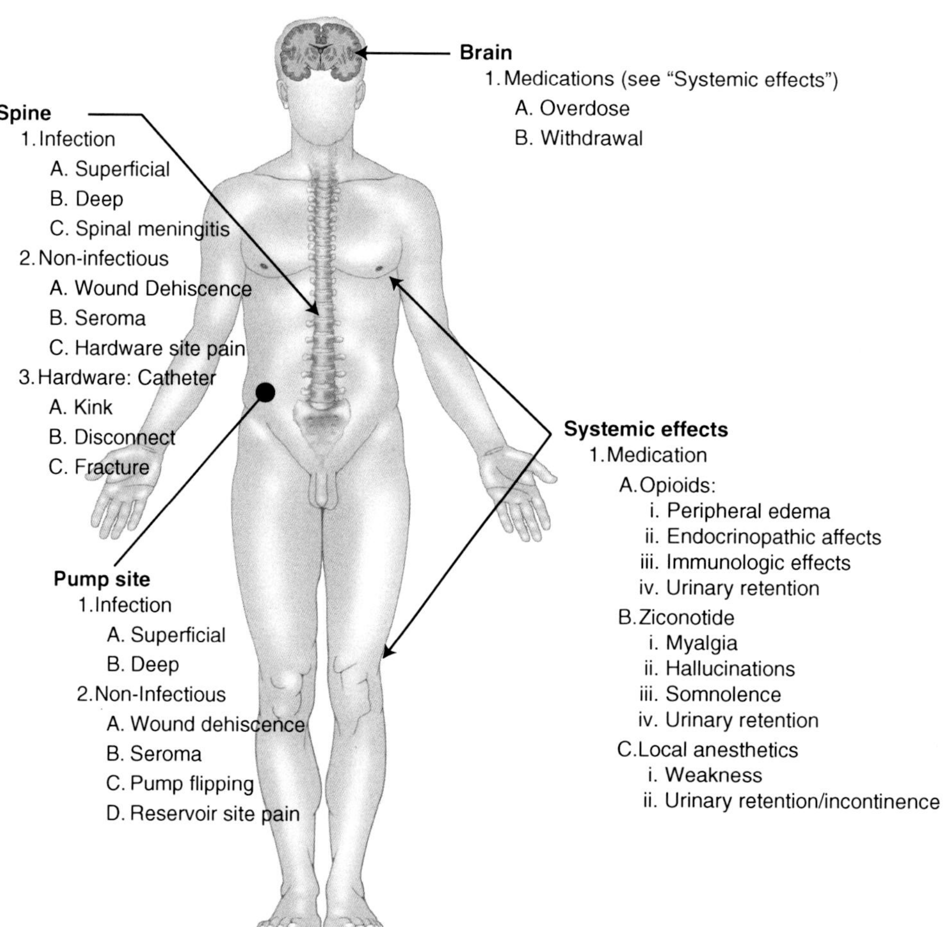

Fig. 43.1 Intrathecal drug delivery may have advantages to systemic drug delivery

43.2 Complications Associated with the Neuraxis

Intrathecal drug delivery involves the placement of a needle and catheter into the thecal sac. This can lead to an injury to the spinal cord, nerve root, or other neuraxial tissue, along with bleeding. Certainly, prior to the consideration of an intrathecal pump placement, the practitioner must consider the complexity of the anatomical spinal space, including spinal stenosis or arachnoiditis, into which the pump is to be implanted because disease pathology, medical characteristics, and variations in spinal anatomy may complicate the procedure.

At the time of placement, it is important to keep the patient as responsive and cogent as possible during needle placement, along with catheter placement, within the intrathecal space. A theoretical risk could include direct injury of the spinal cord; the risk of needle injury is much more likely when the needle entry is above the conus medullaris, which is usually located at L1. Direct needle injury of the spinal cord or the exiting nerves below this level is highly unlikely because the nerves float in the cerebrospinal fluid (CSF) and are usually pushed away by the needle approach, especially if the needle is advanced in the lateral fluoroscopic view and a blunt-tip needle is employed. The catheter can be threaded directly into the conus medullaris or other portions of the spinal cord, causing a new radicular pain, best treated with immediate withdrawal and an attempted repass of the catheter, underscoring the importance of catheter placement in an awake patient, if possible.

Infectious complications are uncommon, but these may include epidural abscess or intrathecal infection/meningitis. Superficial infections may occur at the reservoir site or neuroaxilla near catheter placement and anchoring. Reports of viral-induced transverse myelitis have been reported with pump catheters, but these reports are difficult to differentiate from chemical injury to the tissue. As a precaution perioperative antibiotic use, typically gram-positive coverage, is essential prior to pump placement. Antibiotic irrigation is also used by some practitioners [2]. If an infection is discovered within the neuraxial space (as opposed to a superficial wound infection), it is essential to remove both catheter and pump to prevent ongoing infection or progression and to consult a local infectious disease specialist.

In terms of later postoperative neuraxial complications, it is also possible for neurological sequelae to occur with the formation of granuloma, particularly with long-term use of high-concentration or high-dose opioids. Granuloma is a noninfectious inflammatory mass that appears to be a chronic fibrotic that develops at the tip of the intrathecal catheter with clinical presentations ranging from an asymptomatic problem to a major insult that can cause compressive symptoms. Fortunately, inflammatory masses develop slowly over time and in many cases are detected early based on the development of new clinical signs and symptoms, namely loss of treatment efficacy or new neurological symptoms or signs. The most common clinical presentations are loss of effect, sensory changes, pain in the distribution of the catheter tip, and loss of proprioception. Motor loss usually occurs late in the progression and may increase the urgency of intervention.

The cause of granuloma appears to occur from the long-term use of high-concentration opioids or high daily doses of opioid medications and may represent an example in pharmacokinetic failure based on new insights garnered from CSF hydrodynamics. The most commonly reported opioids are morphine and hydromorphone. In a recent analysis, a consensus panel recommended reducing the drug concentrations when possible to a concentration of morphine not greater than 20 mg/mL and the concentration of hydromorphone not greater than 15 mg/mL, which was increased from the 2007 consensus conference recommendations. In addition to reducing the concentration of opioids, other theories have been developed including using smaller, more lipophilic, molecules such as fentanyl and sufentanil or adding bupivacaine to reduce the dose of opioid required, which has been reflected in the 2012 Polyanalgesic Consensus Conference guidelines (see Chap. 41). Some have theorized a protective effect of clonidine in reducing the formation of granuloma, but this has not been proven prospectively.

There has been one case of granuloma formation with ziconotide reported to the U.S. Food and Drug Administration (FDA) between January 2004 and October 2012 of the 1,753 granuloma formations reported in total, although the case is clouded by prior opioid therapy before ziconotide initiation and granuloma discovery. Thus the relative safety of ziconotide, with regards to granuloma formation, is still quite favorable. In 2010 there is one published case report in the European literature describing a patient who developed two sequential granuloma formations with a ziconotide intrathecal pump within a 10-month period.

The diagnosis of either abscess or granuloma is confirmed by magnetic resonance imaging (MRI), but physical examination and history are very important in making the initial diagnosis. The MRI may be diagnostic with gadolinium depending on the size and location of the mass. Computed tomography (CT) myelogram is an option if the patient has a contraindication to MRI (e.g., cardiac pacemaker, insulin pump, neurostimulator, cochlear implant).

Another complication that can occur is a CSF leak, which may occur in as many as 20 % of patients with intrathecal drug delivery systems [2]. Such leaks may present clinically with symptoms of a post–dural puncture headache (PDPH; e.g., nuchal rigidity, positional headache). Treatment is similar to that of any patient with a PDPH (e.g., caffeine, fluids, conservative management), but interventional epidural blood patch may be pursued with caution to avoid any possibility of intrathecal catheter damage.

43.3 Complications Involving Nonspinal Tissues

Infection of the pump or catheter can lead to explant of the device. The rate of infection varies from practice to practice but is reported from 0 to 4.5 % globally for surgical procedures. Infection is obvious in some cases with redness, purulent drainage, and swelling, but in some cases it may be difficult to differentiate from postoperative skin irritation. The presence of a fever, elevated white blood count with a left shift in neutrophiles, elevated C-reactive protein, and elevated erythrocyte sedimentation rate raises the index of suspicion toward an infectious process. The diagnosis may be confirmed by Gram stain and culture. The diagnosis can be confusing in the immunocompromised patient, such a patient on long-term steroids or a patient with advanced cancer, because the tissue reaction and blood marker elevations may be blunted. In addition to device infection, the clinician should consider other more common sources of fever, such as atelectasis, urinary tract infection, and drug reaction in the acute postoperative, postimplantation period. Vigilance is paramount when managing a suspected infection, and clinical signs and symptoms of an infection are present, it is recommended to manage the patient conservatively and consider explantion of the device.

The noninfectious buildup of serosanguineous fluid, termed seroma, may impede the ability of the wound to heal. This may be very similar to an infection in tissue appearance and may be associated with an elevation of the white blood count. Diagnosis is confirmed by aspiration of straw-colored noninfectious fluid. Seroma formation can be lessened by limited aggressive blunt dissection, the use of sharp dissection, excellent hemostasis, closure of deadspace, and use of compression postoperatively, commonly via an abdominal binder. Treatment may include surgical drainage, simple aspiration, or conservative management.

Although extremely rare, bleeding from the pocket reservoir site or spinal incision can lead to wound dehiscence, pain, and the need for surgical drainage. Diagnosis is made by an expanding wound with pain or by frank bleeding. Small hematoma formation is possible, but an expanding wound may require further intervention. Subdural migration has been reported and can lead to decreased efficacy or in some cases overdose. In addition subdural hematoma is a rare but possible occurrence and presents clinically with severe headache and neurological sequelae requiring urgent surgical intervention. Transverse myelitis has been associated with intrathecal catheters in very rare situations. If a progressive myelopathy develops in the presence of a normal MRI, a neurology consult should be obtained.

The pump can cause pain because of flipping in the tissues, contact with bony landmarks, or erosion of the device through the skin. Erosion is most commonly associated with significant weight loss and a diminished subcutaneous adipose layer. This may develop from an overall decrease in body mass index or by redistribution of fat with aging or diseases. Also, if a pump becomes flipped, this may inhibit the ability to refill the pump with maintenance drug without the use of image guidance and may require acute intervention to prevent medication withdrawal side effects.

43.4 Complications Involving the Catheter

Historically, the most common type of hardware complications in intrathecal drug delivery systems are catheter related. Possible problems seen with intrathecal catheters include kinking, fracture, leak, and migration. Migration of the catheter is rare if proper anchoring and purse-string suturing are utilized. The movement of the catheter out of the spinal canal can lead to loss of pain relief or withdrawal from the infused drug.

Catheter kinking, scarring, and leakage can lead to multiple clinical problems. The problem is suspected with the loss of clinical efficacy, because a higher than suspected volume of the pump reservoir at the time of refill is not clinically reliable. The workup includes a side-port catheter evaluation under fluoroscopy, where an aspiration is attempted from the catheter side port. If 2 mL is able to be withdrawn freely from the catheter, then dye is injected to perform a myelogram surrounding the catheter to inspect for filling defects. If the side-port study suggests a noncongruent system within the intrathecal space, surgical exploration and catheter revision are recommended.

Advancements in catheter technology have remedied some of the historical challenges with catheter malfunctions

43.5 Complications Involving the Implanted Device

Intrathecal pump patients require intermittent refills to continue to deliver drugs, as the reservoir is depleted with slow continuous infusion. This process requires access to the Silastic port. The risks of refill include infection, seroma formation, inadvertent catheter access, inadvertent deposit of drugs outside the pump, termed a "pocket fill," and inability to access the pump. The risk of infection can be significantly reduced by maintaining appropriate sterile technique and using a bactereostatic filter; there may be additional antibacterial effects of local anesthetics themselves when included in the infused agent. Infections appear to be less than 1 in 1,000 when proper technique is used.

Most commonly, the body creates a fibrous pocket around the pump and may stabilize the device. In patients with poor tissue integrity, such as patients with cancer, diabetes, active smokers, and long-term steroid therapy, formation of this pocket may not develop and the device may be prone to flipping and to creating discomfort. These patients may require a Dacron pouch around the pump to establish a localized tissue reaction or placement of "stay sutures" through the suture loops of the device reservoir. Ultimately these patients may require surgical adjustment if the pump is unable to be returned to its proper position.

Rotor failure is a risk of currently approved programmable pumps manufactured by Medtronic (Minneapolis, MN). The problem can be diagnosed by an x-ray after the pump is programmed to give a bolus that will result in a turn of the rotor on films if it is functioning correctly. Motor stalls occur more commonly when off-label medications are employed within the pump, either in combination or as monotherapy. Newly developed devices, such as the Prometra Programmable Infusion Pump system (Flowonix; Mt. Olive, NJ), approved in 2012, employs a valve-gated system that is nonperistaltic and may mitigate the challenges with off-label therapy. Another pump company innovation by Codman (Codman and Shurtleff; Raynham, MA) allows to access the actual volume in the computer without aspirating the pump, as compared with current methods of pump volume as determined by health care provider input. Because this is a relatively newly approved device, complications of these new pump mechanisms are not currently known, and careful observation will be necessary when these products become commercially available.

Typical intrathecal pumps contain a pump side port with a main pump access port entered by noncoring needles that reduce trauma to the materials. These needles are specific to the port of intended refill to reduce the risk of inadvertent refill into the wrong port. Unfortunately, but thankfully very uncommon, the pump can experience failure of the lumen or side port over time that leads to a leakage of drug and a need for a surgical revision.

Patients with drug abuse histories can sometimes be treated successfully with a pump, although pump maintenance and candidacy requires medical compliance. Although intrathecal therapy and use of the patient therapy manager provides the clinician a greater amount of control, all patients with potential risk for drug diversion, secondary gain, or substance abuse should be rigorously screened prior to pump implantation and closely monitored throughout treatment if intrathecal pump implantation is deemed an appropriate therapy.

43.6 Complications Involving Administered Agents

Long-term opioid infusions can lead to complications (Tables 43.1 and 43.2). A multicenter analysis of complications has shown that these complications can affect several body systems. Intrathecally administered opioids cause multiple side effects including nausea and vomiting (25.2 %), pruritus (13.3 %), edema (11.7 %), diaphoresis (7.2 %), weakness (7.2 %), weight gain (5.4 %), and diminished libido (4.9 %).

Peripheral edema is a rare, but bothersome, side effect from opioid infusions. The mechanism appears to be related to a direct effect on the pituitary from intrathecal opioids involving antidiuretic hormone. Clonidine is active at the alpha receptors. This drug can cause hypotension and somnolence. It can be rarely associated with severe rebound hypertension with the sudden withdrawal or reduction.

Ziconotide (SNX-111) is a synthetic analogue of an *N*-type voltage-dependent calcium channel blocker that is the only FDA-approved nonopioid-based medication to treat chronic pain. Common adverse events include dizziness, drowsiness, psychosis, tinnitus, nausea, and fatigue. Caution should be exercised in those patients with a previous history of psychosis or suicidality. Using a slow titration protocol may dramatically reduce the adverse event incidence with this drug.

When refilling the pump, the physician and the nursing staff must be vigilant in ensuring that the drug placed is the intended drug at the intended concentration and dose. Coffey and Burchiel [3] reported increased mortality with intrathecal drug delivery, as compared with spinal cord stimulation or lumbar discectomy, and all events were iatrogenic and included medication programming errors or overdose. Policies and procedures that reduce the risk of this problem should be in place.

Table 43.1 Frequency of complications associated with intrathecal drug delivery

Complication	Reported frequency (%)
Constipation	50
Difficulty urinating	42.7
Nausea and vomiting	24.4–36.6
Impotence	26.8
Nightmares	23.2
Pruritus	13.3–14.6
Edema	6.1–11.7
Diaphoresis	7.2–8.5
Weakness	7.2
Weight gain	5.4
Diminished libido	4.9

Table 43.2 Complications reported with short-term intrathecal infusion of Ziconotide (SNX-111) [4]

	Patients, *n* (%)	
Complication	Ziconotide ($n=72$)	Placebo ($n=40$)
Patients with any adverse event	70 (97.2)	29 (72.5)
Patients with any serious adverse event	22 (30.6)	4 (10.0)
Cardiovascular system	24 (33.3)	4 (10.0)
Postural hypotension	17 (23.6)	2 (5.0)
Hypotension	6 (8.3)	2 (5.0)
Nervous system	60 (83.3)	14 (35.0)
Dizziness	36 (50.0)	4 (10.0)
Nystagmus	33 (45.8)	4 (10.0)
Somnolence	17 (23.6)	3 (7.5)
Confusion	15 (20.8)	2 (5.0)
Abnormal gait	9 (12.5)	0
Urogenital system	23 (31.9)	0
Urinary retention	13 (18.1)	0
Urinary tract infection	7 (9.7)	0

43.7 Treatment of Complications Associated with Implanted Intrathecal Drug Delivery Systems

43.7.1 Treatment of Complications Involving the Neuraxis

Direct trauma to the spine or nerve roots is confirmed by MRI or CT. Once the problem is suspected, immediate neurosurgical consultation and intravenous steroids should be considered. If the catheter is in a location that may cause ongoing trauma, it should be removed when the patient is stable for surgical explant.

Ongoing CSF leak may lead to chronic headache, diplopia, and tinnitus. Treatment includes bedrest, fluids, and caffeine. If the problem persists, a blood patch should be considered, but careful attention should be given to maintain sterile technique, atraumatic needle placement, and avoidance of traumatizing the catheter with the blood patch needle. It is even possible to consider a subdural hematoma related to intrathecal placement.

Once a neuraxial infection is suspected, a workup must be rapidly initiated and treatment initiated. Physical examination should be in detail and with great vigilance. Additional workup includes a sample of CSF, an analysis of the white blood count, and sedimentation rate. Meningitis should be treated by infectious disease in accordance with the documented pathogen. Epidural abscess requires immediate surgical decompression.

Inflammatory mass varies in its presentation and required intervention. In all cases the granulomagenic medication needs to be minimized and discontinued. In small granulomas the management can consist of rotation to a different intrathecal agent and continued observation. As the mass size and clinical presentation become more worrisome, the options for treatment include catheter removal, catheter repositioning, and catheter revision to a new catheter. The need for neurosurgical debridement is rare and is generally only needed when motor symptoms develop.

43.7.2 Treatment of Complications Involving Nonspinal Tissues

The most common reason to replace an intrathecal pump is the battery being at the end of its life, which commonly occurs at approximately 7 years. The procedure seems simple, but if great care and attention is not taken, the outcome can be disastrous. The patient is at risk for drug overdose or withdrawal. In most reported cases of postoperative death, the cause has been a poor estimate of drug dosing. Appropriate attention should be given to careful postoperative respiratory monitoring including oxygen saturation as well as frequent neurological checks. Just as with placement of the device and introduction to the intrathecal route of therapy, intrathecal initiation of opioid-based medications requires 23-h observation. Baclofen withdrawal and opioid overdose are the two most common causes of significant problems in this patient group. Both of these problems can be limited with proper monitoring and patient evaluation.

The use of routine antimicrobial prophylaxis is controversial, but it has become increasingly common (Table 43.3). Treatment of superficial infections may be with oral antibiotics, incision and drainage, and observation. The more extensive infections involving the pocket require device removal.

Seroma treatment includes attention to reducing tissue trauma at the time of the implant. Once a seroma develops, treatment includes pressure to the wound, aspiration of the fluid, or in severe or recurrent cases, tissue exploration and drainage.

Postoperative bleeding can be reduced by preoperative evaluation and management of drugs that may affect blood clotting. Once a bleed occurs, treatment includes pressure to the wound, aspiration of the hematoma, or surgical exploration and evacuation.

Skin irritation from the device can lead to pain, swelling, cellulitis, and eventual loss of the device. Treatment should be aggressive and involves wound exploration, pocket revision, and the consideration of a smaller pump if available.

Table 43.3 Recommended antibiotic prophylaxis prior to implantation of an implanted intrathecal drug delivery system [5]

Antibiotic	Dose and administration
Cefazolin	1–2 g IV 30 min prior to incision
Clindamycin (β-lactam–allergic patients)	600 mg IV 30 min prior to incision
Vancomycin (methicillin-resistant *Staphylococcus aureus* [MRSA] carriers)	1 g IV over 60 min prior to incision

43.7.3 Treatment of Complications Involving the Catheter

Treatments of catheter complications are dependent on the cause of the problem. In most cases the catheter has to be revised, but the scope of revision may vary based on the problem. In the event that the problem is at the spinal incision or in the spine, revision can be performed at that level with a splicing of the catheter from the spine to the existing catheter to the pump. In cases in which the problem is less certain, the revision must involve the entire catheter. In some instances the problem occurs at the pump connector. Although uncommon, this problem is suggested when the pump pocket has swelling in the setting of reduced efficacy in the absence of a seroma and can be identified radiographically. A dye study may be necessary once the revision is completed to ensure no problems exist downstream in the distal catheter. The clinician should open the pocket and, if the problem is at the connector, a revision can occur at the area within the pocket.

43.7.4 Treatment of Complications Involving the Implanted Device

Excessive tension on the margins of the wound, along with inadequate depth of the device, can lead to skin breakdown, cellulitis, erosion, and dehiscence. To prevent this complication, the size of the pocket should be adequate to avoid tissue tension. The wound should be brought together without the need for any forced skin movement. The wound margins should have apposition that is uniform. If proper wound planning and management is performed, a pump can be placed in patients with low body mass index without complications. This group includes patients with malignancy, children with spasticity, and patients with conditions that cause a low protein balance. In this select group, the pump may need to be placed in other locations.

Flipping of the pump can occur resulting in difficulty or impossibility of filling the pump and failure of the catheter secondary to twisting and kinking. The problem can be reduced by proper pocket sizing, anchoring of the pump with suture loops, or sewing in a Dacron pouch. Treatment includes revision of the device and pocket. The most common causes of these problems include weight gain and poor tissue integrity secondary to chronic disease.

Mechanical failure of the pump is a complication that is resolved by pump replacement. Pump replacement is also required if the pump develops a leak from the side port or main port.

43.7.5 Treatment of Complications Involving Administered Agents

The use of intrathecal agents can be very helpful in the majority of patients. As with any route of delivery, a side effect profile exists with drugs even when used properly. This problem cannot be avoided in the patient receiving intrathecal agents, but by using thoughtful algorithmic approaches, the risks can be reduced. When problems develop, the clinician should use techniques to reduce the number of side effects. These techniques include testosterone replacement, diet changes to treat constipation, diuretics, compression stockings for edema, and medications to treat disruptions of sleep.

When the patient experiences side effects from an intrathecal agent, options include dose reduction, addition of an adjuvant drug to produce synergistic effects, drug rotation to an alternative agent, or reduction and removal of all intrathecally administered drugs.

43.8 When to Seek Consultation

Consultation should be considered in the preoperative period to optimize coexisting disease states. Consultation is encouraged with an infectious disease specialist in the high-risk patient or postoperatively should a problem develop. Neurosurgical or neurology consultation should be considered when any change occurs in the neurological function in the postoperative period or over time with continued therapy.

43.9 Risk Assessment

1. Complications are more common in patients with coexisting diseases, such as diabetes, connective tissue disorders, and cancer. Drugs that affect blood clotting can result in neuraxial bleeding or bleeding of the pocket and should be evaluated. Diseases that can affect bleeding should be evaluated with proper laboratory evaluations. Anticoagulation guidelines via the American Society of Regional Anesthesia should be used for appropriate assessment of therapy perioperatively.
2. Skin diseases can lead to a propensity to develop superficial infection, wound dehiscence, and loss of device.
3. Patients with a history of pedal edema, venous varicosities, or vascular disease may be at a higher risk of developing complications of lower extremity swelling from intrathecal drug infusions.
4. Patients who have an equivocal trial are at a high risk of eventual failure. Likewise, patients who are psychologically unstable should be approached with caution.
5. Obese patients are at a higher risk of developing problems with the pocket and have more difficulty in placing catheters into the spinal canal.
6. In emaciated patients, the risk of skin irritation and eventual erosion through the tissue is a high risk.

43.10 Risk Avoidance

1. Any coexisting disease should be optimized prior to moving forward with the device. Because many patients have significant problems, the time to move forward should be decided by the physician managing the disease. In some very ill patients such as those with advanced malignancy, the ability to optimize the disease process may be limited.
2. In patients with a high risk of bleeding, preoperative laboratory evaluation should be carefully reviewed with a focus on platelet function and clotting indices. The primary care physician or cardiologist should be consulted to optimize any disease states and to give an opinion on the management of drugs that may increase the risk of bleeding.
3. When the skin is abnormal in the area of the planned surgery, the procedure should be delayed until proper skin treatment is performed. In some cases the pocket is placed in an area other than the abdomen in order to find a place for an implant.
4. Intrathecal drug delivery has been associated with pedal edema in a small percentage of patients. The patient should be managed closely with limb elevation, compression stockings, and diuretics. The eventual treatment is drug dose reduction or drug change.
5. The intrathecal trial should produce 50 % relief of pain based on the visual analog scale, should produce side effects that are acceptable and manageable, and in noncancer patients should produce an improvement in function. The patient should be cleared by a psychologist or psychiatrist prior to implant. Patients should have concurrent treatment for psychiatric comorbidities, including depression, anxiety, drug abuse, and borderline personality disorder.
6. The obese patient may require longer needles, extended tunneling rods, and pocket modification. The best method of risk avoidance is to plan ahead to prepare for these changes in the procedure. The pocket location may be modified to an area that will be less likely to cause flipping with patient sitting and movement.
7. The patient with low body fat is a challenge for both initial implant and long-term management.

Conclusions

Intrathecal drug delivery is a viable treatment to chronic pain and has proven superior to repeat spinal surgery in many circumstances. Like spinal cord stimulation, intrathecal drug delivery has proven efficacious, cost-effective, and satisfying to many patients with chronic and cancer-related pain. The prevention, recognition, and treatment of complications are a vital part of the successful use of these devices. With proper vigilance, the implanting physician can provide advanced care with outcomes that are acceptable to both the patient and society.

43.11 Supplemental Images

See Figures 43.2, 43.3, 43.4, 43.5, 43.6, 43.7, 43.8, and 43.9.

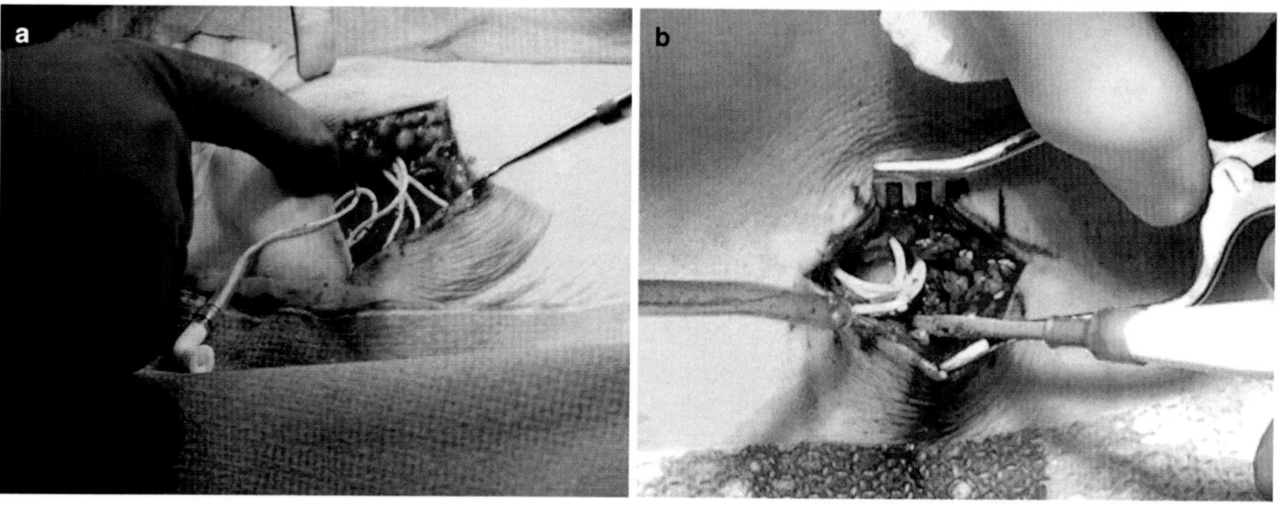

Fig. 43.2 (a) Catheter migration can lead to a malfunction of the system. (b) Catheter migration

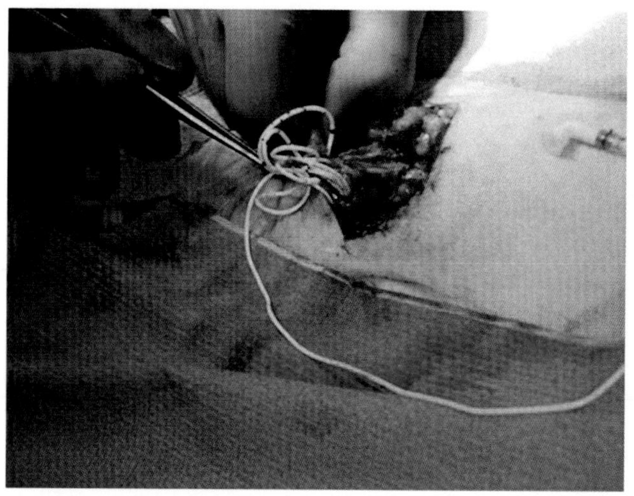

Fig. 43.3 Catheter revision can be difficult when fibrosis develops in the pocket. This may be more extreme in those cases where a Dacron pouch is implanted to add stability to the pump location

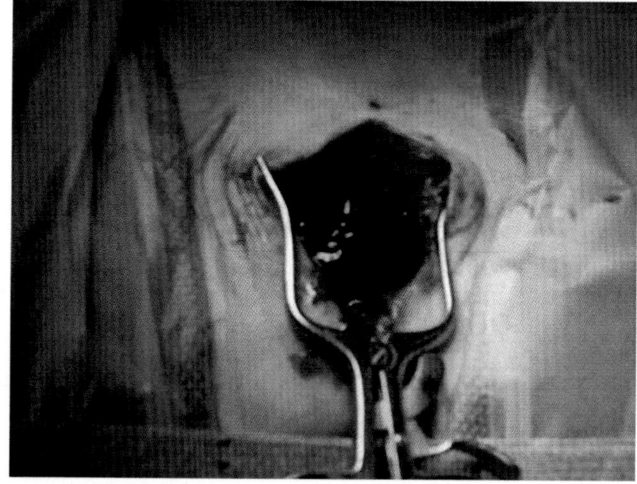

Fig. 43.4 Pocket hematoma can lead to wound swelling and dehiscence. Surgical incision and drainage may lessen the impact of this complication

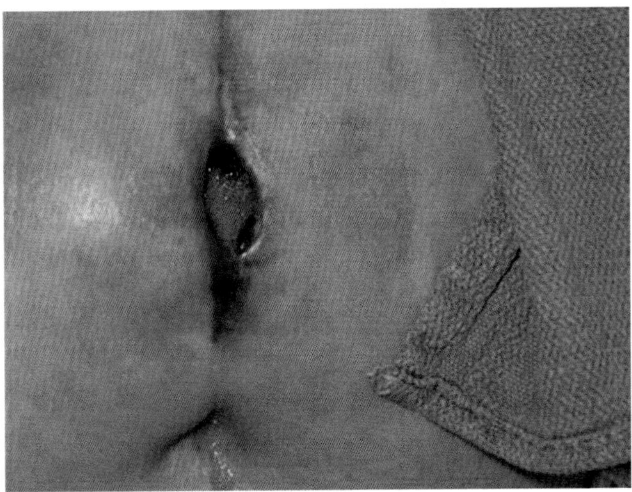

Fig. 43.5 Seroma of a wound can be a subtle finding and may be self-limiting, but if it increases in volume it may lead to wound separation and lead to a secondary infection

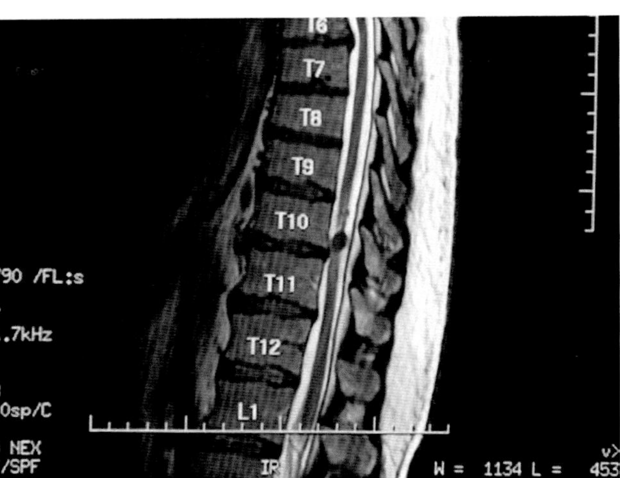

Fig. 43.8 Intrathecal granuloma at T10 creating a space-occupying lesion

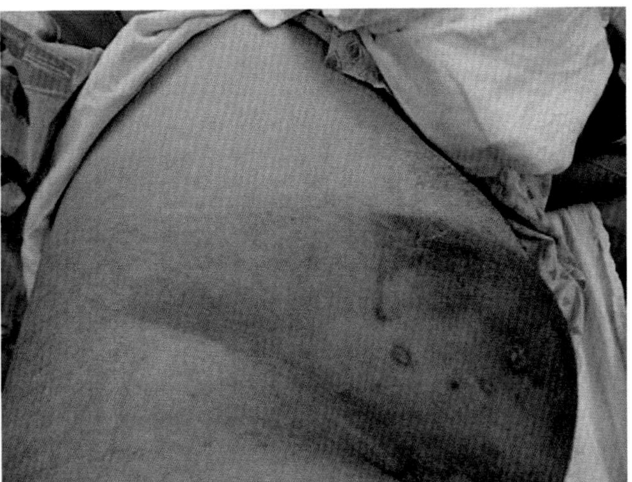

Fig. 43.6 Hematoma is a common occurrence after pump insertion and is normally self-limiting and does not cause longstanding complications

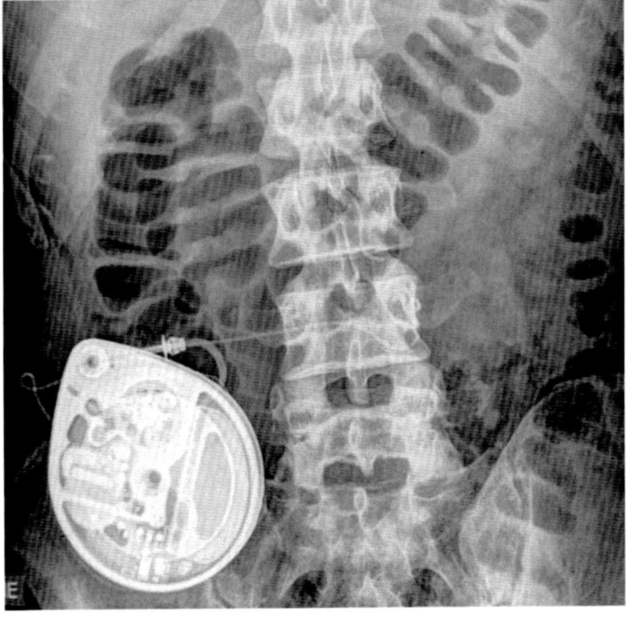

Fig. 43.9 Example of a catheter fracture

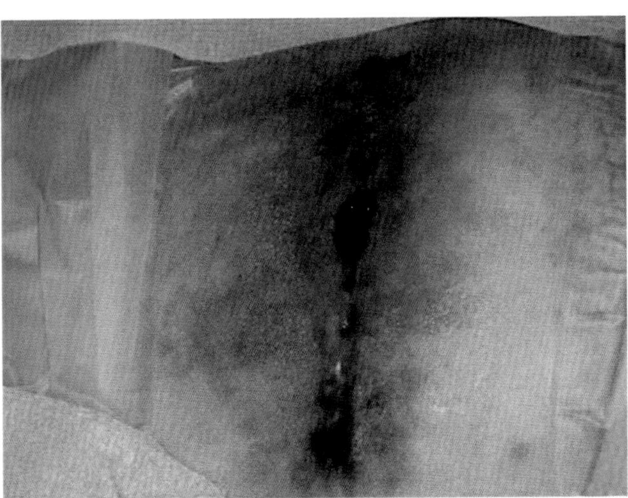

Fig. 43.7 Superficial hematoma may be treated with incision and drainage with preservation of the pump. Once the pump materials are exposed to the environment, the device should be removed

References

1. Hassenbusch SJ. Cost modeling for alternate routes of administration of opioids for cancer pain. Oncology (Williston Park). 1999;13:63–7.
2. Paice JA, Penn RD, Shott S. Intraspinal morphine for chronic pain: a retrospective, multicenter study. J Pain Symptom Manage. 1996;11:71–80.
3. Coffey RJ, Burchiel K. Inflammatory mass lesions associated with intrathecal drug infusion catheters: report and observations on 41 patients. Neurosurgery. 2002;50:78–86; discussion 86–7.
4. Staats PS, Yearwood T, Charapata SG, et al. Intrathecal ziconotide in the treatment of refractory pain in patients with cancer and AIDS. JAMA. 2003;291:62–70.
5. Rathmell JP, Lake TL, Ramundo MB. Infectious risks of chronic pain treatments: injection therapy, surgical implants, and intradiscal techniques. Reg Anesth Pain Med. 2006;31:346–52.

Suggested Reading

Deer T. A prospective analysis of intrathecal granuloma in chronic pain patients. A review of the literature and report of a surveillance study. An original contribution. Pain Physician. 2004;7:225–8.

Deer TR, Smith HS, Burton AW, et al. Comprehensive consensus base guidelines on intrathecal drug delivery systems in the treatment of pain caused by cancer pain. Pain Physician. 2011;14:E283–312.

Deer TR, Smith HS, Cousins M, et al. Consensus guidelines for the selection and implantation of patients with noncancer pain for intrathecal drug delivery. Pain Physician. 2010;13:E175–213.

Follett KA, Naumann CP. A prospective study of catheter-related complications of intrathecal drug delivery systems. J Pain Symptom Manage. 2000;19:209–15.

Harney D, Victor R. Traumatic syrinx after implantation of an intrathecal catheter. Reg Anesth Pain Med. 2004;29:606–9.

Hayek SM, Deer TR, Pope JE, et al. Intrathecal therapy for cancer and non-cancer pain. Pain Physician. 2011;14:219–48.

Huntoon MA, Hurdle MF, Marsh RW, Reeves RK. Intrinsic spinal cord catheter placement: implications of new intractable pain in a patient with a spinal cord injury. Anesth Analg. 2004;99:1763–5, table of contents.

Knight KH, Brand FM, Mchaurab AS, Veneziano G. Implantable intrathecal pumps for chronic pain: highlights and updates. Croat Med J. 2007;48:22–34.

Pope JE, Deer TR. Ziconotide: a clinical update and pharmacologic review. Expert Opin Pharmacother. 2013;14:957–66.

Thimineur MA, Kravitz E, Vodapally MS. Intrathecal opioid treatment for chronic non-malignant pain: a 3-year prospective study. Pain. 2004;109:242–9.

Winkelmuller M, Winkelmuller W. Long-term effects of continuous intrathecal opioid treatment in chronic pain of nonmalignant etiology. J Neurosurg. 1996;85:458–67.

Yaksh TL, Horais KA, Tozier NA. Chronically infused intrathecal morphine in dogs. Anesthesiology. 2003;99:174–87.

Index

A

Abdominal pain
- percutaneous method, epidural stimulation, 130
- postsynaptic dorsal column pathway, 130, 131
- risk assessment, 132
- risk avoidance, 132
- somatic nerves, 130
- surgical procedures, 129
- TAP block procedures, 130, 133
- transversus abdominis plane blocks with locacl anesthetic, 129–131
- ultrasound-guided subcostal approach, 130
- visceral nociceptive pathway, 130
- visceral/somatic, 129

Advanced pain care therapies, 249, 250
- candidates selection, factors of, 114
- chronic orchialgia, 113
- ilioinguinal nerve stimulation, 113, 117
- risk assessment, 119
- risk avoidance, 119
- sacral nerve root stimulation, 113, 115–117
- spermatic nerve stimulation, 113, 114, 117
- vas deferens stimulation, 117–118

American Society of regional anesthesia (ASRA), 16, 17

Anode guarding, 50

ASRA. *See* American Society of regional anesthesia (ASRA)

Auriculotemporal nerve
- artery and vein, 176
- occipital neural stimulation, 236
- PNS, 235
- temporomandibular joint, 176

B

Biomedical engineering, 151

Bioness stimrouter
- carpal tunnel syndrome, 215
- deploying lead anchor, 216
- EPT, 215
- lead implantation, 215–216
- nerves target, 215
- patient programmer, 215
- platinum-iridium alloy lead, 215
- PNS devices, 215
- post-traumatic/postsurgical neuropathic pain, 215
- skin closure, 216
- stimulation probe inserting, 216
- tunneling device inserting, 216

Bion implantable neurostimulator device
- CCH, 214
- chronic headache disorders, 214
- hemicrania continua (HC), 214
- PNS neurostimulation device, 214

Burst stimulation (Burst-SCS)
- advantages, 166
- Barolo mapping, 164
- pain care, 164
- pathway, 165
- risk assessment, 166
- risk avoidance, 166
- studies, 165
- *vs.* tSCS, 164

C

Candidacy for advanced therapies, 12

Catheter placement
- chronic pain, 198
- fascia, 258
- fibrosis, 269
- intrathecal pump, 279
- neuraxis, 303
- purse-string, 258
- resistance, 258
- superficial infections, 303

Cathodal stimulation
- depolarization, 50
- dual anode, 51

Cephalocaudal lumbosacral electrode placement
- coccygeal root, 126
- foot and pelvic root, 125
- individual lower extremity root, 126

Cerebrospinal fluid (CSF)
- catheter, 263
- cephalocaudal lumbosacral, 125
- fibrosis, 269
- headaches, 162
- hemostatic, 264
- hydrodynamics, 303
- needle placement, 255
- spinal cord, 141

Chronic cluster headache (CCH), 214

Chronic infusion
- abdominal wall, 254
- anesthesia technique, 258
- contraindications, 253
- cord injury, 258
- CSF, 258, 259
- decubitus, 254
- flow obstruction, 258
- fluoroscopic imagery, 254
- hemostatic solutions, 259, 260
- Injex deployment system, 260
- intrathecal therapy, 253
- intravenous antibiotics, 259
- long-term delivery, 253

T.R. Deer, J.E. Pope (eds.), *Atlas of Implantable Therapies for Pain Management*, DOI 10.1007/978-1-4939-2110-2

Chronic infusion (*cont.*)
nerve injury, 258
neurostimulator, 254
paraplegia, 258
pump placement, 259
purse-string suture, 260
ventral placement, 258
Chronic orchialgia, 113
Chronic pain, 159
carpal tunnel syndrome, 215
genitofemoral nerves, 176
hyperalgesia and allodynia, 152
iliohypogastric nerves, 176
intrathecal drug delivery, 309
PNS, 69
psychology, 20
sacral transforaminal, 115
SCS, 159
Chronic shoulder pain treatment. *See also* Motor cortex stimulation (MCS)
rotator cuff syndrome, 191
suprascapular nerve, 192
Closed-loop feedback systems, 147
Coagulopathy, 16–17
Coccygeal root placement, 126
Complex regional pain syndrome (CRPS), 7–8, 11, 12, 151
intractable pain, 151
nerve injury, 185
neuropathic pain, 191
SCS, 7
spinal surgery, 7
Contralateral oblique view (CLO), 255, 258
Craniotomy
bone replacement, 230, 233
draping and planning incision, 230, 231
incision exposure, 230, 231
preoperative mapping, 230, 231
skull exposure, 230, 231
Cranium stimulation. *See* Deep brain stimulation (DBS)
C-reactive protein (CRP), 25
CRPS. *See* Complex regional pain syndrome (CRPS)
CSF. *See* Cerebrospinal fluid (CSF)

D

Deep brain stimulation (DBS)
central pain matrix modulation, 225
chronic pain, 225
frame-based/frameless stereotactic approach, 226
hemorrhages, 227
neuromodulation algorithm, 225
neuropathic and nociceptive character, 225
neurosurgical procedures, 227
Parkinson's disease and dystonia, 6
risk assessment, 227
subcutaneous pocket, 226
Dermatographic pain mapping, 182
Device implantation, 20
Device-related complications
device components, erosion of, 97
device flipping and generator pain, 97
lead migration, 97
loss of paresthesia capture, 97
painful/loss of stimulation, 97
Silastic anchor site, 97
Devices, SCS. *See* Needle placement
Disease state indications, SCS, 7, 8
burning/shooting pain, 11
chronic lumbar/cervical radicular pain, 11
congestive heart failure, 12
FBSS and CRPS, 11, 12
neurostimulation, 11
new therapies, 12
pain distributions, 12, 13
pain relief, 11
pelvic, rectal and anal pain, 12
probability, 12, 13
risk of failure, 12
Dorsal root ganglion (DRG)
bilateral L5 DRG placement, 156
biomedical engineering, advances in, 151
bipolar stimulation, 154
contralateral approach, 153
dermatomal organization, 152
dorsal root ganglionectomies, 152
internal pulse generator (IPG), 157
interventional pain therapy, 152
intraspinal lead placement, 154, 156
lead/stylet/sheath system, 153, 155
location, 153, 154
needle trajectory and lead placement, 153, 155
neuropathic pain syndromes, 153
peripheral nerve injury, 152
permanent therapy, 154
preoperative planning, 153
quadripolar DRG neurostimulation, 152, 153, 155
radiculopathies, 152
RF and pulsed RF techniques, 152
risk assessment, 157
risk avoidance, 157
Dorsal root ganglion spinal cord stimulation (DRG-SCS)
life-threatening complications, 157
neurostimulation, 3
PNS, 185
relieving pain, 148
residual limb pain algorithm, 205
stump pain group, 11
Dorsal root ganglion (DRG) stimulation, 109–110
Driving the lead. *See* Lead placement
Drug selection, intrathecal drug delivery
benefits, 290
hydromorphone, 288
morphine and ziconotide, 288
PACC guidelines, 288, 289
physicochemical properties, 288
research and development, 290
risk assessment, 290
risk avoidance, 290–291
safety factors, 288
spasticity, 287
traditional approach, 287

E

Electrical conduction nerve block
HFAC block, 206
inclusion, eligibility criteria, 207
Electrical modeling, 49, 50
Electric fish, 3
ElectroCore gammaCore, 220

Electromyographic (EMG) monitoring. *See also* Sacral root neuromodulation
  intraoperative application, 139
  specific muscles activation, 136
  spine surgery, 135
  SSEPs and MUAPs, 136
Epidural abscess
  diagnosis, 95
  risk factors, 95
  SCS, complications, 95
Epidural hematoma
  bleeding, 95
  diagnosis of, 95
  risk factors, 95
  weakness, 95
Epidural paddle approach, 107, 108
Epidural stimulation method
  guarded array placement, 106, 107
  percutaneous method, 130
  traditional lead placement, 106
Erythrocyte sedimentation rate (ESR), 25
ESR. *See* Erythrocyte sedimentation rate (ESR)
Evoked potentials
  EMG (*see* Electromyographic (EMG) monitoring)
  identification of PM, 136
  SSEP (*see* Somatosensory-evoked potential (SSEP))

F
Failed back surgery syndrome (FBSS), 7, 8, 151
Foot and pelvic root placement, 125
Foot pain. *See* Neuropathic foot pain
Frame-based/frameless stereotactic approach, 226

G
Granuloma
  cause, 303
  diagnosis, 303
  formation, 303
  intrathecal, 311
  medication, 307
Guidelines, 2012 PACC. *See* Polyanalgesic Consensus Conference (PACC)

H
High frequency stimulation
  electrical nerve block, 205, 211
  features, 159–160
  fluoroscope, 161
  frequencies, simulation, 161
  higher pulse rate, 159
  kyphosation, lumbar spine, 161
  lead position, 161
  neuromodulation, 209
  optimal placement, 160
  pain reduction, 206
  patient satisfaction, 159
  puncture, epidural space, 161
  risk assessment, 162
  risk avoidance, 162
  trial leads, 161
  Tuohy needle, 161

I
Ilioinguinal nerve stimulation, 113, 117, 199
  description, 113
  percutaneously access, 117
Implantable programmable generator (IPG), 146, 188, 195
Implantable pulse generator (IPG), 173
Implantable therapies
  DRG (*see* Dorsal root ganglion (DRG))
  SSIs (*see* Surgical site infections (SSIs))
Incision, wound healing, 90, 91
Individual lower extremity root placement, 126
Infection risk reduction, 23
Internal pulse generator (IPG), 77, 157
Intracranial techniques
  DBS, 227
  hemorrhage, 226, 227
Intrathecal catheters
  abdominal pocket, 268
  anchoring, 264
    CSF, 263
    Injex anchor, 265
    ligament/fascia, 263, 266
    long-term migration, 266
    long tubular anchor, 265
    lumbodorsal fascia, 265
    macaroni anchor, 265
    nonabsorbable suture, 269
    purse-string suture, 263, 264, 266
    Silastic anchors, 263
    tunneling, 266
    winged anchor, 265–267
  CSF, 264, 268
  fatty tissue, 264, 269
  fibrosis, 268
  granuloma, 303
  hemostatics, 264
  hygroma, 268
  muscle contraction, 268
  needle placement, 269
  pump placement, 249
  strain-relief loop, 264
  surgical revision, 263
  transverse myelitis, 304
  tunneling, 269, 271–277
Intrathecal drug delivery, 23, 25
  analgesics, 245
  bolus injections, 246
  catheter complication
    fracture, 311
    kinking, scarring and leakage, 304
    migration, 304, 310
    treatments, 308
  chronic diseases, 247
  complications, 301–311
    administered agents, 306, 308
    advantages, 301, 302
    adverse events, 301
    consultation, 309
    hematoma, 311
    implanted device, 305, 308
    intrathecal granuloma, 311
    neuraxis, 303, 307
    nonspinal tissues, 304, 307
    risk assessment and avoidance, 309
    seroma, 311

Intrathecal drug delivery (*cont.*)
- drug selection, 287–291
- hydrocephalus, 246
- infusion systems, 263, 269
- intrathecal pump, 293
- knee pain, 185
- lumbar spine, 246
- morphine, 245
- opioid receptors, 245
- persistent pain, 245
- pocketing, 279–285
- spinal anesthesia, 246
- subcutaneous tissue, 246

Intrathecal medication, 288
Intrathecal pumps
- maintenance, 293
- placement
  - advanced pain care, 249, 250
  - cancer/noncancer, 249
  - implantation, 251
  - infusion systems, 249
  - neuromodulation, 249
  - pain management, 249
  - spasticity, 249

Intrathecal therapy
- management, 288
- pump implantation, 249
- salvage therapy, 291

Invasive techniques, 188, 198
IPG. *See* Internal pulse generator (IPG)
IPG placement, 188, 189

K

Knee pain
- diagnostic nerve block, 187
- innervation, 185, 186, 188, 189
- neuropathic pathology, 185
- PNS, 185, 187
- SCS, 187

L

Laminotomy, 42
Lead fracture
- anterior and posterior views, 101
- risk assessment, 98
- risk avoidance, 100

Lead placement, 28, 30
- anchoring
  - angle of needle, 57
  - Clik™ anchor, 58–60
  - Deer–Stewart anchoring method, 58, 61
  - dual needles, 57, 59
  - fascia and ligament, 57, 59
  - Injex® bi-wing anchor, 58, 60
  - Injex® Bumpy anchor, 58, 60
  - Injex® dispenser tool, 58, 60
  - needle and stylet, 57
  - optimal stimulation, 58
  - patients, category, 57
  - risk assessment and avoidance, 61–62
  - and suturing materials, 61
  - Swift-Lock™ anchor, 58, 60
- angle of, 33
- anterior fusion, 38
- axial, radicular and cervical pain, 38
- bevel of needle, 33, 34
- curved stylet, 33, 35
- epidural obstructions, 34, 35
- hand-held computer screening, 34
- issues, 33, 35
- risk assessment and avoidance, 36
- straight stylet, 33, 35
- thoracic implantation, 37
- T8–10 vertebral bodies, 37
- x-ray, 38

Lumbar catheter techniques, 246
Lumbar transforaminal technique, 115

M

Material engineering, 147
Median nerve stimulation, 192, 193
Meralgia paresthetica syndrome, 177
Migraine
- headaches, 235
- neurostimulator device, 214
- occipital nerve, 5, 148

Miniaturization
- lead fracture/migration, 221
- neurostimulation, 220
- PNS, 213

Minnesota multiphasic personality inventory (MMPI), 20
Mixed paddle approach, 107, 108
MMPI. *See* Minnesota multiphasic personality inventory (MMPI)
Motor cortex stimulation (MCS)
- chronic pain, 229
- complications, 234
- DBS, 229
- dorsal column/peripheral nerve stimulation, 230
- electrophysiological mapping, 232
- epidural exposure, 232
- intracranial bleeding, 234
- lead placement, 232
- monitored anesthesia, 230
- neurological diseases, 229
- neuropathic pain, 234
- pectoralis fascia, 230
- postoperative radiographs, 233
- risk assessment, 234
- sensory cortex, 229
- SSEP waveforms, 231
- stimulation parameters, 230
- trial period stages, 230

Motor unit action potentials (MUAPs), 136, 142

N

Needle placement
- angle of, 28
- bleeding risks, 31
- catheter tunneling, 255, 256
- CLO, 255
- CSF, 255, 257
- epidural space, 28, 29
- fluoroscopic guidance, 28, 30
- granuloma, 255
- hanging drop technique, 28, 29
- headache risk, 31
- infection, 31

intrathecal placement, 255, 257
leads, 28, 30
ligament and fascia, 255
local anesthetic, 28
loss of resistance, 28, 29
nerve injury, 31
paramedian approach, 255
pump connection, 255
vigilance and planning, 27
Nerve root method
caudal approach, 107, 108
electromyogram/nerve conduction study, 107
epidural paddle approach, 107, 108
mixed paddle approach, 107–109
placement, 107, 108
retrograde approach, 107
Nerve targets, PNS
auriculotemporal nerves, 176
axillary nerves, 177
brachial plexus nerves, 177
cluneal and nerves, paravertebral region, 176–177
genitofemoral and iliohypogastric nerves, 176
ilioinguinal nerves, 176
infraorbital nerves, 175–176
intercostal nerves, 176
lateral femoral cutaneous nerves, 177
median nerves, 177
occiput, 175
other mixed nerves, 177
peroneal nerves, 177
radial nerves, 177
saphenous nerves, 177
superficial cervical plexus, 176
supraorbital nerves, 175
suprascapular nerves, 177
sural nerves, 177
tibial nerves, 177
trigeminal neuralgia, 176
ulnar nerves, 177
Neuraxis
epidural abscess, 95
epidural hematoma, 95
gross infection present at generator site, 95, 96
hematoma, 95
neurologic injuries, 95
postoperative cellulitis with early dehiscence, 95, 96
seroma, 95
spinal cord stenosis, 95
tissue trauma, 95
treatment, 96
Neurological dysfunction, 162
Neurological monitoring, spine surgery
EMG monitoring, 135
PMs (*see* Physiological midline (PM))
SSEP, 135
Neurologic injuries, 95
Neuromodulation, 151–152. *See also* Sacral root neuromodulation
anchoring, lead placement, 57–62
"dark ages," 3–4
DBS, 225
device, FDA approval, 6
disease state indications, 11–13
electromagnetic induction, 5
future trends
closed-loop feedback systems, 147
digital medicine, chronic disease, 145
DRG, 148
innovations, SMS, 145, 146
International Neuromodulation Society, 149
IPGs, 146
material engineering, 147
occipital nerve, 148
pain management, features of, 149
SPG, 148
stimulation frequency, 147
supraorbital nerve, 148
vagal nerve stimulation, 148
waveform delivery, 147
indications, SCS, 7–8
intrathecal therapy, 249
lead placement (*see* Lead placement)
MRIs, 9
paddle leads (*see* Paddle leads)
upper extremity, 191
Neuropathic foot pain
conservative measures and advanced techniques, 105
disease cause, 105
DRG stimulation, 109–110
epidural stimulation method, 106–107
lead placement options, 106
nerve root method, 107–109
risk assessment, 111
risk avoidance, 111
SCS, 105
Neuros Altius
HFAC block, 218
HFAC stimulator, 219
neurostimulation, 218
post-amputation nerve pain, 218
Neurostimulation. *See also* Abdominal pain
ancient/classical age, 3
axillary nerve, motor and sensory function, 192, 194
batteries, 4
bluetooth innovation, 3
cardioversion, 5
chronic shoulder pain treatment, 192
"electreat," 5
electrical current, 5
electrical force and distance, 4
electricity, 3–4
electromagnetism, 3
harnessing energy, 3–4
high-frequency stimulation, 5
infectious disease cures, 5
magnetic electrical machine, 5
magnetism, 5
median nerve stimulation, 192, 193
mesenchymal stem cells, 220
miniaturization, 220
modern, 6
peripheral ulnar nerve stimulation, 192
PNS, 191
radial nerve stimulation, 192
risk assessment, 195
SCS, 191
suprascapular nerve stimulation, 192, 194
torpedo fish, 4
in United States, 4
voltage alterations, 5
Neurosurgical laminotomy approach, 117

O

Occipital nerve stimulation, 148, 199, 200
Occipital neuralgia. *See* Peripheral nerve stimulation (PNS)
Optimization
- disease comorbidities, 15
- outcome, 210
- tonic stimulation therapies, 15

Overdose
- lumbar discectomy, 306
- opioid, 307
- pump programming, 295

P

PACC. *See* Polyanalgesic Consensus Conference (PACC)
Paddle leads
- axial and foot pain, 45
- configurations, 42, 43
- epidural space, 42, 43
- fluoroscopic guidance, 42, 43
- gluteal pocket, 42, 43
- indications, 41
- lumbar radiculopathy, 46
- risk assessment and avoidance, 44
- strain-relief loop, 42
- types, 42, 43

Paddle placement. *See* Paddle leads
Paresthesia
- direct nerve stimulation, 175
- IPG, 173
- joint, covering, 177
- PNfS, 174
- SCS, 176
- spinal lead, 173

Paresthesia free method, Burst-SCS, 164, 166
Paresthetic montage creation methods, 173
Patellar branch nerve stimulation, 177, 187
Patient comorbidities, 15, 20
Patient indications
- intrathecal pumps, 251
- nerve trauma, 190
- patient selection (*see* Patient selection, SCS)
- pump placement, 249

Patient selection, SCS
- indications, 7–8
- neuroaxial imaging, 9
- pain syndrome, 9
- pain types, 9
- pelvic, rectal and anal pain, 9
- risk of failure, 9

PDPH. *See* Post–dural puncture headache (PDPH)
Pelvic pain. *See* Advanced pain care therapies
Percutaneous implantation, 174–175
Percutaneous lead placement, 111
Percutaneous trialing methods, 173
Perioperative precautions, infection control. *See* Surgical site infections (SSIs)
Peripheral nerve field stimulation (PNfS)
- implantation, 178
- nerve targets (*see* Nerve targets, PNS)
- occipital/facial nerves, 174
- paresthesia, 174
- SCS anchors, 174
- skin infection, 177
- targets, placement, 172

Peripheral nerve stimulation (PNS), 77. *See also* Pocketing generator, peripheral nerve stimulation
- abnormal nerve function, 187
- advancements, 220, 221
- anterolateral thigh, lead placement, 182
- anteroposterior (AP), 236, 238
- bilateral knee pain, 181
- bion, 214
- central nervous system, 218
- cervical radiculitis, 235
- chronic postoperative knee pain, 181
- cryotherapy, 235
- cuff lead placement, 192
- A delta and C fibers, 173
- dermatographic pain mapping, 182
- direct nerve contact, 111
- DRG-SCS, 185
- electrocore system, 213
- experimental trial, 188
- fascia, anchoring, 180
- fascial graft creation, 188
- fluoroscopy, 236
- Halo technique, 239, 241
- headaches, 235
- hemostasis, 236
- humeral head trauma, 192
- infraorbital stimulation, 236, 239, 241
- internal pulse generator, 242
- invasive approach, 188, 209
- lead placement, 111, 199
- local anesthetic placement, 179, 236
- musculoskeletal treatment, 242
- nerve block, relief, 215
- nerve targets (*see* Nerve targets, PNS)
- neuroanatomy, 236, 237
- neuromodulation, 205, 209
- neuropathic knee pain, 185
- neuropathic pain, mapping, 179
- neurostimulation, 213
- occipital nerve, 175
- patient marking, 179
- pectoral pocketing, 180
- percutaneous leads insertion, 179
- pinpoint method, 198
- pocket creation, 179
- proximity, axillary nerve, 182
- PRP, 220
- recovery time reducing, 221
- regenerative treatments, 220
- risk assessment, 177, 190
- selecting candidates, 172
- seroma infection, 190
- skin disorders, 242
- skin infection, 132, 177
- skin integrity, 190
- spinal-based systems, 191
- supratrochlear stimulation, 239, 240
- targets, placement, 172
- TRD, 188
- tunneling, 180
- ultrasound-guided (*see* Ultrasound guidance)
- upper extremity, 192
- zygomaticofacial nerve, 239

Peripheral ulnar nerve stimulation, 192
Periventricular grey matter (PVG)
- dorsal nucleus, thalamus, 225
- limbic system, 225

nociceptive pain, 225
single-lead stimulation, 226
Personality disorders, 20
Phantom limb pain, 7, 11, 205, 229
Physiological midline (PM)
EMG activation, specific muscles, 136
intraoperative electrophysiological monitoring equipment, 136
intraoperative EMG, SCS placement, 136
SSEPs and MUAPs, 136
thoracic paddle lead implantation, 136
Platelet-rich plasma (PRP), 220
PM. *See* Physiological midline (PM)
PNS. *See* Peripheral nerve stimulation (PNS)
PNS, advancements, 220, 221
PNS, implantation technique
cuff placement, 209
IPG, lead placement, 210
meticulous attention, 209
neuromodulation, 209
Pocket formation
blunt dissection, 280–281
body habitus, 281
collagen fibers, 280
electrocautery, 284
electrothermal dissection, 280
fascia, 280
fluoroscopy, 280, 283
gluteal incision, 43
hemostasis, 57, 59, 281
iliac spine, 280
implantation, 285
incision length, 285
intercostal nerves, 176
intrathecal pump, 279
Langer's lines, 280, 282
local infection, 280
monofilament suture, 280
pelvis, 284
PNS (*see* Pocketing generator, peripheral nerve stimulation)
renal disease, 280
reservoir placement, 285
seroma, 281
skin incision, 280
skin turgor, 280
sterile surgical tapes, 280
subcutaneous tissue, 279
trigeminal neuralgia, 176
tunneling, 279
wound dehiscence, 284
Pocketing generator, peripheral nerve stimulation
blunt dissection technique, 69
decision-making, 69
hemostasis, 70
incision depth, 69
Langer's lines, 69, 72
pocket site selection information, 69–71
posterior flank incision, 74
risk assessment and avoidance, 73–74
tunneling procedure, 70, 72
wound closure, 70, 75
wound healing, 75
Polyanalgesic Consensus Conference (PACC)
intrathecal agents
maximum concentration, 288
maximum dose, 289
starting doses, 288
neuropathic pain, 289
nociceptive pain, 289
Post-amputation pain
electrical nerve block, 205
HFAC block, 207
neuroma, 205
peripheral mechanisms, 206
phantom limb pain, 205
residual limb pain, 205
Post–dural puncture headache (PDPH)
chronic, 36
inadvertent dural puncture with, 95
risk-avoidance procedures, 31
Postmastectomy syndrome, 176
Postoperative cellulitis with early dehiscence, 95, 96
Post-operative surgical course, 89
Postsynaptic dorsal column (PSDC) pathway, 130, 131
Postthoracotomy syndrome, 176
Preimplantation testing
local anesthetic block, 208
neuroma, 208
palpation technique, 208
placebo effect, 208
ultrasound guidance, 208
upper extremity amputations, 208
Preoperative considerations
SCS
allergies, 18
cardiac issues, 18
coagulopathy, 16–17
cognition, 20
dermatological diseases, 18
diabetes mellitus, 18
education, 20
hypertension, 18
infection, 15–16
optimization, 15
physical, 19
prescriptions, 20
psychiatric and psychological, 20
radiological evaluation, 19
recommendations, 19
surgical procedure, 15
tonic stimulation therapies, 15
SSIs
risk factors, 24
Staphylococcus aureus, 24
weight-based dosing, antibiotics, 24
Programming, SCS
anode-driven hyperpolarization, 50
basics, 49
cathode-driven depolarization, 50
clinical example, 51–53
components, 50
lead placement, 49
risk assessment and avoidance, 54
waveform innovations, 55
PSDC. *See* Postsynaptic dorsal column (PSDC) pathway

R

Radial nerve stimulation, 192, 193
Radiofrequency (RF) and pulsed RF techniques, 152
Recalcitrant cases, 177
Rectal pain. *See* Advanced pain care therapies

Refills, intrathecal pump
computer telemetry, 296
evaluations, 293
fluoroscopic/ultrasound imaging, 294
intermittent aspiration and filling, morphine, 298
laser-guided fluoroscopy, 296
maintenance, 293
medication, 294
nonprogrammable, 294
Prometra pump, 294, 298
risk assessment and avoidance, 295
securing, needle, 297
skin abnormalities, 296
sterile drapes, abdomen, 296
sterile dressings, 296
sterile kits, 294
telemetry, 293
template, 297
tubing, 298
vigilance, 293
Reflex sympathetic dystrophy (RSD), 7, 11
Reservoir site, 303, 304
Residual limb pain, 205
Retrograde insertion
dual electrodes, 121, 124
dual epidural "lateral" approach, 121, 123
dual L2/3 needle tips, steep caudal view, 121, 123
electrode crossing midline level, 121, 122
electrode directed caudally, 121, 122
electrode posterior, 121, 123
electrode rotated to foramen, 121, 123
needle tip in steep caudal view, 121, 122
Retrograde technique, 115
Risk prevention
DBS, 227
MCS, 234
neurostimulation, 195
PNS, 178, 190
ultrasound guidance, 203

S
Sacral hiatus/caudal approach technique, 116
Sacral nerve root stimulation
description, 113
lumbar transforaminal technique, 115
neurosurgical laminotomy approach, 117
retrograde technique, 115
sacral hiatus/caudal approach technique, 116
sacral transforaminal technique, 115
Sacral root neuromodulation
bilateral pelvic stimulation, 142
conus medullaris, 141
EMG activation with postoperative-induced paresthesia-sacral paddle, 142, 143
permanent retrograde implantation, 142, 143
SSEP and EMG monitoring, 141
treatment, 141
Sacral transforaminal technique, 115
Selective nerve root stimulation (SNRS)
"anterograde" SCS, 121
cephalocaudal lumbosacral electrode placement, 125–126
"retrograde" electrode placement, 121–124
Seroma, 95, 98
Silastic anchor site, 97
SNRS. *See* Selective nerve root stimulation (SNRS)
Somatosensory-evoked potential (SSEP). *See also* Sacral root neuromodulation
recording
dermatomal testing, 135
functional integrity, nervous system, 135
and MUAPs, 136
Spermatic nerve stimulation, 113, 114, 117
SPG. *See* Sphenopalatine ganglion (SPG)
Sphenopalatine ganglion (SPG), 148
Spinal cord stenosis, 95
Spinal cord stimulation (SCS). *See also* Neuraxis; Neuropathic foot pain; Selective nerve root stimulation (SNRS)
Burst-SCS (*see* Burst stimulation (Burst-SCS))
chronic pain, 93
complications of, 93, 94
device-related complications, 97
disease state indications, 11–13
dorsal root ganglion, 3, 6
DRG (*see* Dorsal root ganglion (DRG))
education and training, 57
facial lead, 176
high-frequency (*see* High frequency stimulation)
indications, 7–8
innovations in, 146
lead placement, 33–38, 57–62
low-frequency, 159
needle placement, 27–31
neuromodulation, 172
neuropathic limb pain, 176
paddle leads, 41–46
paresthesia, 176
patient selection, 7–9
persistent back and leg pain management, 159
PM (*see* Physiological midline (PM))
PNfS, 174
pocketing generator, 69–75
pocket proximity, 174
preoperative considerations, 15–20
programming, 49–55
recalcitrant cases, 177
risk assessment
bleeding risks, 98
device flipping, loss of pain relief, 98
inadvertent dural puncture, 98
lead fracture, 98
lead migration, 98
neural injury during implantation, 98
pain at generator site, 98
perioperative comorbidities, 98
proper stimulation paresthesia, loss of, 98
seroma, 98
stenosis development, 98
wound infections, 98
risk avoidance
hematoma, 99
lead fracture, 100
lead migration, 99–100
medications, 98
pain at generator site, 99
pain relief, loss of, 100
paresthesia, loss of, 99
patient education and cooperation, 99
PDPH, risk reductions, 99
preimplant imaging, 99
preoperative antibiotics, 98
seroma formation, 99
vigorous irrigation, 99
wound infections, 99

SSIs, 23
tripolar paddle (*see* Tripolar paddle)
t-SCS (*see* Tonic spinal cord stimulation (t-SCS))
tunneling, 63–67
wound closure, 77–78
Spinothalamic tract (STT), 130
SSEP. *See* Somatosensory-evoked potential (SSEP)
STT. *See* Spinothalamic tract (STT)
Supraorbital nerve, 148
Suprascapular nerve stimulation, 192, 194
Surgery
auriculotemporal, 176
bleeding, 16–17
cervical spinal, 11
epidural hematoma, 95
infection, 24
intercostal nerves, 176
PNS, 213
radiation therapy, 90
SCS, 7
SSEP, 135
SSIs (*see* Surgical site infections (SSIs))
superficial cervical plexus, 90
Surgical leads. *See* Paddle leads
Surgical site infections (SSIs)
C-arm cover, 25
chlorhexidine gluconate, 25
healthcare costs, 23
implantable pain therapy, methods, 23
medical morbidity, 23
postoperative, 25
povidone-iodine, 25
preoperative, 24
Surgical techniques
wound closure (*see* Wound closure, suturing technique)
wound healing, 89–91
Suture abscess, 101

T

TAP. *See* Transversus abdominis plane (TAP)
Targeted drug delivery. *See* Intrathecal drug delivery
Targeting, driving the lead. *See* Lead placement
Techniques
anchoring, lead placement, 57–62
paddle placement (*see* Paddle leads)
sterile, 305, 307
tunneling, 63–67
Technologies
Bioness stimrouter, 213
Bion implantable neurostimulator device, 213
ElectroCore gammaCore, 220
electrocore system, 213
Neuros Altius system, 213
Thoracolumbar spinal cord stimulation. *See* Neurological monitoring, spine surgery
Tonic spinal cord stimulation (t-SCS)
deficits, 166
lateral pathway activation, 165
vs. Burst-SCS, 164
Traditional lead placement, 106
Transformed migraine, 175, 235–242
Transversus abdominis plane (TAP)
block procedure, 130, 133
stimulation, 130
Treatment-resistant depression (TRD), 188
Tripolar paddle
initial placement of, 137
lead placement and alignment, midline, 137, 138
T-SCS. *See* Tonic spinal cord stimulation (t-SCS)
Tunneling
anchoring, 63
angle of, 64
approaches, 63
decubitus position, 65, 66
depth, adipose tissue, 63
devices, 63
fluoroscopy, 63
initiation, lead insertion site, 64
intrathecal catheters
abdominal abnormalities, 271
analgesia, 272
bupivacaine, 272
cerebral spinal flow, 272
cluneal neuralgia, 272, 277
dorsal incision, 271
hematoma, 276
incision, 272
intrathecal pumps, 276
lead Placement, 272, 275
lidocaine, 272
local anesthetic placement, 272, 273
muscular fascia, 277
platelet function, 277
posterior pump placement, 276
pump pocket, 271, 272
skin marking, 272, 273
spinal canal, 271
spinal incision, 272, 274
landmarks, 64
lead position, generator pocket, 65
lead wiring, 70, 72
local anesthesia, 63, 64
muscle, abdominal cavity and pleura, 64
palpation, 65
posterior flank incision, 70, 73
risk assessment, 66
risk avoidance, 66–67
sterile technique, 64
wire strain relief loop, 73, 74

U

Ultrasound guidance
central neuraxis injury, 197
closed proximity, 199
common peroneal nerves, 199
electrode positioning, 203
fascia, nonabsorbable suture, 203
HFAC block, 208
ilioinguinal nerve stimulation, 199, 200
intercostal nerve, 197
invasive techniques, 198
occipital nerve stimulation, 199, 200
peripheral nerve targets, 199
permanent device implantation, 203
PNS lead placement, 199
posterior tibial nerves, 199
procedures, invasiveness, 198
risk assessment, 203
saphenous nerves, 199
transducer approach, 200

Upper extremity pain
neuropathic pain, 191
neurosurgical interventions, 195
PNS, 192
SCS, 191
ulnar nerve stimulation, 192
US-guided images
ilioinguinal nerve, 200
occipital nerve, 200
saphenous nerve, 200

V

Vagal nerve stimulation, 148
Vas deferens stimulation
pocket placement, sacral nerve stimulation, 117, 118
spermatic nerve stimulation, 117
Ventral posterior lateral thalamus (VPL), 226
Visceral nociceptive pathway, 130

W

Waveforms, 147
strategy, SCS. *See* Burst stimulation (Burst-SCS)
Withdrawal
baclofen, 307
catheter, 303
hypertension, 290, 306
opioid, 295
Wound closure, suturing technique
absorbable and non-absorbable sources, 79, 80
elimination, dead space, 77, 78
horizontal mattress stitch, 85
knot tying, 82, 83
needle types, 79, 81
peripheral nerve stimulation, IPG, 77
postoperative appearance, 77
simple interrupted stitch, 84
simple running stitch, 84
steri-stripes and staples, 87
vertical mattress stitch, 86
Wound healing
aging, 89
blood supply, 90
chronic disease, 90
dehydration, 90
factors, adverse effect, 40, 89
immune responses, 90
nutritional status, 90
old scar, 90
phases, 89, 91
radiation therapy, 90
tensile strength, 89
tissues, 89
weight, 89–90